PCEP

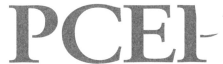

Perinatal Continuing Education Program

Maternal and Fetal Evaluation and Immediate Newborn Care

BOOK I

American Academy
of Pediatrics

DEDICATED TO THE HEALTH OF ALL CHILDREN™

The original version of these self-instructional books was developed in 1978 at the University of Virginia under contract (#N09-HR-2926) from the National Heart, Lung, and Blood Institute. Subsequent versions have been developed independently by the authors and, for the current edition, an editorial board.

PCEP Original Authors
John Kattwinkel, MD
Lynn J. Cook, RNC, MPH
Hallam Hurt, MD
George A. Nowacek, PhD
Jerry G. Short, PhD

Primary authors for the original obstetrical content
Warren M. Crosby, MD
Lynn J. Cook, RNC, MPH

Several different approaches to specific perinatal problems may be acceptable. The PCEP books have been written to present specific recommendations rather than to include all currently acceptable options. The recommendations in these books should not be considered the only accepted standard of care. We encourage development of local standards in consultation with your regional perinatal center staff.

Library of Congress Control Number: 2012937490

ISBN: 978-1-58110-657-2

The PCEP books are one part of a larger perinatal program. Information about the books, and the educational program, may be obtained by visiting the PCEP Web site at www.pcep.org and by obtaining the *PCEP Implementation Manual* CD, available through www.aap.org/bookstore. Information about obtaining CME and CEU credit (up to 54 hours) for book study may be obtained by visiting www.cmevillage.com.

Brand names are furnished for identification purposes only. No endorsement of the manufacturers or products mentioned is implied.

Every effort has been made to ensure that the drug selection and dosage set forth in this text are in accordance with the current recommendations and practice at the time of publication. It is the responsibility of the health care provider to check the package insert of each drug for any change in indications and dosage and for added warnings and precautions.

The publishers have made every effort to trace the copyright holders for borrowed material. If they have inadvertently overlooked any, they will be pleased to make the necessary arrangements at the first opportunity.

Printed in the United States of America

PC0009
5-262/0512

1 2 3 4 5 6 7 8 9 10

Perinatal Continuing Education Program, 2nd Edition

Textbook Editorial Board

Continuing Education Credit

Continuing education credit is available for every perinatal health care provider who studies the Perinatal Continuing Education Program (PCEP) books. The American Medical Association's *AMA PRA Category 1 Credit(s)™* or contact hours/continuing education units (CEUs) are available to physicians, nurses, nurse practitioners, nurse midwives, respiratory therapists, and any other professional who provides care to pregnant women or newborn babies.

Accreditation and Designation Statements

The University of Virginia School of Medicine is accredited by the Accreditation Council for Continuing Medical Education (ACCME) to provide continuing education for physicians.

The University of Virginia School of Medicine designates this enduring material for a maximum of 54 *AMA PRA Category 1 Credit(s)™*. Physicians should claim only the credit commensurate with the extent of their participation in the activity.

The University of Virginia School of Medicine awards 0.1 CEU per contact hour to each nonphysician participant who successfully completes this educational activity. The CEU is a nationally recognized unit of measure for continuing education and training activities that meet specific educational planning requirements. The University of Virginia School of Medicine maintains a permanent record of participants who have been awarded CEUs.

Disclosure of Financial Relationships

All the authors and editorial board members listed on the previous pages have disclosed that they have no relevant financial relationships with any commercial interest.

AMA PRA Category 1 Credit(s)™ or Contact Hour Credit
Credit is given only for complete books, not individual educational units. Possible hours: Book I, 14.5; Book II, 15.5; Book III, 16.5; Book IV, 7.5.

To register for education credits, visit www.cmevillage.com.

BOOK I

Maternal and Fetal Evaluation and Immediate Newborn Care

For more information, see the other books in the PCEP series.

Book II: Maternal and Fetal Care

Book III: Neonatal Care

Book IV: Specialized Newborn Care

What You Need to Know

1. What Is Perinatal Care?

2. What Are the Goals of Perinatal Care?

3. Why Are Community Hospitals So Important in Perinatal Care?

4. What Attitudes Lead to Effective Perinatal Care?

5. How Should You Interpret the Content of the PCEP Books?

6. How Are the PCEP Books Organized?
A. Written Material
B. Skill Units
C. Participants
D. Time Frame
E. Glossary
F. Recommended Routines
G. Continuing Education Credit
H. Conversion Charts

Table 1. Fluid Conversion
Table 2. Temperature Conversion
Table 3. Weight Conversion

Objectives

In this introduction you will learn
A. The purpose of the Perinatal Continuing Education Program (PCEP)
B. How the PCEP books are organized and what materials are included
C. What you need to know to participate in PCEP
D. What you need to do to earn credit for study of the PCEP books
E. How to convert between metric and English measurements

1. What Is Perinatal Care?

Perinatal means "the time surrounding a baby's birth." It includes the latter part of pregnancy and the first month of a baby's postnatal life. Perinatal care is the prenatal and postpartum health care of a woman, her unborn fetus, and her newly born baby.

Prenatal or *antenatal* (before birth) and *antepartum* (before delivery) refer to the care of a woman and her fetus. *Postpartum* (after delivery) refers to the care of the mother. *Postnatal* (after birth) refers to the care of the baby. The first month of postnatal life is called the *neonatal* period. A baby 1 month or younger is called a *neonate*.

The Perinatal Continuing Education Program (PCEP) focuses on the recognition of risk factors and illness in perinatal patients, stabilization, and short-term intensive care. The program was originally designed for the medical and nursing staff providing perinatal care in community hospitals, where most babies are born. Today, many regional referral centers also use PCEP within their institutions. The Perinatal Continuing Education Program does not address long-term intensive care or highly specialized therapies provided in maternal/fetal and neonatal intensive care units.

2. What Are the Goals of Perinatal Care?

The goals of perinatal care are to reduce maternal, fetal, and neonatal *mortality* (death) and *morbidity* (complication or damage that results from an illness).

Because the infant mortality and morbidity rates in the United States are higher than in many other developed countries, there is a critical need to make health care available to all women and babies and to improve all aspects of perinatal care, prenatal maternal/fetal care, postnatal newborn care, and postpartum maternal care.

3. Why Are Community Hospitals So Important in Perinatal Care?

They are vitally important because far more babies are born and cared for in community hospitals than in regional medical centers. Serious complications can develop suddenly, even in low-risk pregnant women.

 Every hospital with a delivery service, regardless of hospital size or number of deliveries, should be competent in the management of obstetrical emergencies and in carrying out neonatal resuscitation.

Perinatal care provided in community hospitals can dramatically influence maternal and neonatal outcome, even for patients transferred to a regional center for intensive care. The hours of initial assessment and stabilization in a community hospital may make a decisive impact on maternal, fetal, and/or neonatal outcome. Days or weeks of intensive care provided in a regional subspecialty center may not be able to overcome problems created by inadequate initial care.

4. What Attitudes Lead to Effective Perinatal Care?

The most important attitude regarding pregnant women is the understanding that prenatal care involves the care of 2 patients: the woman and the fetus. For optimal outcome, the health of both patients must be reassessed repeatedly throughout pregnancy.

The most important attitude regarding newborns is the belief that prompt, effective action can improve a baby's long-term healthy development. When perinatal mortality decreases because of appropriate action taken by health care providers, the morbidity of survivors also decreases. With proper care, more than 90% of all babies born preterm grow up with no sign of damage or problems.

5. How Should You Interpret the Contents of the PCEP Books?

Several different approaches to particular perinatal problems may be acceptable. The PCEP books have been written to present specific recommendations rather than include all currently acceptable options.

The recommendations in these books should not be considered the only accepted standard of care. We encourage development of local standards in consultation with your regional perinatal center staff.

Self-test

Now answer these questions to test yourself on the information in the last section.

A1. Perinatal care involves care of the
- **A.** Pregnant woman
- **B.** Fetus
- **C.** Newborn
- **D.** All of the above

A2. "Morbidity" refers to
- **A.** Death
- **B.** Complication or damage that results from an illness

A3. When perinatal mortality decreases, morbidity among the survivors _____
- **A.** Increases
- **B.** Decreases
- **C.** Remains the same

A4. When given proper care, more than __ of all babies born preterm will grow up with no sign of problems.
- **A.** 10%
- **B.** 30%
- **C.** 60%
- **D.** 90%

A5. The infant mortality rate in the United States is _____ than in many other developed countries.
- **A.** Higher
- **B.** Lower

A6. **True   False**

For babies born in community hospitals, the brief period of care prior to neonatal transfer is as important to the baby's outcome as is the care given in the regional intensive care nursery.

Answers are given on the last page of this section.

6. How Are the PCEP Books Organized?

A. Written Material

The PCEP books contain educational units, or chapters, organized in sequence. Some of these units deal primarily with maternal and fetal care, others with newborn care. You can select to study the books most suitable to your specialty. Many people, however, work through all the books. The books and suggested audience are as follows:

Book Number	Cover Color	Audience
I: Maternal and Fetal Evaluation and Immediate Newborn Care	Green	All perinatal care providers
II: Maternal and Fetal Care	Orange	Obstetric care providers
III: Neonatal Care	Blue	Neonatal care providers
IV: Specialized Newborn Care	Purple	Neonatal care providers (Some units will not apply to all hospitals.)

Another way of looking at this is to follow a study track.

- PCEP Maternal/Fetal Track (2 books): Book I and Book II (for those who provide prenatal, intrapartum, postpartum, and immediate newborn care)
- PCEP Neonatal Track (2 books): Book I and Book III (for those who provide immediate and post-birth newborn care)
- PCEP Perinatal Track (3 books): Book I, Book II, and Book III (for those who provide prenatal, intrapartum, immediate newborn, and post-birth maternal and newborn care)
- PCEP Specialized Neonatal Care Track (3 books): Book I, Book II, and Book IV (for those who provide immediate and post-birth specialized newborn care)
- PCEP Complete Series Track (4 books): Book I, Book II, Book III, and Book IV (a comprehensive, easy-to-use reference source for all hospitals with a delivery service; some hospitals will want their staff to be familiar with the content of all 4 books)

B. Skill Units

Many skills, such as sterile speculum examination for pregnant women and blood pressure measurement for neonates, are included in the program. If your hospital is participating in PCEP through a regional medical center in your area using the program for outreach education, 2 nurses from your hospital would have been trained as local PCEP coordinators.

These PCEP coordinators learned how to perform and how to teach the skills included in the program. Together with the outreach education staff from your regional center, the coordinators will organize the program for your hospital. They will schedule skill practice sessions to coincide with your study of the written material. During these skill sessions, the coordinators will demonstrate the skills and you will practice them.

If you are studying the books individually, outside an organized implementation of the complete program, read the skill units carefully. They are written as step-by-step instructions.

C. Participants

This educational program is useful for everyone who cares for pregnant women and newborns, including obstetricians, registered nurses, nursing assistants, pediatricians, family physicians, respiratory therapists, licensed practical nurses, nursing supervisors, nurse midwives, nurse practitioners and, in some cases, anesthetists and/or anesthesiologists and other professional staff members. One of the particularly valuable benefits of PCEP is that all perinatal team members participate in the same program. This enhances communication between medical and nursing staff and between obstetric and neonatal care providers.

D. Time Frame

You will read and study the books at your own pace; however, try to pace yourself so that you complete one book every 4 to 6 weeks. This has been found to be a comfortable pace for study of the written material and practice of the corresponding skills.

E. Glossary

A glossary is included at the end of this book. It defines words and phrases used in the PCEP books that may be unfamiliar to you. In some cases, it includes tidbits of information not given elsewhere in the books.

F. Recommended Routines

A list of recommended routines is given near the end of most of the educational units. These routines are based on material presented in the unit and specify procedures and policies that can lead to delivery of optimum perinatal care.

The routines are written to help you put the information in the unit into daily practice in your bedside care of pregnant women and newborns. You will be asked to consider each routine and decide whether it is already part of your hospital's standard operating procedure or whether implementation of the routine needs to be discussed by your staff.

G. Continuing Education Credit

The PCEP books were originally released in 1978, with repeated updating and revised editions since then. The most recent date for revision and update of book content is 2012. See page III for details of PCEP authors and 2012 editorial board.

AMA PRA Category 1 Credit(s)™ or contact hours are available to all perinatal health care professionals: physicians, nurses, respiratory therapists, nurse practitioners, nurse midwives, and all others who care for pregnant women or newborns.

AMA credits can only be granted by the institution where a program was developed. For this reason, Physician Recognition Award AMA category 1 credit(s)™ are available *only* from University of Virginia (UVA). Nursing credits may be obtained from UVA, or a center may choose to apply for credits locally. Some centers provide credits to nurses that include credits for practice and demonstration of the skills presented in the skill units, as well as credits for the cognitive units.

Credits are by book, not by individual unit within the books. Available credits for completion of each book are as follows:
Book I: 14.5 credits
Book II: 15.5 credits
Book III: 16.5 credits
Book IV: 7.5 credits

One contact hour is equivalent to 0.1 CEU, making 54 contact hours the same as 5.4 CEUs. It is possible to submit some books for credit in 1 year and other books in the next year, thus accommodating different accreditation and licensing cycles.

Please see additional information on page V in this book and at www.pcep.org. Credit for study of this edition of the PCEP books is approved through July 2015.

Testing is online at www.cmevillage.com or www.cmevillage.org. A participant can take each post-test, for each unit, as many times as desired. These post-tests are considered practice quizzes, and no fee is charged for completion of these quizzes, regardless of the number of times they are taken.

To obtain credits, a book exam must be completed and passed at 80% correct. Each book exam has test items taken from the individual unit post-tests and includes about 110 test questions each for Book I, II, and III, with fewer questions for Book IV.

When you are ready, go to www.cmevillage.com or www.cmevillage.org and click the PCEP link on the lower left side of the page. You will need to complete 3 steps:
1. Registration to create online ID and password
2. Complete book exam, scoring 80% correct
3. Complete book evaluation form and pay fee ($15 per book)

After successful book exam completion, a certificate, listing the number of credits earned, can be downloaded and printed.

H. Conversion Charts

Some hospitals (and most medications) use metric measurement, such as milliliters (mL), centigrade (°C), grams (g), milligrams (mg), and kilograms (kg). Other hospitals use English measures, such as ounces (oz) and Fahrenheit (°F).

The metric system is used with increasing frequency and is used throughout this program. You should be able to convert from one system to the other by using conversion charts like those in the following tables.

Table 1. Fluid Conversion

Ounces (oz)		Milliliters (mL)	Ounces (oz)		Milliliters (mL)	Ounces (oz)		Milliliters (mL)
0.25	=	7.5	2.25	=	67.5	4.25	=	127.5
0.5	=	15	2.5	=	75	4.5	=	135
0.75	=	22.5	2.75	=	82.5	4.75	=	142.5
1.0	=	30	3.0	=	90	5.0	=	150
1.25	=	37.5	3.25	=	97.5	5.25	=	157.5
1.5	=	45	3.5	=	105	5.5	=	165
1.75	=	52.5	3.75	=	112.5	5.75	=	172.5
2.0	=	60	4.0	=	120	6.0	=	180

Table 2. Temperature Conversion

°F	°C	°F	°C	°F	°C	°F	°C	°F	°C
70	21.1	84.0	28.8	89.0	31.6	94.0	34.4	99.0	37.2
71	21.6	84.2	29.0	89.2	31.7	94.2	34.5	99.2	37.3
72	22.2	84.4	29.1	89.4	31.8	94.4	34.6	99.4	37.4
73	22.7	84.6	29.2	89.6	32.0	94.6	34.7	99.6	37.5
74	23.3	84.8	29.3	89.8	32.1	94.8	34.8	99.8	37.6
75	23.8	85.0	29.4	90.0	32.2	95.0	35.0	100.0	37.7
76	24.4	85.2	29.5	90.2	32.3	95.2	35.1	100.2	37.8
77	25.0	85.4	29.6	90.4	32.4	95.4	35.2	100.4	38.0
78	25.5	85.6	29.7	90.6	32.5	95.6	35.3	100.6	38.1
79	26.1	85.8	29.8	90.8	32.6	95.8	35.4	100.8	38.2
80	26.6	86.0	30.0	91.0	32.7	96.0	35.5	101.0	38.3
81	27.2	86.2	30.1	91.2	32.8	96.2	35.6	101.2	38.4
82	27.7	86.4	30.2	91.4	33.0	96.4	35.7	101.4	38.5
83	28.3	86.6	30.3	91.6	33.1	96.6	35.8	101.6	38.6
		86.8	30.4	91.8	33.2	96.8	36.0	101.8	38.7
104	40.0	87.0	30.5	92.0	33.3	97.0	36.1	102.0	38.8
105	40.5	87.2	30.6	92.2	33.4	97.2	36.2	102.2	39.0
106	41.1	87.4	30.7	92.4	33.5	97.4	36.3	102.4	39.1
107	41.6	87.6	30.8	92.6	33.6	97.6	36.4	102.6	39.2
		87.8	31.0	92.8	32.7	97.8	36.5	102.8	39.3
		88.0	31.1	93.0	33.8	98.0	36.6	103.0	39.4
		88.2	31.2	93.2	34.0	98.2	36.7	103.2	39.5
		88.4	31.3	93.4	34.1	98.4	36.8	103.4	39.6
		88.6	31.4	93.6	34.2	98.6	37.0	103.6	39.7
		88.8	31.5	93.8	34.3	98.8	37.1	103.8	39.8

Table 3. Weight Conversion

Ounces

Pounds	0	1	2	3	4	5	6	7	8	9	10	11	12	13	14	15
0	0	28	57	85	113	142	170	198	227	255	283	312	340	369	397	425
1	454	482	510	539	567	595	624	652	680	709	737	765	794	822	850	879
2	907	936	964	992	1,021	1,049	1,077	1,106	1,134	1,162	1,191	1,219	1,247	1,276	1,304	1,332
3	1,361	1,389	1,417	1,446	1,474	1,503	1,531	1,559	1,588	1,616	1,644	1,673	1,701	1,729	1,758	1,786
4	1,814	1,843	1,871	1,899	1,928	1,956	1,984	2,013	2,041	2,070	2,098	2,126	2,155	2,183	2,211	2,240
5	2,268	2,296	2,325	2,353	2,381	2,410	2,438	2,466	2,495	2,523	2,551	2,580	2,608	2,637	2,665	2,693
6	2,722	2,750	2,778	2,807	2,835	2,863	2,892	2,920	2,948	2,977	3,005	3,033	3,062	3,090	3,118	3,147
7	3,175	3,203	3,232	3,260	3,289	3,317	3,345	3,374	3,402	3,430	3,459	3,487	3,515	3,544	3,572	3,600
8	3,629	3,657	3,685	3,714	3,742	3,770	3,799	3,827	3,856	3,884	3,912	3,941	3,969	3,997	4,026	4,054
9	4,082	4,111	4,139	4,167	4,196	4,224	4,252	4,281	4,309	4,337	4,366	4,394	4,423	4,451	4,479	4,508
10	4,536	4,564	4,593	4,621	4,649	4,678	4,706	4,734	4,763	4,791	4,819	4,848	4,876	4,904	4,933	4,961
11	4,990	5,018	5,046	5,075	5,103	5,131	5,160	5,188	5,216	5,245	5,273	5,301	5,330	5,358	5,386	5,415
12	5,443	5,471	5,500	5,528	5,557	5,585	5,613	5,642	5,670	5,698	5,727	5,755	5,783	5,812	5,840	5,868
13	5,897	5,925	5,954	5,982	6,010	6,039	6,067	6,095	6,124	6,152	6,180	6,209	6,237	6,265	6,294	6,322
14	6,350	6,379	6,407	6,435	6,464	6,492	6,521	6,549	6,577	6,606	6,634	6,662	6,691	6,719	6,747	6,776
15	6,804	6,832	6,861	6,889	6,917	6,946	6,974	7,002	7,031	7,059	7,088	7,116	7,144	7,173	7,201	7,229

Grams (inside the boxes)

Self-test

Practice using the conversion charts.

Fluid Conversion

B1. A 3½-oz feeding is equal to __ mL.

B2. A 60-mL feeding is equal to __ oz.

B3. 75 mL is equal to __ oz.

B4. 1½ oz is equal to __ mL.

Temperature Conversion

B5. A temperature of 98.6°F is __°C.

B6. A temperature of 97.0°F is __°C.

B7. A room temperature of 72.0°F is __°C.

Weight Conversion

B8. An 8-lb, 8-oz baby weighs __ g or __ kg.

B9. A 5-lb, 7-oz baby weighs __ g or __ kg.

B10. A 3,005-g baby weighs __ lb __ oz.

B11. A 2,000-g baby weighs __ lb __ oz.

Check your answers with those on the next page.

Self-test Answers

These are the answers to the self-test questions. Please check them with the answers you gave and review the information in the Introduction wherever necessary.

A1. D

A2. B

A3. B

A4. D

A5. A

A6. True

B1. 105 mL

B2. 2 oz

B3. 2½ oz

B4. 45 mL

B5. 37.0°C

B6. 36.1°C

B7. 22.2°C

B8. 3.856 g; 3.856 kg

B9. 2,466 g; 2.466 kg

B10. 6 1b, 10 oz

B11. 4 1b, 6½ oz (Note: 2,000 g does not appear on the chart. The answer is an estimate to the nearest half ounce.)

Unit 1: Is the Mother Sick? Is the Fetus Sick?

Objectives

In this unit you will learn

A. What is meant by high-risk or at-risk pregnancy or delivery

B. How to classify a pregnant woman as well, at risk, or sick

C. How to classify a fetus as well, at risk, or sick

D. Why it is important to decide if a pregnant woman or fetus is well, at risk, or sick

E. That fetal health and maternal health need to be evaluated separately from each other

F. The general measures you should take for every pregnant woman or fetus who is at risk or sick

G. That the health of a pregnant woman or fetus may change unexpectedly, and frequent reevaluation throughout the pregnancy and labor is essential

H. What to do when a pregnant woman telephones with concerns or symptoms

I. What is important to include in the initial evaluation of every woman in labor, regardless of her risk status

Obstetric care is strengthened by knowing the consequences that maternal health and treatment have for the fetus and newborn.

Neonatal care is strengthened by knowing the implications that maternal and fetal health and antenatal care have for postnatal health and care of the newborn.

Unit 1 Pretest

Before reading the unit, please answer the following questions. Select the *one* best answer to each question (unless otherwise instructed). Record your answers on the test and check them against the answers at the end of the book.

1. Which of the following is an appropriate way to provide prenatal care to a woman with a high-risk pregnancy?

   Yes   No

   ____ ____   By the woman's primary care physician, in consultation with a specialist

   ____ ____   By the woman's primary care physician, until she enters labor

   ____ ____   Jointly, by the woman's primary care physician and a specialist, with prenatal visits by the woman to both

   ____ ____   Transfer of the woman's care entirely to a specialist at a regional medical center

2. Which of the following should be done for *every* pregnant woman evaluated for labor?

   Yes   No

   ____ ____   Ask the woman about recent intake of prescription and nonprescription drugs.

   ____ ____   Check fetal heart rate.

   ____ ____   Assess frequency, duration, and quality of contractions.

   ____ ____   Review the course of previous labors and deliveries.

   ____ ____   Assess fetal position and estimate fetal weight.

3. All of the following should be done for every high-risk patient during labor, *except:*

   A. Start an intravenous fluid line in the pregnant woman.

   B. Notify nursery personnel of maternal and fetal condition as soon as the woman is admitted.

   C. Provide intensive fetal heart rate and uterine contraction monitoring.

   D. Insert a Foley catheter.

4. **True   False**   All women with high-risk pregnancies deliver sick babies.

5. **True   False**   A healthy woman will always have a healthy fetus.

6. **True   False**   When a fetus has a congenital anomaly that will require neonatal intensive care, but the pregnancy is otherwise uncomplicated and the woman is healthy, there is no benefit to transferring the woman for delivery at a regional medical center.

7. **True   False**   If there is evidence of late-pregnancy vaginal bleeding, a vaginal examination should be done immediately.

8. **True   False**   Nearly 100% of high-risk pregnancies can be identified before the onset of labor.

9. **True   False**   A woman with a high-risk condition during her pregnancy may develop another, unrelated, high-risk condition during labor.

10. **True   False**   Every hospital with a delivery service should be capable of beginning an emergency cesarean section within 30 minutes, at any time.

11. Which of the following findings indicate that a fetus is sick or at risk?

Yes   No

____   ____   Decreased fetal movement for 1 day, at 34 weeks' gestation

____   ____   Occasional periods of bradycardia (heart rate <110 beats per minute)

____   ____   Premature rupture of membranes

____   ____   A woman with gestational hypertension

12. Which of the following maternal conditions pose an increased risk(s) for a pregnant woman or her fetus?

Yes   No

____   ____   Gonorrhea

____   ____   Stable renal disease

____   ____   Abnormal glucose tolerance

____   ____   Maternal age of 13 years

1. What Does *High Risk* or *At Risk* Mean?

A high-risk *pregnancy* is one in which risk factors indicate an increased likelihood of illness or death for the fetus and/or the pregnant woman. Risk factors are conditions identified by history, psychosocial findings, physical findings, ultrasound examination, and/or laboratory tests.

The presence of a risk factor does not mean that a woman or her fetus will always develop a problem. A risk factor simply increases the likelihood that a particular problem will develop. More than one risk factor, for the same or different problems, may be present.

 A well fetus or pregnant woman may become at risk or sick at any time during pregnancy. Systematically reexamine the status of both the woman and her fetus at each prenatal visit. While many risk factors may be identified before the onset of labor, care providers must remain vigilant for change in maternal status during labor or even postpartum.

When a pregnancy is high risk, the danger the pregnancy imposes on the pregnant woman and the fetus must be weighed against the danger delivery would impose on the woman and the fetus. Potential complications may change as pregnancy advances. The relative risks to both the woman and the fetus must be reweighed each time patient status is reevaluated. Risks that need to be balanced to decide whether a fetus should be delivered at any point include the risk to the

- Woman of continuing or ending the pregnancy
- Fetus of intrauterine compromise or death
- Newborn of being born prematurely

A high-risk *delivery* is one that poses a serious threat of injury or illness to the woman and/or the fetus. The increased risk may be due to a factor(s) identified during pregnancy or due to a problem(s) that develops during labor. Risk factors that occur during labor may or may not be related to risk factors identified during pregnancy. A woman with an uncomplicated pregnancy and no identified risk factors may still develop a serious problem(s) during labor.

 Careful, thorough evaluation of maternal and fetal status throughout labor is essential. Despite careful prenatal evaluations, some high-risk conditions may not be known, or may not become apparent, until after the onset of labor.

The management of all pregnancies and deliveries requires a team approach for optimal outcome. For many patients, that team will be entirely within your hospital. Other patients will require the full resources of a regional network of care.

High-risk patients may not develop difficulties until labor is too advanced to allow safe transfer to another hospital for delivery. Low-risk patients can develop emergent conditions suddenly during labor. Teams ready and fully capable of attending to the emergent needs of a woman and of a newborn need to be available at all times, within every hospital that has a delivery service. The woman and her fetus may be sick at the same time, so response to maternal and neonatal emergencies may be needed at the same time.

There is one standard for emergency perinatal care. Regardless of size or delivery rate, every facility with a delivery service should be capable of

- *Beginning a cesarean delivery within 30 minutes of the decision to operate, at any time of the day or night.**
- *Providing resuscitation of a pregnant or postpartum woman, at any time of the day or night.*
- *Providing resuscitation of a newborn, at any time of the day or night.*

2. What Factors Make a Pregnancy or Delivery At Risk or High Risk?

Risk factors can be obstetric conditions (either problems experienced in previous pregnancies or new conditions identified during the current pregnancy); preexisting medical or psychological conditions in the woman; adverse social, economic, or work situations; or complications that develop during labor. Some antenatal risk factors carry a more serious health threat than others. Various systems of weighing the relative risk of different factors have been devised. You may find these a helpful guide in reviewing all risk factors, but no system is perfect in predicting risk. You will need to weigh the hazard of each risk factor for each specific woman and fetus.

The following list includes conditions that may pose significant risks to a pregnant woman and/or her fetus during pregnancy or delivery. Some conditions also pose risks to a woman and/or her baby following delivery.

Some women with uncommon health conditions will have risk factors not included in this list. Every condition listed is discussed in other units within the Perinatal Continuing Education Program books.

Maternal Medical Conditions

- Cardiovascular disease
  - Hypertension—chronic and/or gestational hypertension
  - Cardiac disease
- Metabolic/endocrine disease
  - Diabetes mellitus/abnormal glucose tolerance
  - Thyroid disease
  - Obesity
- Infectious disease
  - Sexually transmitted infections (STIs) that may affect a fetus
    - Chlamydia
    - Gonorrhea
    - Herpes simplex virus
    - Human immunodeficiency virus
    - Human papillomavirus
    - Syphilis

---

*Some indications for a cesarean delivery can be appropriately accommodated in longer than 30 minutes. Conversely, some indications (eg, hemorrhage from placenta previa, abruptio placentae, prolapse of the umbilical cord, or uterine rupture) may mandate a more expeditious delivery. American Academy of Pediatrics, American College of Obstetricians and Gynecologists. Intrapartum and postpartum care of the mother. In: American Academy of Pediatrics Committee on Fetus and Newborn, American College of Obstetricians and Gynecologists Committee on Obstetric Practice. *Guidelines for Perinatal Care.* 6th ed. Elk Grove Village, IL: American Academy of Pediatrics; 2007:159.

   – Other (non-STI) maternal infections that may affect a fetus
     ○ Cytomegalovirus
     ○ Hepatitis B virus
     ○ Listeriosis
     ○ Parvovirus B19 (fifth disease or erythema infectiosum)
     ○ Rubella (German measles)
     ○ Streptococci colonization (Group B streptococci [GBS])
     ○ Toxoplasmosis
     ○ Tuberculosis
     ○ Varicella-zoster virus (chicken pox)
   – Sites of maternal infections with a variety of causative organisms
     ○ Bacterial vaginosis
     ○ Urinary tract infection and acute pyelonephritis
     ○ Chorioamnionitis
     ○ Puerperal endometritis
     ○ Puerperal mastitis
 • Hematologic disease
   – Severe anemia
   – Hemoglobinopathies (sickle cell disease [SS, SC, and S-ß thalassemia])
   – Thrombocytopenia
 • Immunologic disease
   – Systemic lupus erythematosus
   – Antiphospholipid antibody syndrome
 • Renal disease
 • Neurologic disease
   – Seizure disorder
 • Respiratory disease
   – Asthma
   – Cystic fibrosis

Other Factors That Can Adversely Affect a Pregnancy
 • Maternal age
 • Psychological maladaptation to pregnancy
 • Substance use
 • Adverse socioeconomic factors

Past Obstetric and Family History
 • Previous uterine surgery
 • Previous macrosomic newborn
 • Previous perinatal death, including stillborn baby
 • Previous fetus with congenital malformation(s) or hereditary disease
 • High parity
 • Previous cesarean section
 • Previous blood group incompatibility

Current Pregnancy Conditions
 • Early antenatal testing (not a risk factor; rather, testing is used to evaluate risk)
   – Screening tests
   – Diagnostic tests

- Multifetal gestation
- Abnormal volume of amniotic fluid
  - Hydramnios
  - Oligohydramnios
- Growth-restricted fetus
- Large-for-gestational-age fetus
- Preterm labor and delivery
- Premature rupture of membranes
- Post-term fetus
- Obstetric hemorrhage
  - Early pregnancy bleeding
    - Ectopic pregnancy
    - Spontaneous abortion
  - Late pregnancy bleeding
    - Placental bleeding
      - Placenta previa
      - Abruptio placentae
    - Cervical bleeding
    - Vaginal bleeding of unknown origin
- Abnormal labor progress and difficult deliveries
  - Prolonged labor
  - Forceps or vacuum extraction delivery
  - Precipitate labor
  - Meconium-stained amniotic fluid
  - Fetal heart rate abnormalities
  - Maternal analgesia and/or anesthesia
  - Prolapsed umbilical cord
  - Shoulder dystocia
- Abnormal third stage of labor

3. Why Is It Important to Decide if a Pregnant Woman or Her Fetus Is Well, At Risk, or Sick?

Determining fetal condition, and the condition of a pregnant woman, will help you decide how to manage the woman and her fetus. It also will help you anticipate problems the baby may have after birth.

- If a pregnant woman is WELL, and if evidence indicates a fetus is WELL:

  You continue to *evaluate* both the woman and the fetus at *regular intervals*.

- If a pregnant woman is AT RISK, or if factors place a fetus AT RISK:

  You *anticipate* problems, *investigate* suspicious findings, and *frequently reevaluate* both maternal and fetal well-being.

- If a pregnant woman is SICK, or if evidence indicates a fetus is SICK:

  You *intervene promptly* to correct the problem(s) that can be corrected, and *closely monitor* the condition of both the woman and the fetus.

Regardless of initial risk status, *every* pregnant woman and fetus need a

1. Comprehensive examination to identify risk factors.
2. Review of risk factors (if any) and patient status at every prenatal visit.
3. Determination of pregnancy dates as early and as accurately as possible.

If a pregnancy that is initially low risk becomes high risk, gestational age can be a crucial factor in detecting problems (such as fetal growth restriction or large for gestational age), interpreting test results (such as maternal serum alpha fetoprotein or amniotic fluid index), determining treatment choices, and/or selecting timing and route of delivery.

 Establish pregnancy dates as accurately as possible for every pregnancy.

4. How Do You Know a Pregnant Woman Is Well?

A healthy pregnant woman has *all* of the following:

• Normal vital signs
• Normal weight gain
• Normal laboratory findings
• No medical illnesses
• No past or present obstetric complications
• No substance use
• No severely adverse social, economic, work, or psychological conditions

 Risk factors can change throughout pregnancy or may not develop until labor occurs. It is vital to reevaluate risks and your plan of care for each patient at every prenatal visit and during labor.

5. How Do You Know a Pregnant Woman Is At Risk?

A pregnant woman whose health is at risk has *one or more* of the following:

• Abnormal vital signs, particularly blood pressure elevated to 140/90 mm Hg or higher
• Abnormal weight gain or weight loss
• Abnormal laboratory findings
• Well-controlled medical illness
• Obstetric complication in previous pregnancy
• Stable obstetric complication in current pregnancy
• Substance use
• Severely adverse social, economic, work, or psychological conditions
• Psychiatric illness
• Exposure to infectious diseases that may adversely affect the fetus

 An at-risk pregnant woman needs careful monitoring, anticipation of problems, investigation of suspicious findings, and either prevention of problems or timely treatment.

6. How Do You Know a Pregnant Woman Is Sick?

A pregnant woman who is sick has *one or more* of the following:

- Abnormal vital signs, particularly blood pressure elevated above 160/110 mm Hg
- Abnormal laboratory findings
- Medical illness in poor control
- Unstable obstetric complication in current pregnancy

 A sick, pregnant woman needs prompt investigation of abnormal findings and may require immediate intervention to correct a serious threat to maternal and/or fetal health. Depending on fetal gestational age and the severity of maternal illness, emergency delivery may be required.

7. Why Is It Important to Assess Fetal Well-being?

The fetus of a healthy woman may be well, at risk, or sick. Likewise, the fetus of a sick or at-risk woman may be relatively unaffected by maternal complications, or may be seriously ill as a result of maternal disease.

 Maternal health and fetal well-being need to be evaluated separately.

It is not always possible to determine with certainty whether a fetus is well or sick. Ongoing monitoring of risk status is necessary to individualize patient care.

Fetal activity determinations, also called kick counts, should be done by low- and high-risk pregnant women. Other than fetal activity determinations, antenatal testing of fetal well-being should be tailored to the individual patient, and may include the following:

- *Nonstress test* (assessment of spontaneous fetal heart rate accelerations that occur with fetal activity)
- *Contraction stress test* (assessment of fetal heart rate response during a brief period of either spontaneous or induced uterine contractions)
- *Biophysical profile* (score based on 5 indicators of fetal health: nonstress test, amniotic fluid volume, fetal movement, fetal muscle tone, and fetal respirations)
- *Modified biophysical profile* (assessment using nonstress test and amniotic fluid volume)

While weekly testing beginning at 26 to 28 weeks may be used as a starting point, the timing and frequency of the testing of fetal well-being will depend on the specific maternal and/or fetal condition. For example, the specific cause of previous perinatal death needs to be considered. Regular testing beginning before 28 weeks would be appropriate for a woman with diabetes mellitus who experienced a previous fetal death at 28 weeks. Testing 2 or more times a week may be needed. However, a woman whose previous fetus died at term from bacterial sepsis may not need weekly testing, or testing starting as early as 28 weeks. Gestational age of the fetus should be considered when evaluating results of some tests. Specific tests to evaluate fetal age and well-being are described in detail in the next 2 units in this book.

8. What Findings Indicate That a Fetus Is Well?

A fetus that has *all* of the following is likely to be well:

- Normal fundal height for gestational age
- Normal fetal growth
- A Category I fetal heart rate tracing (See Unit 3, Fetal Well-being, in this book.)
- Normal fetal heart rate
- Normal fetal activity
- Normal volume of amniotic fluid
- Normal fetal anatomy
- Normally located placenta
- A healthy mother

 Rarely, a fetus will be sick even when the results of all maternal and fetal evaluations are normal.

9. How Do You Know a Fetus Is At Risk?

An at-risk fetus has *one or more* of the following:

- Abnormal fundal height for gestational age
- Abnormal fetal growth
- A Category II fetal heart rate tracing (See Unit 3, Fetal Well-being, in this book.)
- Abnormal fetal activity
- Abnormal ultrasound findings: decreased or increased amniotic fluid volume, fetal malformation, and/or placenta previa
- A mother with one or more risk factors

 An at-risk fetus needs careful monitoring, anticipation of problems, investigation of suspicious findings, and either prevention of problems or timely treatment.

10. What Makes You Suspect a Fetus Is Sick?

A fetus that is sick is likely to have *one or more* of the following:

- A decrease or unexpected increase in fundal height
- Decreased fetal activity
- A Category III fetal heart rate tracing (See Unit 3, Fetal Well-being, in this book.)
- Fetal growth restriction
- Abnormal fetal anatomy
- Abnormal ultrasound findings (decreased or increased amniotic fluid volume, poor fetal muscle tone, no movement, and/or no respirations)
- A seriously ill mother

 A sick fetus requires prompt investigation and may need immediate intervention to correct a serious threat to the health of the fetus and/or the pregnant woman. Depending on fetal gestational age and the severity of maternal illness, emergency delivery may be required.

If the problem(s) is not correctable in utero, such as a congenital malformation, fetal condition should be frequently evaluated so delivery can be timed appropriately and preparations can be made for neonatal care.

11. What Should You Do for Every Pregnant Woman or Fetus Who Is At Risk or Sick?

- Anticipate and screen for fetal problems according to the woman's history. Monitor fetal growth and well-being.
- Schedule more frequent prenatal visits. Reassess maternal and fetal risk factors at each visit and during labor.
- Consider consultation with obstetric and pediatric specialists, and/or other specialists (ie, cardiology, neurology, etc), depending on maternal illness, fetal condition, and probable neonatal condition. Discuss anticipated care with nursing staff and support services, such as respiratory therapy and clinical laboratory. Distance and ease of transportation to a regional perinatal center, resources available (24 hours a day) within your hospital, and severity of the woman's illness or fetal condition may influence when and with whom consultation is obtained.

Care of a high-risk pregnant woman is managed in any of the following ways:

- By the woman's primary care physician, with initial or continuing consultation with a specialist at a regional center
- Through comanagement by the woman's primary care physician and a specialist, who examines the patient periodically during her pregnancy
- With transfer of the care of the patient to a specialist at a regional center

Ideally, the most appropriate place for delivery is planned in advance as a joint decision of the patient, the primary care provider, and the specialist. This decision should *not* be based entirely on the woman's condition. If a woman's condition is stable, but if intensive care of the baby is anticipated, transfer of the woman before delivery to a hospital with an intensive care nursery is recommended. Predelivery transfer of a woman in stable condition (in utero transport of the fetus) is generally much less stressful than neonatal transport would be to the baby. It has been shown that sick or premature babies born in a hospital with an intensive care nursery do better than those transferred after birth.

- Discuss pregnancy complications, fetal status, anticipated neonatal condition, and possible need for specialized neonatal care with pediatric physicians and neonatal nurses (at your hospital and, depending on the situation, at the regional center) *prior* to delivery.
- Discuss, and periodically review, pregnancy complications, fetal status, anticipated neonatal condition, and care options with the pregnant woman, her family, and other support persons of her choosing.

12. Why Is it Advisable to Consult With Regional Center Experts as Soon as a High-Risk Fetus Is Identified?

- If delivery at a regional center has been planned, but labor occurs and progress is such that travel to the regional center is not considered prudent, intrapartum management in the community hospital by community hospital providers and regional center consultants can be better coordinated if all practitioners know the woman, her condition, and the condition of her fetus.
- In some instances (eg, certain types of congenital heart disease, diaphragmatic hernia, etc), the fetus may be in good health in utero, but will be quite ill as a newborn. Early involvement of the regional center staff will allow initial neonatal management to be planned and to go more smoothly than if it were unanticipated.
- Regional center staff, those who may provide care to the woman or her newborn, can get to know the parents before the birth occurs.

- The woman and her family can meet the neonatologists, nurse practitioners, and neonatal intensive care unit (NICU) nursing staff members and have the anticipated care of their baby explained, thus making their baby's illness and care after birth, as well as their introduction to the NICU, less traumatic.

 Anticipation of possible problems and coordination of the management of high-risk pregnancies between obstetric and pediatric caregivers is critical to optimal outcome for a pregnant woman and her baby.

Consultation with regional center specialists is highly recommended.

13. What Should You Do if a High-Risk Woman Will Deliver at Your Hospital?

If delivery at a regional center is advisable, but labor is too far advanced to allow safe transfer, provide the following during labor for all women with high-risk pregnancies:

- Start an intravenous (IV) line for hydration of the pregnant woman and for infusion of volume expanders and medications, as needed.
- Provide intensive fetal heart rate and uterine contraction monitoring.
- Position the woman on her side to avoid compression of the inferior vena cava (which can restrict venous blood return to the heart) and allow maximum placental perfusion.
- Inform nursery personnel of the maternal and fetal condition as soon as the woman is admitted.
- Arrange to have personnel skilled in neonatal resuscitation, and responsible only for the care of the baby (not the mother), attend the delivery.
- Be prepared, with anesthesia and surgical support personnel, to begin a cesarean delivery within 30 minutes of the time the decision to operate is made, at any time of the day or night.
- Consult with a regional center specialist(s) regarding management during labor and neonatal stabilization for problems specific to this pregnancy and anticipated neonatal condition.
- Prepare for the safe postnatal transfer of the woman and/or the baby to a higher level of care.

Self-test

Now answer these questions to test yourself on the information in the last section.

For each of the cases in A1 through A3, decide if the woman and the fetus are well, at risk, or sick, and what action you should take.

Actions include

    A. Evaluate the woman and fetus at regular intervals.

    B. Anticipate problems, investigate suspicious findings, and reevaluate frequently.

    C. Intervene promptly to investigate and/or correct the problem(s).

A1. A healthy, 20-year-old woman who is pregnant with her second child comes for a routine prenatal visit at 35 weeks. She has normal vital signs, weight gain, and increase in uterine size. You note a baseline fetal heart rate of 174 beats per minute.

The woman is: _____

The fetus is: _____

You should: _____

A2. A healthy, 26-year-old woman who is pregnant with her first child has a brief episode of vaginal bleeding at 35 weeks. A placenta previa is diagnosed by ultrasound. The fetus has normal activity, growth, and heart rate.

The woman is: _____

The fetus is: _____

You should: _____

A3. A 30-year-old woman with compromised but stable kidney function is pregnant at 26 weeks' gestation with her first child.

The woman is: _____

The fetus is: _____

You should: _____

At 32 weeks' gestation, the woman's renal function begins to deteriorate. Fetal growth has been normal; fetal activity and heart rate are normal.

The woman is now: _____

The fetus is now: _____

You should: _____

A4. A high-risk pregnant woman's care plan includes delivery at a regional perinatal center, but she presents in labor that is too far advanced to allow safe transfer. What should you do for her?

_____

_____

_____

_____

_____

_____

_____

_____

_____

A5. What are the advantages of early consultation when a high-risk fetus is identified?

_____

_____

_____

_____

Check your answers with the list that follows the Recommended Routines. Correct any incorrect answers and review the appropriate section in the unit.

14. When Should a Pregnant Woman Go to a Hospital for Evaluation?

Patients who think they are in labor or who have concerns about symptoms they are experiencing often telephone to ask when they should go to the hospital. *ALWAYS recommend that she talk with her obstetric practitioner or come to the hospital for evaluation.*

 A woman's perception of her condition may be dramatically different than your direct clinical assessment of it.

DO NOT TRY TO PROVIDE DEFINITIVE ASSESSMENT OR SUGGEST TREATMENT OVER THE TELEPHONE.

Some information from the woman may be useful in identifying the urgency of the situation. Ask the woman, "What problem are you having?" If her concerns relate to her pregnancy, it is generally useful to gather and record the following information:

1. When is your due date?
2. Are you having contractions (labor pains)?
   If she answers "No" and the pregnancy is preterm, ask about other symptoms of preterm labor (watery vaginal discharge, low backache, sense of heaviness or pressure in her lower abdomen or perineum, and/or feeling of "gas pains" or menstrual cramps).
3. Have your membranes ruptured? (Did your water break?)
4. Are you bleeding from your vagina?
5. Do you have headaches, blurred vision, or spots before your eyes?
   - Do you have a marked and/or sudden increase in the swelling in your hands or feet?
   - Do you have less urine than usual?
   - Do you have abdominal pain (particularly right upper quadrant pain)?
6. Is the baby moving less than usual?

 A positive answer to any of these questions indicates the possibility of an urgent condition.

Advise the patient to come to the hospital IMMEDIATELY for evaluation.

It may be appropriate to call the woman's obstetrical care provider to relay the patient's concerns as well as the information you obtained, and to notify him or her that the patient was advised to seek further evaluation. Each perinatal unit should establish a protocol for notifying the provider.

15. What Is Important to Include in the Evaluation of a Woman Who *May* Be in Labor?

Some women will not be in labor and can safely go home after evaluation. For this reason, outpatient evaluation in an obstetrical care area is recommended. Hospital admission can be arranged for women in labor or who require further care after the period of observation and assessment.

A. Review the Prenatal Record.
   Obstetric practitioners usually send a copy of each patient's record to the labor and delivery area during the third trimester. Electronic health records that are available to all perinatal team members are ideal. *One standard form* used by all obstetric practitioners at a hospital is recommended. A standard form
   - Allows information to be located quickly
   - Provides a simple way to be sure comprehensive, consistent information is available for all patients

Because most women are healthy, a checklist style is useful for initial history and for periodic status review. If problems are identified, their evaluation and management can be recorded separately.

B. Establish Priorities for Care.

Make a brief, targeted assessment of maternal and fetal well-being to identify urgent conditions needing immediate attention.

1. Obtain immediate history.
   - Evidence of vaginal bleeding
   - Time of onset of contractions (or other symptoms if preterm)
   - Frequency, duration, and quality of contractions
   - Degree of pain with contractions, need for analgesia
   - Whether membranes have ruptured; if ruptured, time of rupture and description of fluid
   - Recent fetal movement or lack of activity

   Be sure to ask: "Do you have any other questions or concerns?"

2. Check maternal vital signs.

   Ask about recent activity, intake of food, alcohol, medications and other drugs, etc.

3. Monitor fetal heart rate and pattern.

   Monitoring of fetal heart rate and uterine contractions may continue while other aspects of the evaluation are carried out. If any findings are worrisome, investigate further. Be sure the woman and fetus are stable before proceeding with complete history, physical examination, and laboratory tests.

4. Determine if the pregnancy is preterm or term.
   - If preterm, see Book II: Maternal and Fetal Care, Unit 7, Preterm Labor, for evaluation details.
   - If term, determine if labor is true, false, or prodromal. (See Book II: Maternal and Fetal Care, Unit 9, Abnormal Labor and Difficult Deliveries.)

C. Obtain complete history. If prenatal record is not available or is incomplete, obtain history from the patient.

1. Current pregnancy history
   - Problems encountered and treatment given
   - Drugs (prescription, nonprescription, and illicit [what, when, how much], allergies and sensitivities)
   - Intimate partner violence: frequency and nature of episodes, current safety of woman (and children, if present)

2. Obstetric history
   - Number and course of previous pregnancies, length of gestation
   - Course of labor and delivery
     - Length of labor(s)
     - Problems encountered
     - Type of delivery (spontaneous vaginal, operative vaginal, cesarean section)
   - Postpartum course
   - Previous neonatal status
     - Birth weight
     - Outcome (sick, healthy, anomaly, etc)

3. Medical history
   - Cardiovascular disease/status
   - Metabolic/endocrine disease/status
   - Infectious disease(s)/treatment status
   - Hematologic disease/status

- Immunologic disease/status
- Renal disease/status
- Neurologic disease/status
- Respiratory disease/status
- Family history of inherited diseases, chromosomal abnormalities, or congenital anomalies (if not already in the prenatal record)

   4. Psychosocial and lifestyle history

If prenatal care was inadequate (late entry to care or missed appointments), pay particular attention to factors that might have interfered with the woman obtaining care (cultural, financial, lifestyle, intimate partner violence, employment, child care obligations, addictions, institutional health care barriers, and/or other factors).

D. Perform Physical Examination.
1. General condition.
2. Determine fetal presentation. (See the skill unit that follows this unit.)
3. Uterine examination.
   - Fundal height.
   - Areas of tenderness or pain.
   - Consistency between contractions (soft, firm, rigid, etc).
   - Nature of contractions.
   - Estimate fetal weight and record your findings. (At a minimum, note whether the fetus is small or large.)
4. Vaginal examination.

 Do NOT perform a vaginal examination if there is
- *Bleeding (until placenta previa has been ruled out)*
- *Premature rupture of membranes*

   - Check for presence of skin lesions (condylomata, herpes, syphilis, etc).
   - Determine whether membranes are ruptured. (See Book II: Maternal and Fetal Care, Premature Rupture and/or Infection of the Amniotic Membranes, skill units.)
   - Examine cervix (dilatation, effacement, consistency). (See Book II: Maternal and Fetal Care, Unit 8, Inducing and Augmenting Labor.)
   - Determine fetal station and identify presenting part.

E. Obtain Laboratory Tests.
1. All patients
   - Test urine for protein and glucose.

   If not available from prenatal care record or if patient status has changed, obtain a
   - Complete blood count.
   - Platelet count.
2. Women with prenatal tests not obtained or results not available, obtain the following:
   - Urinalysis with urine culture
   - Cervical cultures for gonorrhea and chlamydia
   - Lower vaginal and rectal cultures for GBS
   - Serologic test for syphilis
   - Rh and antibody screen (major blood group is not necessary, unless obstetric bleeding is present)

3. Women with risk factors and/or abnormal findings on physical examination
   • Obtain tests as indicated by history and examination findings (eg, finger stick blood glucose for women with diabetes mellitus or gestational diabetes).

F. Identify the Woman's Questions and Concerns.
   1. *If in labor,* determine the woman's preparation for childbirth and her preferences regarding analgesia, anesthesia, and other aspects of intrapartum care.
   2. *If not in labor,* assess need for patient education regarding continued care and treatment.
   3. *Birth plan:* If one is available, review it with the woman. If the woman has not established a plan, discuss options with her.

16. How Do You Proceed?

A. Record Your Findings.

   Document your findings in the patient's chart. Note any differences from previous examinations, if the prenatal record is available. Follow institutional protocol to relay findings of the assessment to an appropriate provider who may diagnose false or true labor.

B. Make a Plan.
   1. *Determine the care that needs to be delivered and establish priorities* based on your findings and the patient's preferences.
   2. *Decide if maternal/fetal transfer* to the regional center for delivery is advisable for the health of the woman and/or her fetus. Then decide if transfer can be done safely. If not, refer to Section 13 for intrapartum care needed by all high-risk women.
   3. *Discuss implementation strategies and expected outcomes* with the
      • Patient and the patient's family (if present)
      • Other members of the care delivery team

C. Monitor Patient Status and Review Plan of Care.

   Compare patient status with expected outcome. Be alert for possible development of new, unexpected changes in the condition of the woman or the fetus. Systematically review your plan of care to assess whether it meets the health care goals and the patient's needs. Readjust your plan, as appropriate, to meet changes in patient status.

Is the Mother Sick? Is the Fetus Sick?

Recommended Routines

All the routines listed below are based on the principles of perinatal care presented in the unit you have just finished. They are recommended as part of routine perinatal care.

Read each routine carefully and decide whether it is standard operating procedure in your hospital. Check the appropriate blank next to each routine.

Procedure Standard in My Hospital   **Needs Discussion by Our Staff**

_____	_____	1. Establish a record-keeping system that includes • Use of a single, standard prenatal record form by all obstetric practitioners. • Identification of risk status. • Reliable availability to labor and delivery staff of all prenatal records for all patients.
_____	_____	2. Develop a system that allows outpatient evaluation, in an obstetric care area, of women who may or may not be in labor until it is determined that discharge home or hospitalization is appropriate.
_____	_____	3. Establish a system for notification of nursery personnel regarding any risk factor as soon as a pregnant woman is admitted to the hospital.
_____	_____	4. Establish a system of prenatal consultation and/or referral for high-risk patients.
_____	_____	5. Provide fetal heart rate and uterine contraction monitoring for all patients during labor.
_____	_____	6. Establish a system whereby an emergency cesarean delivery can be started within 30 minutes of the decision to operate, at any time of the day or night.
_____	_____	7. Establish a system whereby personnel and equipment are available to provide resuscitation to a pregnant or postpartum woman, at any time of the day or night.
_____	_____	8. Establish a system whereby equipment and personnel for resuscitation of a newborn are available for every delivery.
_____	_____	9. Establish a protocol for documentation of telephone contact with patients, including history to be obtained, standard advice offered, and instructions given for communication with their obstetrical care providers.

Self-test Answers

These are the answers to the self-test questions. Please check them with the answers you gave and review the information in the unit wherever necessary.

A1. The woman is: well
     The fetus is: at risk
     You should: B. Investigate the fetal tachycardia.*

A2. The woman is: at risk
     The fetus is: at risk
     You should: B. Anticipate problems, reevaluate woman and fetus frequently.*

A3. The woman is: at risk
     The fetus is: at risk
     You should: B. Anticipate problems, reevaluate the woman and fetus frequently.*
     The woman is now: sick
     The fetus is now: at risk
     You should: C. Intervene promptly to investigate the cause of worsening renal function and reevaluate fetal condition.*

A4. • Start an intravenous line.
     • Provide intensive fetal heart rate and uterine contraction monitoring.
     • Position the woman on her side.
     • Notify nursery personnel of maternal and fetal condition immediately, and labor progress.
     • Arrange for personnel skilled in neonatal resuscitation to attend the delivery.
     • Have staff and equipment prepared to perform a cesarean delivery, within 30 minutes, if that becomes necessary.
     • Consult with regional center maternal/fetal medicine subspecialists and neonatologists regarding labor management and neonatal stabilization.
     • Prepare for postnatal/postpartum transfer of the woman and/or baby to more specialized care.

A5. • Intrapartum management can be better coordinated, if delivery at your hospital becomes necessary, if the woman is known to the regional center staff.
     • In utero transfer is less stressful to the fetus than neonatal transport is likely to be for the baby.
     • Regional center staff can get to know the woman and her family before the birth, and the same for the woman becoming familiar with the regional center staff.
     • The baby's anticipated care can be explained and introduction to the neonatal intensive care unit can be made, thus making the situation less traumatic for the parents.

*Consultation with a specialist(s) also may be appropriate for the patients. In some cases, referral to a regional center for continued care and delivery may be recommended. More details regarding management of specific conditions are given in the units that follow.

Unit 1 Posttest

If you are applying for continuing education credits, a posttest for this unit is available online. Completion of unit posttests and the book evaluation form are required to achieve continuing education credit. For more details, go to www.cmevillage.com.

SKILL UNIT

Determining Fetal Presentation With Leopold's Maneuvers

This skill unit will teach you a systematic method to determine fetal presentation by palpation of the maternal abdomen. Not everyone will be required to learn and practice this skill. Everyone, however, should read this unit and attend a skill session to learn how the examination is carried out.

Study this skill unit, then attend a skill demonstration and practice session.

An abdominal palpation manikin (optional) is available from several companies. One company with a suitable manikin is

> www.childbirthgraphics.com
> Phone: 800/299-3366, ext 287

To master the skill, you will need to demonstrate each of the steps listed below correctly. A manikin may be used to practice the skill, but you will be asked to demonstrate your proficiency with patients who need to be examined.

1. Explain the procedure and be able to answer questions a pregnant woman might ask about the examination.
2. Prepare and position the woman for the examination.
3. Demonstrate the 4 steps that comprise Leopold's maneuvers.
4. Correctly identify fetal presentation and estimate fetal weight for 3 different patients.
5. Record your findings.

Note: Illustrations in this skill unit from Olds SB, London ML, Ladewig PA. *Maternal-Newborn & Women's Health Care Nursing.* 7th ed. Reprinted by permission of Pearson Education Inc., Upper Saddle River, NJ.

PERINATAL PERFORMANCE GUIDE

Leopold's Maneuvers

ACTIONS	REMARKS

Deciding When to Use Leopold's Maneuvers

1. What are the indications for an examination? • Is the fetal presentation unknown or in doubt?	Leopold's maneuvers are used to identify fetal lie and presentation. Generally, they are used only in the third trimester but, in some women, it is possible to feel fetal parts in the second trimester. This examination is used in conjunction with a sterile vaginal examination (if appropriate) to determine the presenting part.
• Is the fetus large or small? What is the estimated fetal weight?	Estimation of fetal weight by clinical examination has been shown to be as accurate as that provided by ultrasound examination.
• Is there a need to identify the fetal back?	Fetal heart tones are generally easiest to obtain through the abdominal wall overlying the fetal back. Auscultation of the fetal heart rate, as well as placement of an external fetal heart rate monitor, is facilitated when the position of the fetal back is known.
Yes: Employ Leopold's maneuvers. No: There is no indication for Leopold's maneuvers.	Abdominal palpation to determine fetal position and estimate fetal weight has been used for centuries. The 4 steps of this systematic examination were described in 1894 by Leopold and Sporlin.

Preparing for the Examination

2. Explain the purpose of the examination to the patient.	
3. Ask the woman to empty her bladder.	The examination is easier to perform and more comfortable for the woman when her bladder is empty.
4. Ask the woman to rest on her back, with her knees bent and the soles of her feet flat on the bed or examination table. Place a pillow under her head and shoulders.	This position helps to relax the muscles of the abdominal wall.
5. Wash your hands in warm water before beginning the examination.	Mineral oil or lotion applied to your hands may make them slide more easily over the woman's abdomen.
6. Ask the patient to bare her abdomen.	

24

ACTIONS   REMARKS

Preparing for the Examination (continued)

7. Stand facing the patient on the side most comfortable for you. The first 3 maneuvers are done facing the patient's head. With the fourth maneuver, the position is reversed and the examiner faces the patient's feet.

The maneuvers may be done in any order. It is important, however, that they be done *systematically*. The sequence of steps taught in this skill unit is the sequence used most commonly.

Performing Leopold's Maneuvers

8. Keep in mind what you are trying to locate.
   • What part of the fetus (head or breech) is in the fundus?
   • Where is the fetal back? The extremities?
   • What part of the fetus is presenting in the pelvis? Does this match with what was found in the fundus?
   • What is the estimated size of the fetus?

Maternal obesity, hydramnios (excess amount of amniotic fluid), tumors, and placental implantation in the anterior of the uterus may make it difficult or impossible to determine fetal presentation.

9. First Maneuver
   Gently palpate the fundus with the fingertips of both hands.

   • **Head:** Harder, rounder, and smoother than the breech

   • **Breech:** Less well-defined, less movable than the head; more irregular and softer than the head

   If the fetal head or the breech is found in the fundus, the fetus is in longitudinal lie (maternal and fetal spinal columns are parallel with each other).

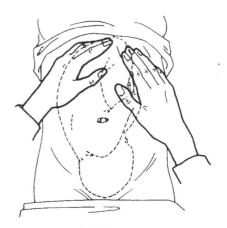

First Maneuver

Second Maneuver
a. Slide your hands down so the palms are on either side of the abdomen.

b. Exert gentle but deep, steady pressure with one hand to hold the fetus in place, while palpating the opposite side of the uterus with the other hand.

c. Reverse the hand applying pressure and the hand palpating.

   • **Extremities:** Softer, knobby, smaller, irregular, mobile parts with more "give"; fetal movement may be felt

   • **Back:** Long, firm, smooth; it may be possible to determine which way the back is turned (anterior, posterior, etc)

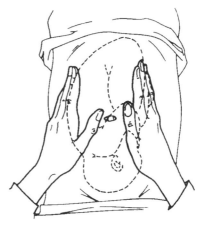

Second Maneuver

25

ACTIONS

REMARKS

Performing Leopold's Maneuvers (continued)

Third Maneuver

a. Grasp the lower portion of the maternal abdomen, just above the symphysis pubis, with the thumb and fingers of one hand.

   • **Not engaged:** Presenting part will be movable

   • **Engaged:** Presenting part will not be movable

b. Palpate the presenting part to determine if it is the head or the breech. (Refer to the descriptions given for the first maneuver to decide which part is presenting.)

c. Ask yourself: Does what I'm finding here fit with what I found in the fundus?

If the vertex and breech cannot be identified in the fundus and lower uterine segment, consider that the lie is transverse (fetus horizontal across the maternal abdomen, rather than aligned vertically). This is a rare situation. Instead of the vertical oval shape of a pregnant uterus with a fetus in longitudinal lie, the oval may appear to lie crossways, at a right angle to the long axis of the woman. If you suspect transverse lie, try to locate the fetal head along either side of the uterus.

Your other hand may be placed on the fundus to steady the fetus (not shown).

An unengaged head moves more than an unengaged breech.

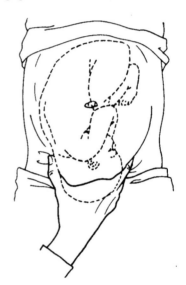

Third Maneuver

ACTIONS   **REMARKS**

Performing Leopold's Maneuvers (continued)

Fourth Maneuver

a. Turn and face the woman's feet.

b. Press firmly with the tips of the first 3 fingers of both hands to outline the fetus, as you move your hands downward, toward the pelvic inlet.

c. Applying deep pressure, move your hands symmetrically along the fetal sides. In vertex presentations, the hard, round head can be identified in the pelvis.

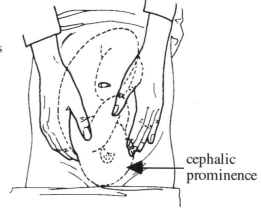

cephalic prominence

Fourth Maneuver

d. When a fetus's head is well-flexed, the cephalic prominence will be on the side opposite the fetal back (see illustration).

If you cannot locate the cephalic prominence by abdominal palpation, the head may be deep in the maternal pelvis. Confirm this with vaginal examination.

If the cephalic prominence is found on the same side as the back, the head may be de-flexed as with brow or face presentation.

If you cannot find the cephalic prominence by abdominal or vaginal examination or if it seems to be on the same side as the fetal back, and labor progress is delayed, consider ultrasound examination to identify fetal presentation and position.

Recording Your Findings

10. Record the results of the examination, including

   • Fetal presentation

   • Whether the presenting part is engaged in the pelvis

   • Location of cephalic prominence, if vertex presentation

   • Estimation of fetal weight

   • Any unusual findings

If you are not sure of your findings, indicate your uncertainty with a note describing the question(s) you have.

Notify appropriate personnel of unusual or questionable findings.

When this examination is done, you may detect the presence or absence of fetal movement.

ACTIONS	REMARKS
What Can Go Wrong?	

1. Maternal abdominal muscles may not be relaxed enough to feel the fetal parts.

   Make sure the woman is as comfortable as possible before the examination begins. If anxious, answer her questions and try to define and address her concerns. Abdominal relaxation also is aided when a woman's knees are bent and there is a pillow under her head and shoulders.

2. Maternal obesity, hydramnios, maternal intolerance to the examination, and/or an anterior placenta make it difficult to identify fetal parts.

   It may not be possible to use Leopold's maneuvers effectively in these situations.

3. An inexperienced examiner may not have confidence in his or her findings.

   Practice and experience are required to become proficient with this skill. If in doubt, ask a second person to perform an examination. Compare your findings and, if differences exist, review those aspects of the examination.

4. Findings from Leopold's maneuvers may not be consistent with findings from a sterile vaginal examination.

   If the presenting part or relative size of the fetus is not completely clear, consider obtaining an ultrasound evaluation of fetal presentation and position and an estimation of fetal weight.

Unit 2: Fetal Age, Growth, and Maturity

Objectives

In this unit you will learn

A. Why assessment of fetal age, growth, and maturity is important

B. What tests are used to evaluate fetal age, growth, and maturity

C. How gestational age and growth are assessed
   - Clinical findings
   - Ultrasound measurements

D. How pulmonary maturity is assessed

E. When fetal maturity should be assessed

Unit 2 Pretest

Before reading the unit, please answer the following questions. Select the *one best* answer to each question (unless otherwise instructed). Record your answers on the test and check them against the answers at the end of the book.

1. All the following measures are used to assess fetal gestational age, *except:*
  A. Fundal height of the uterus
  B. Maternal serum estriol level
  C. Menstrual history
  D. Time at which fetal heart tones can first be heard with a non-amplified fetoscope

2. Which of the following criteria is used to estimate the pulmonary maturity of a fetus?
  A. Presence of phosphatidyl glycerol in amniotic fluid
  B. Biparietal diameter
  C. Urinary estriol concentration
  D. Crown-rump length

3. All of the following influence fundal height, *except:*
  A. Uterine tumors
  B. Maternal obesity
  C. Hydramnios
  D. Maternal age

4. **True** **False** Estimation of gestational age using ultrasound measurement of fetal crown-rump length is most reliable during the first trimester.

5. **True** **False** A fetus determined to be small by ultrasound or fundal height measurements may actually be term and have mature lungs.

6. **True** **False** If phosphatidyl glycerol is present in the amniotic fluid, the fetus's lungs are almost always mature, even in women with diabetes mellitus.

7. **True** **False** Recent use of oral contraceptives does not interfere with menstrual dating of a pregnancy.

8. **True** **False** Quickening often occurs earlier in a primigravida than in a multigravida.

9. Which of the following is most helpful in determining fetal gestational age?
  A. Serial biparietal diameter measurements, starting before 24 weeks' gestation
  B. Date of quickening
  C. Presence or absence of distal femoral epiphyses on x-ray
  D. Level of phosphatidyl glycerol in the amniotic fluid

10. All of the following are possible with ultrasound, *except:*
  A. Detect all structural abnormalities of the fetus.
  B. Assess relative volume of amniotic fluid.
  C. Determine fetal heartbeat.
  D. Evaluate fetal respiratory activity.

11. **True** **False** The pregnant uterus can first be felt in the abdomen, at the symphysis pubis, at 8 weeks' gestation.

12. **True** **False** Following amniocentesis, there is a 10% chance of serious complications, including spontaneous abortion and rupture of membranes.

13. **True** **False** A lecithin-sphingomyelin ratio of greater than 2.0 may not indicate fetal lung maturity in women with abnormal glucose tolerance.

14. **True** **False** The lamellar body count measures the concentration of the surfactant complex in the amniotic fluid, which increases with advancing lung maturity.

1. Why Is Evaluation of Fetal Age, Growth, and Maturity Important?

As noted in the previous unit, early and precise documentation of gestation length is important for all pregnancies. Situations can arise in late pregnancy in which accurate knowledge of the length of gestation is critical to optimal management. Determining length of gestation is best done in early pregnancy, when the changes from week to week are more definitive.

Assessment of fetal growth can help identify a sick or at-risk fetus. Evaluation of fetal maturity can help determine the best time to deliver the baby for women with high-risk pregnancies.

2. What Tests Are Used to Evaluate Fetal Age, Growth, and Maturity?

A. Last Menstrual Period (LMP)

The LMP is used to determine when conception most likely occurred. Length of gestation is calculated from the first day of the LMP.

B. Serum Pregnancy Test

Human chorionic gonadotropin (hCG) is detectable in a woman's serum within 2 weeks of conception. It may be used to confirm a pregnancy and to help establish the length of gestation.

C. Quickening

Fetal movement is usually first felt by the pregnant woman at 16 to 20 weeks. The date of quickening helps to confirm length of gestation.

D. Fundal Height

The uterus usually grows at a predictable rate, corresponding to normal fetal growth and gestational age.

E. Fetal Heart Tones

Heart tones of the fetus can first be heard with a Doppler device at 10 to 12 weeks and with a non-amplified fetoscope at 18 to 22 weeks. The date heart tones are first heard helps to confirm length of gestation.

F. Ultrasound Measurements

Fetal biparietal diameter, abdominal circumference, crown-rump length, femur length, and calculations of fetal weight are used to assess fetal growth over time and length of gestation. These measures, however, may not correspond to fetal lung maturity.

G. Amniotic Fluid Analyses

The lecithin-sphingomyelin (L/S) ratio, phosphatidyl glycerol (PG), lamellar body count, and other tests are used to assess fetal lung maturity and to predict whether a baby would develop respiratory distress syndrome (RDS) if delivered at the time the test is obtained.

Self-test

Now answer these questions to test yourself on the information in the last section.

A1. Determining length of gestation is best done _____ in pregnancy.

A2. Length of gestation should be determined as precisely as possible for _____ pregnancies.

A3. List at least 3 tests or criteria used to assess fetal length of gestation.

_____

_____

_____

A4. List at least 2 tests used to assess fetal lung maturity.

_____

_____

Check your answers with the list that follows the Recommended Routines. Correct any incorrect answers and review the appropriate section in the unit.

3. What Is Gestational Age?

The gestational age of a fetus is the age (in weeks) from the first day of the woman's LMP to the point in time at which you assess it. Various gestational ages are associated with different problems. The lower the gestational age, the more problems there are associated with immaturity. There are also significant problems associated with post-maturity. It is important to establish gestational age early in pregnancy. In particular, the physical examination of the pregnant woman in late pregnancy may not accurately reflect fetal age.

Not all fetuses who seem small by physical examination of the pregnant woman are preterm. They may be term and growth restricted.

Not all fetuses who seem large by physical examination of the pregnant woman are term. They may be large for their gestational age and still be preterm and have immature lungs. This is especially true for fetuses of women with diabetes mellitus or abnormal glucose tolerance.

4. How Are Clinical Findings Used to Determine Gestational Age?

A. Menstrual History

Most pregnancies will deliver approximately 280 days (40 weeks) from the first day of the LMP. This is how a woman's estimated date of delivery (EDD) is calculated. These calculations assume that a woman has regular 28-day cycles, and ovulated and became pregnant on the 14th day of her cycle.

For women with longer, but regular cycles, the conception date should be calculated 14 days prior to the next expected menstrual period.

Although an EDD is calculated for 40 weeks' gestation, babies born between 37 weeks, 0 days and 42 weeks, 0 days gestation are considered term. However, although 37 to 38 weeks are technically considered "term," because of the increased risk of respiratory distress in the newborn, elective induction or operative delivery is not recommended prior to 39 weeks unless there are medical indications.

Potential problems in interpretation of menstrual history include the following:

- The dates for a woman's last menstrual cycle may be incorrect.
- There is wide variability in the length of women's menstrual cycles.
- Ovulation may not occur exactly 2 weeks after the first day of menses.
- Ovulation may be delayed while breastfeeding.
- Ovulation also may be delayed after a woman stops taking oral contraceptives. When the last menstrual cycle occurred in association with taking oral contraceptives, menstrual dating is less reliable than if a woman's periods were spontaneous.
- A significant proportion of pregnancies are unplanned; women with unplanned pregnancies may not keep as accurate menstrual records as those who are planning a pregnancy.

B. Quickening History

Fetal movement may first be seen by ultrasound as early as 10 weeks. Quickening is the term applied to the sensation a pregnant woman feels when the fetus first moves strongly enough for her to notice it. In a primigravida, this usually occurs between 16 and 20 weeks. When a woman has had a previous pregnancy, she is often aware of fetal movement earlier than with her first baby. In a multigravida, quickening may be detected as early as 14 or 16 weeks.

Quickening is a subjective sign that is dependent on the woman's ability and willingness to feel it. Women who deny the existence of an unwanted pregnancy may only admit to feeling the baby move much later in pregnancy. Women who have a strong desire for pregnancy may believe they have felt quickening much earlier in pregnancy. For most women, quickening occurs between 16 and 20 weeks' gestation.

Potential problems in interpretation of quickening history include the following:

- Quickening is a subjective sign that cannot be felt by the examiner.
- Perception of quickening varies from woman to woman and with the number of children a woman has borne.

C. Fetal Heart Tones

Fetal heart tones can first be heard with a *non-amplified fetoscope* at 18 to 22 weeks' gestation. If fetal heart tones have been heard non-amplified for a period of 20 weeks, the baby is likely to be term. In the same way, the date of term gestation can be calculated by adding 20 weeks to the date at which non-amplified fetal heart sounds are *first* heard. This assumes the patient was examined the week before and fetal heart tones could not be heard at that time. Non-amplified fetoscopes are no longer commonly used in obstetric practice.

Fetal heart tones can first be heard with a *Doppler ultrasound device* (amplified) at 10 to 12 weeks. Doppler ultrasound detects the movement of fetal blood through the umbilical cord (whoosh-whoosh sound) or the ventricular contraction of the fetal heart (galloping horse sound). Occasionally, some of the Doppler sounds created by blood flow through large vessels in the maternal pelvis are misinterpreted as fetal heart tones. If there is uncertainty about the origin of the sounds, check the maternal pulse and compare it to the rate of the sounds heard with the Doppler device. The maternal heart rate should be much slower than the fetal heart rate; the normal range of the fetal heart rate is 110 to 160 beats per minute.

Potential problems in interpretation of fetal heart tones include the following:

- Different examiners have varying abilities to hear fetal heart tones. Some people may not be able to hear non-amplified heart tones until later than 20 weeks' gestation.

- The concept that a fetus is at term if fetal heart tones have been audible for 20 weeks applies only to fetal heart tones heard with a non-amplified fetoscope.
- Conditions that affect the relationship of the fetal back to the maternal abdomen (fetal position, hydramnios, maternal obesity, etc) may delay the detection of fetal heart tones.

 The most common reasons for not finding fetal heart tones at the expected time are

- *Dates are wrong.*
- *Pregnant woman is extremely obese.*
- *Fetus is dead or was spontaneously aborted.*
- *Patient is not pregnant.*

D. Uterine Size and Fundal Height

Gestational age may be determined based on assessment of uterine size by pelvic and/or abdominal examination. The accuracy of this method increases when the first pelvic examination is done at the earliest possible time during pregnancy and then is followed by periodic examinations.

1. First trimester

During the first trimester, there is a dramatic increase in the size of the uterus, making a uterus at 12 weeks easily distinguishable from a uterus at 8 weeks (Table 2.1).

Table 2.1. Palpable Characteristics of the Uterus in the First Trimester		
Weeks (description)	**Uterine Size**	
4 (same as non-pregnant size)	6-8 cm	Palpable with bimanual pelvic examination
6 (slightly enlarged)	8-10 cm	
8 (clearly enlarged)	10-12 cm	
10 (size of a large orange or grape-fruit)	12-15 cm	
12 (size of a cantaloupe)	at symphysis pubis	Palpable abdominally

2. Second and third trimesters

As the fetus grows, the height of the fundus (top part of the uterus) increases. Fundal height is measured from the symphysis pubis to the top of the fundus.

The gestational age of the fetus correlates roughly with fundal height, in centimeters. For example, when the fundus is at the level of the umbilicus (fundal height of 20 cm) most pregnancies have reached 20 weeks. Between 20 and 34 weeks, there is usually a difference of less than 2 cm between fundal height and the number of weeks of gestation. Figure 2.1 illustrates the size of the uterus at 4-week intervals during the second and third trimesters.

Note: The top of the uterus may recede during the last 4 weeks of pregnancy as the fetus "drops" into the pelvis (sometimes called "lightening"). This is shown by the dashed line labeled 40 weeks in Figure 2.1.

There are several acceptable methods for measuring fundal height. Regardless of the method used, consistency of measurement is essential for accurate results.

Ideally, fundal height should be measured by the same examiner at each prenatal visit. If that is not possible, all examiners should use the same technique.

Figure 2.2 illustrates one reliable method for measuring fundal height. In this technique, fundal height is measured from the top of the symphysis pubis in a straight line to the point over the abdomen where the highest part of the fundus is felt. Note: Some clinicians measure around the curvature of the uterus.

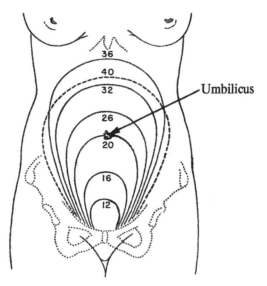

Figure 2.1. Fundal Height at Different Weeks of Gestation.
Adapted with permission from Danforth's *Obstetrics and Gynecology*, 4th ed. Philadelphia, PA: Lippincott Williams & Wilkins; 1982: 362.

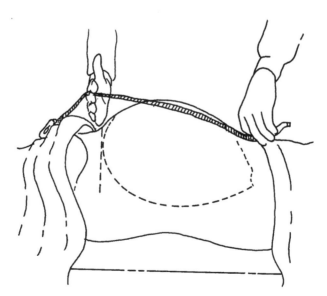

Figure 2.2. Measurement of Fundal Height.
Adapted with permission from Danforth's *Obstetrics and Gynecology*, 4th ed. Philadelphia, PA: Lippincott Williams & Wilkins; 1982:362.

37

Potential problems in interpretation of fundal height include the following:

- A growth-restricted fetus may be term, but have poor increase in fundal height.
- A large fetus may have consistent or even accelerated increase in fundal height, but still be preterm.
- Fundal height is more difficult to determine in obese women.
- Fibroids in the uterus may make measurement of uterine size unreliable in determining fetal growth.
- Multiple gestation, and conditions such as oligohydramnios and hydramnios, will affect fundal height and not necessarily reflect the size of the fetus(es).
- During the third trimester, the height of the fundus may vary from woman to woman at the same week of gestation.
- Measurements of fundal height can vary between examiners.

5. What Do You Do When Clinical Findings and Pregnancy Dates Do Not Match?

When clinical findings indicate a fetus larger or smaller than expected by the dates of the pregnancy, there is a size-date discrepancy. A discrepancy may exist between any of the clinical findings and pregnancy dates. Some minor discrepancies can be explained by normal variation in fetal and uterine growth.

A. Significant Size-Date Discrepancies

The following discrepancies are sufficiently important enough to require additional investigation:

- The uterus feels smaller or larger than would be expected based on the date of the LMP.
- Quickening occurs before 16 weeks or not until after 20 weeks.
- Fetal heart sounds cannot be heard with a Doppler ultrasound device until more than 12 weeks have elapsed.
- Fetal heart sounds may not be audible with a non-amplified fetoscope until more than 22 weeks have elapsed.
- Between 20 and 34 weeks, there is a difference of 2 to 3 cm or more between fundal height and the number of weeks of pregnancy, when the measuring method described previously is used. For example, a fundal height measurement of 28 cm (using the method described) in a pregnancy at 32 weeks' gestation needs investigation.

B. Investigation of Size-Date Discrepancy

- Review the maternal history and clinical findings for high-risk conditions likely to cause abnormal fetal or uterine growth, such as
  - Hypertension, smoking, congenital infection, etc (small-for-gestational-age fetus)
  - Maternal diabetes, previous large babies, etc (large-for-gestational-age fetus)
  - Multifetal gestation, hydramnios, etc (abnormal uterine growth)
- Obtain ultrasound evaluation for estimation of fetal size and gestational age, amniotic fluid volume, and other factors that could affect uterine size.

Self-test

Now answer these questions to test yourself on the information in the last section.

B1. Quickening is likely to occur _____ in a primigravida than in a multigravida.

B2. Give 2 common reasons fetal heart tones may not be heard when first expected.

_____

_____

B3. **True** **False** The estimated date of confinement is calculated as 280 days from the first day of the last menstrual period.

B4. **True** **False** The usual time of quickening occurs between 22 and 26 weeks.

B5. **True** **False** Quickening is a subjective sign that may be influenced by the woman's state of mind.

B6. **True** **False** Fetal size may not indicate fetal age or maturity.

B7. Inaccurate determination of a woman's estimated date of delivery may be due to which of the following?

Yes	**No**	
____	____	Inaccurate date of last menstrual cycle
____	____	Use of oral contraceptives immediately preceding the pregnancy
____	____	Delayed ovulation
____	____	Irregular menstrual periods

B8. Non-amplified fetal heart tones are usually first heard at _____, while fetal heart tones amplified with a Doppler device are usually first heard at _____.

B9. During the second and third trimester, fundal height is measured from the _____ to the _____.

B10. A pregnancy is 24 weeks by last menstrual period dates. Non-amplified fetal heart tones have been heard for 5 weeks. You measure a fundal height of 31 cm. What action, if any, would you take?

_____

_____

B11. A pregnancy is 24 weeks by last menstrual period dates. Amplified fetal heart tones have been heard for 6 weeks, but non-amplified heart tones cannot be heard. What action, if any, would you take?

_____

_____

B12. A pregnant uterus the size of a cantaloupe on bimanual examination is palpable abdominally at the symphysis pubis. This most likely represents a pregnancy of _____ weeks' gestation.

Check your answers with the list that follows the Recommended Routines. Correct any incorrect answers and review the appropriate section in the unit.

6. How Is Ultrasonography Used to Evaluate a Pregnancy?

Ultrasound imaging, also called ultrasonography, sonography, and sonogram, is an imaging technique using high-frequency sound waves. A transducer placed on the maternal abdomen or in the vagina transmits these sound waves through maternal tissue. The sound waves are reflected by the structures they encounter. The reflected sound waves are received by the transducer and "translated" into images on the video monitor. Rapid cycling of the sound waves allows imaging to occur in "real time."

A. Tests That Can Be Done With Ultrasonography

- Determine the presence of a gestational sac.
- Determine the presence or absence of a fetal heartbeat.
- Determine the number of fetuses.
- Determine gestational age by measurement of the
  - Fetal crown-rump length
  - Biparietal diameter of the fetal skull
  - Fetal head circumference
  - Fetal abdominal circumference
  - Fetal femur length
- Determine placental location and size.
- Determine fetal position.
- Evaluate the presence or absence of some congenital malformations.
- Estimate relative volume of amniotic fluid.
- Evaluate fetal muscle tone, body movements, and respiratory activity.
- Evaluate the uterus, cervix, and ovaries.

B. Types of Ultrasonography

1. Basic

   Basic ultrasound examination is used to identify gestational sac location and fetal heart motion, perform measurements to determine the gestational age, perform a basic fetal anatomic evaluation, and determine fetal number and position.

2. Comprehensive

   Comprehensive ultrasound examination is a much more time-consuming and detailed examination of each fetal organ system. It is used only when a basic ultrasound examination has suggested an abnormality of fetal development, or when the clinical history suggests such a problem. Much greater experience and skill are needed to perform and interpret a comprehensive ultrasound than a basic ultrasound examination.

 Fetal abnormalities may be missed or misinterpreted by even the most experienced ultrasonographer, and some abnormalities cannot be detected by ultrasound. The absence of an ultrasound-detectable abnormality is not a guarantee of an anatomically normal baby.

7. How Is Ultrasonography Used to Determine Gestational Age?

Because the growth pattern of a fetus varies throughout pregnancy, the accuracy of a particular measurement and its usefulness in determining gestational age and growth changes with each trimester (Table 2.2).

A. First Trimester

   Normal variation in size is minimal during the first 12 weeks of pregnancy.
   Measurements made at this time are accurate within 1 week 95% of the time.

   1. Gestational sac

      This is first seen in a pregnancy at 5.0 to 5.5 weeks.

   2. Crown-rump length

      This is the distance from the top of the fetal head to the bottom of the fetal spine. It
      is most accurate as a measure of gestational age between 6 and 12 weeks. After that,
      other measurements are more reliable.

B. Second Trimester

   1. Biparietal diameter (BPD)

      This is the distance between one side of the fetal head and the other, as measured
      between the 2 parietal bones. When measured between 14 and 24 weeks, it gives an
      accurate estimate of gestational age within 2 weeks. It is less accurate when the head
      shape is not normal (eg, the elongated "dolichocephalic" head in the breech fetus).

   2. Femur length (FL)

      Used alone, femur length is most reliable as an estimation of gestational age between
      14 and 24 weeks. It is used throughout pregnancy, however, as a second indicator of
      fetal growth.

   3. Head circumference (HC)

      The head circumference is measured at the same level as the BPD and has the same
      degree of accuracy, with the advantage of being independent of head shape in its abil-
      ity to assess gestational age.

   4. Abdominal circumference (AC)

      The abdominal circumference is the measurement most affected by variations in fetal
      growth, and has the largest range of error late in pregnancy when compared with
      other ultrasound measurements.

C. Third Trimester

   1. All ultrasound measurements after 30 weeks' gestation are subject to a range of error
      of +/- 3 weeks. Composite biometry and serial measurements better estimate gesta-
      tional age than a single measurement of a single structure.

   2. Modern ultrasound equipment has software packages that use the measurements to
      estimate gestational age and fetal weight. A composite of the above measurements
      is considered preferable to a single measurement in estimating fetal weight. Multiple
      measurements partially compensate for a single inaccurate measurement as well as the
      inherent range of error in ultrasound measurements.

8. How Do the Accuracy of Clinical Findings and Ultrasound Measurements Compare in Assessing Gestational Age?

Table 2.2. Clinical Findings Versus Ultrasound Measurement in Estimating Gestational Age	
Range of Accuracy in Weeks (based on a single measurement)	**Clinical Finding or Ultrasound Measure**
	Clinical Finding
2-6	• Last menstrual period*
4-6	• Quickening
4-6	• Non-amplified fetal heart tones heard
2	• First trimester physical examination by skilled examiner
2-3	• Fundal height measurement between 20 and 24 weeks
	Ultrasound Measure
1	• Gestational sac before 7 weeks
1	• Crown-rump length between 6 and 11 wks
1-2	• Femur length between 14 and 24 weeks
1-2	• Biparietal diameter before 20 weeks[†]
2-3	• Biparietal diameter between 20 and 30 wks
3-4	• Biparietal diameter after 30 weeks
3	• Femur length after 30 weeks

*Variation depends on regularity of cycles, ability to recall period date, no birth control pills for previous 3 months, and whether the mother is breastfeeding.

[†]Serial ultrasound examinations, with the first one obtained before 20 weeks, allow the clinician to judge the gestational age within 1 to 2 weeks in late pregnancy.

Self-test

Now answer these questions to test yourself on the information in the last section.

C1. True False Ultrasound measurements of the fetus evaluate fetal maturity.

C2. True False A comprehensive ultrasound examination is much more detailed than a basic ultrasound examination.

C3. True False In skilled hands, it is possible to identify all fetal malformations by ultrasound.

C4. True False During the third trimester, biparietal diameter may be used to estimate fetal weight.

C5. True False When only biparietal diameter measurements are available, serial ultrasound measurements, with the first one obtained before 20 weeks, is the most reliable way to estimate gestational age.

C6. True False First trimester ultrasound measurements are accurate to within 1 week of fetal age 95% of the time.

C7. When is ultrasound measurement of femur length most accurate for estimation of gestational age?
   A. Between 7 and 14 weeks
   B. Between 14 and 24 weeks
   C. Between 24 and 32 weeks

C8. Crown-rump length gives a reliable estimation of fetal gestational age during the _____ trimester.

C9. During the third trimester, abdominal circumference may be used together with _____ to estimate gestational age.

C10. List at least 4 tests that can be done with ultrasonography.

_____
_____
_____
_____

Check your answers with the list that follows the Recommended Routines. Correct any incorrect answers and review the appropriate section in the unit.

9. How Is Pulmonary Maturity Assessed?

Many things about a preterm baby may be immature, but the most important organ system in determining whether the baby lives or dies is the pulmonary system. If a newborn's lungs are very immature, there may be little or no surfactant present. Surfactant is composed of substances (proteins and phospholipids) that help to keep the alveoli (air sacs in the lungs) open at the end of expiration. A preterm baby with too little surfactant will develop respiratory distress syndrome and thus require additional oxygen, and perhaps assisted ventilation, until the lungs become mature enough to make their own surfactant.

When preterm birth is unavoidable, corticosteroids given to the pregnant woman can help accelerate fetal pulmonary maturity. After birth, surfactant deficiency can be treated by endotracheal administration of a commercially available surfactant preparation. While these therapies have been proven beneficial, neither can be guaranteed to eliminate serious lung disease in a preterm baby.

A fetus estimated to be near term may still have immature lungs, particularly if the woman has diabetes mellitus or abnormal glucose tolerance.

  A. When Is Pulmonary Maturity Determined?

    1. *Before induction of labor or cesarean delivery prior to the onset of spontaneous labor,* if there is a question of fetal size or pregnancy dates, or if a discrepancy exists between obstetrical history and clinical examination.

2. *When early delivery of the fetus may be necessary,* either for the woman's or fetus's well-being, as may be the case in certain high-risk pregnancies. Repeated amniocenteses may be done to determine when the fetal lungs are mature enough to minimize the chance that the baby will develop breathing difficulties.

3. *Pregnancies complicated by diabetes mellitus* when delivery is anticipated prior to 39 weeks or the spontaneous onset of labor.

B. How Do You Test for Lung Maturity?

Tests for lung maturity are done with amniotic fluid. Amniocentesis is performed to obtain the amniotic fluid. Before amniocentesis is done, the placenta and fetus are located by ultrasonography. During the procedure, ultrasound guidance is used while a needle is inserted, under sterile conditions, through the maternal abdominal wall and into the uterus. A syringe attached to the needle is used to withdraw amniotic fluid.

C. What Are the Risks of Amniocentesis?

- Spontaneous abortion (uncommon; less than 0.5% at 15 weeks' gestation or later)
- Puncturing the placenta, which may cause fetal bleeding (rare)
- Puncturing the cord (rare)
- Puncturing the fetus, which may cause fetal death (rare)
- Infection (rare)
- Rupture of membranes (uncommon; occurs in approximately 1% in late pregnancy)
- Onset of labor (uncommon)
- Sensitization of an Rh-negative woman carrying an Rh-positive fetus

Note: Rh immune globulin should be given to all Rh-negative women following amniocentesis, unless delivery is anticipated within 72 hours. If delivery occurs within 72 hours, the baby's blood group can be determined to learn if Rh immune globulin is actually needed.

 In experienced hands, amniocentesis is a useful, reliable, and safe technique with a complication rate of 1% or lower.

D. What Tests Are Done to Estimate Pulmonary Maturity?

Several tests of amniotic fluid are used to determine pulmonary maturity. These tests are performed late in pregnancy when determination of fetal lung maturity is important in decision making related to timing of delivery.

1. Lecithin-sphingomyelin ratio (L/S)

Mature fetal lungs secrete a group of substances called surfactants. These substances are made up in part of lecithin and sphingomyelin. As the fetal lungs mature, the amount of lecithin increases in the amniotic fluid during the third trimester, while the amount of sphingomyelin remains about the same. The increase in lecithin is associated with increasing fetal lung maturity.

The pulmonary maturity of a fetus can be estimated by taking a sample of amniotic fluid and measuring the amount of lecithin compared to the amount of sphingomyelin. This is called the L/S ratio. Because the amount of sphingomyelin remains relatively constant, the L/S ratio is usually given as a single number indicating the proportion of lecithin present. For example, an L/S ratio of 1.3 indicates the fetus's lungs are immature, while a ratio of 3.0 indicates fetal lung maturity.

The Table 2.3 illustrates the relationship between L/S ratio and fetal lung maturity.

Table 2.3. Relationship Between Lecithin-Sphingomyelin (L/S) Ratio and Fetal Lung Maturity	
L/S Ratio	**Interpretation**
0.0–1.0	The lungs are immature and the baby will likely develop respiratory distress syndrome.
1.0–1.5	The lungs are more mature, but the baby may develop respiratory distress syndrome.
1.5–2.0	The lungs are almost mature, but approximately 20% of babies will still have respiratory distress syndrome.
>2.0	This is generally associated with mature lungs with <2% of babies having breathing problems from respiratory distress syndrome.
Note: The L/S ratio associated with pulmonary maturity may vary for different laboratories. Check the category ranges for your laboratory.	

The major exception to this interpretation of L/S ratio is for women with diabetes mellitus or abnormal glucose tolerance. In these women, an L/S ratio of 2.0 or higher may still be associated with immature fetal lungs. Caution should be used in the interpretation of L/S ratio in women with diabetes mellitus.

Blood or meconium in the amniotic fluid may decrease the accuracy of the L/S ratio; however, if the L/S ratio indicates lung maturity, this is usually reliable.

While an L/S ratio provides relatively detailed information about fetal lung maturity, several hours are required to run the test and obtain results. A high level of technical proficiency is required on the part of the laboratory staff. In certain clinical situations, therefore, other measures of fetal pulmonary maturity that provide results more quickly may be more useful from a practical standpoint.

2. Phosphatidyl glycerol (PG)

The measurement of the presence or absence of another surfactant substance, PG, in the amniotic fluid also may be helpful in determining fetal lung maturity. Phosphatidyl glycerol begins to be produced by the fetal lungs at approximately 36.5 weeks' gestation. When PG is present, there is a less than 0.5% chance of the baby developing respiratory distress syndrome, regardless of the L/S ratio or gestational age. Levels of PG are generally not reported. Phosphatidyl glycerol is either present or absent. Blood or meconium in the amniotic fluid will not affect the accuracy of PG determination.

Determination of PG can be particularly helpful in assessing lung maturity in pregnancies of diabetic women, where the L/S ratio is less predictive. In women with diabetes mellitus or abnormal glucose tolerance during pregnancy, the presence of PG indicates fetal lung maturity.

3. Lamellar body count

Lamellar bodies are the stored form of surfactant protein within type II pneumocytes in the fetal lung, and their concentration in amniotic fluid increases with advancing gestational age. Lamellar body counts are easily performed on a hematology analyzer due to their similarity in size to a platelet. A lamellar body count of $50,000/mm^3$ or higher predicts the absence of RDS with a high negative predictive value. Lamellar body counts of less than 40,000/mm^3 are associated with a high rate of RDS. Since lamellar bodies and platelets are similar in size, the presence of blood in the sample will make interpretation difficult.

E. What Can Be Done to Accelerate Pulmonary Maturity?

The administration of corticosteroids to the pregnant woman has been shown to accelerate maturation of several organ systems and tissues in preterm fetuses. While primarily used to speed up the process of fetal lung maturation, corticosteroids also accelerate the maturation of cardiovascular, nervous, and gastrointestinal tissue in preterm fetuses. This reduces the frequency of respiratory distress syndrome, intraventricular hemorrhage (bleeding into the ventricles of the brain), and deaths in preterm newborns born between 24 and 36 weeks' gestation. Administration of corticosteroids should be considered whenever preterm delivery is unavoidable or is necessary for the well-being of either the woman or the fetus.

See Book II: Maternal and Fetal Care, Unit 7, Preterm Labor, for more details and recommendations regarding antenatal use of corticosteroids.

Self-test

Now answer these questions to test yourself on the information in the last section.

D1. In a preterm newborn, the organ system most important in determining whether the newborn lives or dies is _____.

D2. When phosphatidyl glycerol is present in the amniotic fluid, there is a less than _____ chance of the baby developing respiratory distress syndrome.
  A. 0.5%
  B. 5%
  C. 15%
  D. 50%

D3. **True   False**   The concentration of lecithin in the amniotic fluid increases as the fetus's lungs become more mature.

D4. **True   False**   Ultrasonography should be used while an amniocentesis is performed.

D5. What maternal condition interferes with the usual interpretation of lecithin-sphingomyelin ratios?
_____

D6. Sometimes corticosteroids are given to the pregnant woman to help _____.

D7. To obtain accurate results from a lamellar body count test, the amniotic fluid must be free of
_____.

D8. Which of the following tests are used to evaluate fetal lung maturity?

Yes	No	
___	___	Lecithin-sphingomyelin ratio
___	___	Alpha fetoprotein
___	___	Phosphatidyl glycerol
___	___	Lamellar body count
___	___	Femur length
___	___	Fundal height

D9. Match the following lecithin-sphingomyelin ratios with their usual interpretation.
  ___ 1.8   **A.** Immature fetal lungs
  ___ 2.3   **B.** Nearly mature fetal lungs
  ___ 0.8   **C.** Mature fetal lungs
  ___ 1.2
  ___ 3.0

Check your answers with the list that follows the Recommended Routines. Correct any incorrect answers and review the appropriate section in the unit.

10. Which Tests Should Be Performed Before a Planned Delivery?

Planned delivery, whether by induction of labor or cesarean delivery, should not occur before 39 weeks' gestation unless a valid medical or obstetrical reason is present. Situations exist where delivery is necessary before 39 completed weeks' gestation due to pregnancy complications that threaten maternal and/or fetal well-being. In these cases, determination of fetal lung maturity prior to delivery may not be necessary. Planned delivery, whether by cesarean section or induction of labor, also carries the risk of incorrect estimation of fetal gestational age. The baby may be born preterm and immature.

Assessment of fetal maturity is important whenever delivery is planned to occur before the spontaneous onset of labor. Induction of labor carries with it an increased risk for overstimulation of uterine contractions, abnormal fetal heart rate patterns, and need for cesarean section. Induction of labor should have a stated indication, one in which the expected benefits outweigh the risks (Book II: Maternal and Fetal Care, Unit 8, Inducing and Augmenting Labor).

Of the many ways to estimate fetal age and maturity, some tests, and some combinations of tests and clinical findings, are more reliable than others. The following guidelines will help you determine the best date for a planned delivery:

1. Fetal heart tones have been heard for 20 weeks by non-amplified fetoscope or for 30 weeks by Doppler ultrasound.

2. Thirty-six weeks have elapsed since positive results were obtained from a serum or urine hCG test performed by a reliable laboratory.

3. Ultrasound measurement of crown-rump length, obtained at 6 to 11 weeks, supports a gestational age of 39 weeks or more.

4. Clinical history, plus physical and ultrasound examinations obtained between 12 and 20 weeks, support a gestational age of 39 weeks or more.

In women with normal menstrual cycles, and no immediately antecedent use of oral contraceptives, any 1 of the 4 findings outlined above may be used to confirm menstrual dating of fetal age.

Fetal lung maturity also should be confirmed for any pregnancy elected to be delivered before 39 weeks' gestation, unless there are contraindications to amniocentesis.* However, because no test of fetal lung maturity can completely eliminate the possibility of respiratory distress syndrome or other neonatal complications, these risks must be weighed against the risk of continuing the pregnancy.

---

*American Academy of Pediatrics, American College of Obstetricians and Gynecologists. Intrapartum and postpartum care of the mother. In: *Guidelines for Perinatal Care*. 6th ed. Elk Grove Village, IL: American Academy of Pediatrics; 2007:160.

Fetal Age, Growth, and Maturity

Recommended Routines

All the routines listed below are based on the principles of perinatal care presented in the unit you have just finished. They are recommended as part of routine perinatal care.

Read each routine carefully and decide whether it is standard operating procedure in your hospital. Check the appropriate blank next to each routine.

Procedure Standard in My Hospital	Needs Discussion by Our Staff	
_____	_____	1. Develop a system for ensuring frequent and appropriate evaluation of each high-risk pregnancy throughout gestation.
_____	_____	2. Ensure that each high-risk pregnancy has access to each of the following, as needed: • Amniocentesis • Comprehensive ultrasonography • Laboratory evaluation for fetal lung maturity • Maternal-fetal medicine subspecialist
_____	_____	3. Establish a routine for consistent measuring and recording of fundal height at each prenatal visit.
_____	_____	4. Use a system to ensure that fetal maturity has been documented prior to a planned delivery.

Self-test Answers

These are the answers to the self-test questions. Please check them with the answers you gave and review the information in the unit wherever necessary.

A1. Early

A2. All

A3. Any 3 of the following:
- Last menstrual period
- Human chorionic gonadotropin
- Quickening
- Fundal height
- Fetal heart tones
- Ultrasound measure of
  - Biparietal diameter
  - Abdominal circumference
  - Crown-rump length
  - Femur length
  - Estimate of fetal weight

A4. Any 2 of the following:
- Lecithin-sphingomyelin ratio
- Phosphatidyl glycerol
- Lamellar body count

B1. Later

B2. Any 2 of the following:
- Menstrual dates are wrong
- Dates of the pregnancy were miscalculated
- Early fetal death
- Spontaneous abortion
- Extreme maternal obesity
- Hydramnios

B3. True

B4. False. Quickening usually occurs between 16 and 20 weeks, although it may occur earlier in a multigravida.

B5. True

B6. True

B7.

Yes	No	
X	____	Inaccurate date of last menstrual cycle
X	____	Use of oral contraceptives immediately preceding the pregnancy
X	____	Delayed ovulation
X	____	Irregular periods

B8. Non-amplified: 18 to 22 weeks
Amplified: 10 to 12 weeks

B9. Symphysis pubis, top of the uterus.

B10. Remeasure fundal height. If unchanged, obtain ultrasound evaluation because fetal heart tones are consistent with last menstrual period dates, but uterine size is considerably larger than what would be expected.

B11. Recheck dates and consider doing an ultrasound. It is most likely that the dates are wrong and the pregnancy is less than 24 weeks.

B12. 12 weeks

C1. False. Ultrasound measurements are used to assess fetal age and monitor growth, but are not reliable indicators of fetal maturity.

C2. True

C3. False. Some fetal abnormalities cannot be detected by ultrasound. In addition, even the most expert of ultrasonographers may miss, or misinterpret, some abnormalities.

C4. True

C5. True

C6. True

C7. B. Between 14 and 24 weeks

C8. First

C9. Biparietal diameter

C10. Any 4 of the following:
- Determine the presence of a gestational sac.
- Determine the presence or absence of a fetal heartbeat.
- Determine the number of fetuses.
- Measure the biparietal diameter of the fetal skull.
- Measure the length of the fetal femur.
- Measure the fetal crown-rump length.
- Estimate the fetal head circumference.
- Estimate the fetal abdominal circumference.
- Determine placental location and size.
- Determine fetal position.
- Evaluate the presence or absence of certain congenital malformations.
- Estimate relative volume of amniotic fluid.
- Evaluate fetal muscle tone, body movements, and respiratory activity.
- Evaluate the uterus and surrounding structures.

D1. Pulmonary system or lungs

D2. A. 0.5%

D3. True

D4. True

D5. Diabetes mellitus or abnormal glucose tolerance

D6. Mature the fetus's lungs

D7. Blood

D8.

Yes	No	
X		Lecithin-sphingomyelin ratio
	X	Alpha fetoprotein
X		Phosphatidyl glycerol
X		Lamellar body count
	X	Femur length
	X	Fundal height

D9.
B	1.8
C	2.3
A	0.8
A	1.2
C	3.0

Unit 2 Posttest

If you are applying for continuing education credits, a posttest for this unit is available online. Completion of unit posttests and the book evaluation form are required to achieve continuing education credit. For more details, go to www.cmevillage.com.

Unit 3: Fetal Well-being

Objectives

In this unit you will learn

A. How fetal well-being is assessed during pregnancy
  - Fetal activity determination
  - Nonstress test
  - Contraction stress test
  - Biophysical profile
  - Modified biophysical profile

B. What actions to take if abnormal test results are obtained

C. How fetal well-being is assessed during labor
  - Intermittent auscultation of fetal heart tones
  - Continuous electronic monitoring of fetal heart rate and uterine contractions
  - Fetal scalp stimulation
  - Fetal acoustic stimulation

D. How to interpret electronic monitoring results during labor
  - Uterine activity
  - Baseline fetal heart rate
  - Periodic or episodic rate changes
  - Fetal scalp stimulation
  - Fetal acoustic stimulation

E. What actions to take if abnormal monitoring results are obtained

Unit 3 Pretest

Before reading the unit, please answer the following questions. Select the *one best* answer to each question (unless otherwise instructed). Record your answers on the test and check them against the answers at the end of the book.

1. An abnormal contraction stress test means that, within a 10-minute period,
    A. One uterine contraction occurred.
    B. The oxytocin level fell to an acceptable range.
    C. Repeated early decelerations of fetal heart rate occurred.
    D. Repeated late decelerations of fetal heart rate occurred.

2. All of the following are part of a biophysical profile, *except:*
    A. Contraction stress test
    B. Amniotic fluid volume estimation
    C. Fetal muscle tone assessment
    D. Fetal respiration evaluation

3. For which of the following pregnant women would a nonstress test be *most* useful?
    A. Woman with her third pregnancy at 37 weeks' gestation
    B. Woman with diabetes mellitus
    C. Woman with a previous preterm delivery
    D. Woman with low phosphatidyl glycerol level in the amniotic fluid

4. A woman has been recording fetal activity. She says the baby has moved much less often than usual that day. You check the fetal heart rate and find it is 136 beats per minute. What else should be done?
    A. Reassure her that it is normal for a fetus to have "sleepy" days.
    B. Ask her to continue to chart the fetal activity.
    C. Prepare for her to have a nonstress test the same day.
    D. Obtain a lecithin-sphingomyelin ratio.

5. The contraction stress test is used to assess the
    A. Maturity of the fetus
    B. Size of the fetus
    C. Gestational age of the fetus
    D. Well-being of the fetus

6. All these statements about biophysical profile testing are accurate, *except:*
    A. Scores of 4 or lower indicate fetal distress and usually require immediate delivery.
    B. When used to evaluate high-risk pregnancies, it is generally started at 28 weeks' gestation.
    C. Scores of 8 or higher indicate fetal distress and usually require immediate delivery.
    D. It includes nonstress testing and ultrasound evaluation.

7. **True   False**   Fetal heart rate response to auditory stimulation may be used as an indication of fetal well-being.

8. **True   False**   A contraction stress test can be done only after the membranes have ruptured.

9. **True** **False** Turning a woman on her side may correct an abnormal fetal heart rate pattern.

10. **True** **False** Variable fetal heart rate decelerations are probably due to compression of the umbilical cord.

11. **True** **False** Early fetal heart rate decelerations are usually not associated with fetal distress.

12. **True** **False** An abnormal nonstress test should be followed by a contraction stress test or biophysical profile.

13. **True** **False** A normal nonstress test occurs when there are no fetal heart rate accelerations with fetal activity.

14. **True** **False** Fetal bradycardia is a baseline heart rate less than 110 beats per minute.

15. **True** **False** Fetal heart rate accelerations with a scalp stimulation test indicate that the fetus is acidotic.

16. In which of the following is internal fetal monitoring contraindicated?
    A. Twins
    B. Placenta previa
    C. Post-term pregnancy
    D. Vaginal birth after cesarean delivery

17. Fetal tachycardia, without accompanying decelerations, may be due to
    A. Narcotics given to the laboring woman
    B. Fetal hypothyroidism
    C. Maternal fever
    D. Post-term fetus

18. Loss of fetal heart rate variability may be due to all of the following factors, *except:*
    A. Fetal activity
    B. Barbiturates or tranquilizers given to the mother
    C. Fetal acidosis
    D. Chronic fetal hypoxia

19. In which of these situations would fetal activity determinations be *most* helpful?
    A. Contracted maternal pelvis
    B. First trimester rubella infection
    C. Previous macrosomic baby (>4,000 g)
    D. Woman with chronic hypertension

1. Why Is It Important to Determine Fetal Well-being?

As described in the first unit in this book, a pregnant woman may be well, at risk, or sick. A fetus also may be well, at risk, or sick. The health of either a woman or a fetus may change during pregnancy and/or labor. Ongoing reevaluation of both maternal and fetal health is essential for optimal perinatal care and informed decision making.

2. How Is Fetal Well-being Assessed?

A. Fetal Activity Determination (FAD)

Fetal activity determination (also called fetal movement or kick counts) is a simple, cost-free measure that does not require any special equipment. For a specified period every day, a pregnant woman records the number of times her fetus moves. Every fetus has its own pattern of movements. Most show some diurnal variation, with more movements in the early morning and late evening. Except when there are very few daily movements, there is no significance to the number of movements, provided that the number of movements remains within a constant range for that fetus. The woman's perception of a decrease in fetal movement is more important than any set guideline for the number of movements. Any significant decrease in the number of movements is a warning sign.

Fetal activity determination is a useful screening tool to identify fetuses at risk in high- and low-risk pregnancies. Abnormal FAD results are an indication for further antenatal testing.

Fetal activity determination is particularly helpful in high-risk pregnancies that may result in chronic fetal stress, such as maternal hypertension or diabetes mellitus, suspected post-maturity, etc. If *in utero* death occurs in pregnancies with such chronic stress, it is often preceded by a decrease in fetal movement (in some cases, for several days). During this time, baseline fetal heart rate usually remains within the normal range.

Fetal activity determination is *not* useful in the detection or management of acute changes in fetal status, such as that which may occur with cord prolapse or abruptio placentae.

1. Indications
    *   All known high-risk pregnancies, starting at approximately 28 weeks' gestation.
    *   May be used in all low-risk pregnancies, because even these pregnancies may have unanticipated fetal death.

2. Description

    The most commonly used method is for the woman to count fetal movements during a period of up to 2 hours.

    Ask the woman to lie on her side and begin counting the fetus's movements at approximately the same time each day. Count for 2 hours or until 10 distinct fetal movements have been felt. After 10 fetal movements have been noted, the count for that day may be stopped.

3. Interpretation
    a. Reassuring: A minimum of 10 movements in 2 hours.
    b. Non-reassuring.
       *   Fewer than 10 movements in 2 hours
           or
       *   A decrease in the total number of movements, or a significant increase in the length of time required to reach 10 movements.

    4. Implications

        a. Reassuring results: Continue other routine testing.

        b. Non-reassuring results: Arrange for the patient to be seen the *same day* and have further antenatal testing.

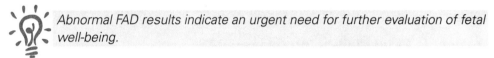 *Abnormal FAD results indicate an urgent need for further evaluation of fetal well-being.*

    5. Complications: None

    6. Contraindications: None

B. Nonstress Test (NST)

The NST is used to evaluate fetal well-being by assessing spontaneous fetal heart rate accelerations that occur with fetal activity in a normally resting woman. The NST has the advantages of requiring no intravenous medication, may be performed quickly, and has no contraindications to its use.

Generally, weekly testing is started when fetal risk is first detected, or before the point in time when a problem developed in a previous pregnancy. For some pregnancies, testing starts as early as 26 weeks, while, for others, it may not be needed until 38 weeks or later.

    1. Indications

- Suspected post-term pregnancy
- Suspected intrauterine growth restriction
- History of previous fetal death
- Maternal medical disorders, such as hypertension, diabetes mellitus, sickle cell disease, collagen vascular diseases, etc
- Obstetric disorders, such as multifetal gestation, Rh isoimmune disease, oligohydramnios, etc
- Abnormal fetal activity determination
- Any other condition where there is a risk for uteroplacental insufficiency

    2. Description

- The woman rests on her side in a semi-recumbent position. Her blood pressure is recorded periodically to be sure it is normal.
- Fetal heart rate and uterine activity are monitored externally.
- Baseline fetal heart rate and maternal pulse are obtained.
- A 20-minute observation period is initiated, during which fetal heart rate is recorded externally. The period may be extended for an additional 20 minutes (total 40 minutes) to accommodate variations in the typical fetal sleep-wake cycle.

    3. Interpretation

        a. Normal (reactive): During a 20-minute observation period, the occurrence of at least 2 fetal heart rate accelerations lasting at least 15 seconds from baseline to baseline and with an increase of at least 15 beats per minute (bpm), with or without fetal movement, is considered reactive or normal.

        b. Abnormal (nonreactive): If fetal heart rate accelerations are less than 15 bpm, last less than 15 seconds, or are less than 2 in a 40-minute period, the results are considered nonreactive or abnormal.

        If fetal sleep is thought to be the reason for an abnormal (nonreactive) NST, acoustic stimulation (lasting 1 second) may be used. If a fetal heart rate acceleration of at least

15 bpm and lasting at least 15 seconds occurs in response to acoustic stimulation, the NST is considered normal. If no acceleration occurs, or one fewer than 15 bpm and lasting less than 15 seconds, the NST is considered abnormal. Acoustic stimulation also may be used safely to reduce testing time.

There is a high falsely abnormal (nonreactive) rate with NST, particularly in preterm fetuses. The fetal heart rate reactivity increases with advancing gestational age. Before 32 weeks, fetal heart rate accelerations may last 10 seconds from start to return to baseline and increase 10 bpm. As many as 15% of fetuses at less than 32 weeks' gestation will have a nonreactive NST but will be healthy. An abnormal NST by itself should *not* be an indication for delivery.

If recurrent variable decelerations (more than 3 in 20 minutes) occur during the NST, further evaluation of fetal well-being is indicated. This includes ultrasound evaluation for decreased amniotic fluid volume. Variable decelerations during an NST are particularly concerning in a post-term pregnancy, and prompt delivery should be seriously considered.

Regardless of fetal gestational age, if ultrasound evaluation reveals oligohydramnios, the clinical situation requires careful evaluation because delivery may be indicated.

4. Implications
   a. Normal (reactive): An NST is usually conducted 1 or 2 times a week, depending on the clinical situation. If the clinical situation worsens, more frequent testing may be necessary.
   b. Abnormal (nonreactive): This is a warning sign that there may be abnormal placental function. The fetus is at risk. A contraction stress test (CST) or biophysical profile (BPP) should be performed after *every* abnormal NST.

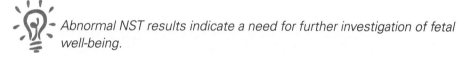 *Abnormal NST results indicate a need for further investigation of fetal well-being.*

5. Complications: None.

6. Contraindications: None.

C. Contraction Stress Test (CST)

The CST is used to evaluate fetal well-being when uteroplacental insufficiency is suspected. The test consists of a brief period during which fetal heart rate and uterine contractions are monitored.

Uterine contractions may be either spontaneous or induced with oxytocin or breast stimulation. If induced with oxytocin, the test is called an oxytocin challenge test (OCT); if induced with breast stimulation, the test is called a nipple stimulation test. (Note: A nipple stimulation test is *not* the same as NST described above.)

1. Indications: Abnormal (nonreactive) NST and desire for a provocative test that may unmask placental insufficiency

2. Description
   • The woman rests on her side in a semi-recumbent position. Her blood pressure is recorded periodically to be sure it is normal.
   • Fetal heart rate and uterine contractions are monitored externally. A baseline tracing of the fetal heart rate is made for 10 to 20 minutes.

- If at least 3 uterine contractions of 40 seconds or longer do not occur spontaneously within 10 minutes, contractions may be induced by either of 2 methods.
  - Self-stimulation of one nipple by gentle massage through her clothing for 2 minutes may cause contractions. When contractions begin, stop nipple stimulation. If an inadequate contraction pattern results, self-stimulation may be repeated after 5 minutes. This cycle of stimulation until a contraction starts, then cessation of stimulation, then 5 minutes' rest, may be repeated until an adequate pattern is achieved.

  OR

  - If nipple stimulation does not produce adequate contractions or if the woman prefers the use of oxytocin, a low-dose intravenous (IV) infusion may be used. If IV oxytocin is used, it is necessary to use an infusion pump for precise control of the infusion rate. The recommended dose of oxytocin is 0.5 to 1.0 milliunits (mU) per minute to start, increased every 15 to 20 minutes until a pattern of 3 contractions each 40 seconds or longer in a 10-minute period occurs.

3. Interpretation
   a. Normal (negative): *No* late or significant variable decelerations in fetal heart rate occur. This indicates adequate uteroplacental function at the time of the test.
   b. Abnormal (positive): Late decelerations follow 50% or more of contractions, even if there are fewer than 3 contractions in 10 minutes. This indicates inadequate uteroplacental function at the time of the test.
   c. Suspicious
      - Intermittent late or significant variable decelerations occur.
      - Fetal heart rate decelerations occur in the setting of contractions occurring more often than every 2 minutes or last longer than 90 seconds.
        Note: Excessive uterine activity can occur with either nipple stimulation or oxytocin infusion, and may require retesting for correct interpretation.
   d. Unsatisfactory
      - Fewer than 3 contractions in 10 minutes or an uninterpretable tracing

4. Implications
   a. Positive (abnormal): This is a danger sign.
      - If the fetus is near term, delivery is usually indicated.
      - If the fetus is preterm, delivery may be necessary immediately or in the near future. Consider administration of corticosteroids.
      - Consider consultation with regional center staff.

 An abnormal CST usually indicates the fetus is sick. Consultation with and/or referral to maternal-fetal medicine specialists at a regional perinatal center is recommended.

   b. Suspicious: Repeat the test in 24 hours. Other tests of fetal well-being and maturity may be appropriate. Consider consultation with maternal-fetal medicine specialists.
   c. Unsatisfactory: Consider other methods of testing
   d. Normal: Continue antenatal testing at predetermined interval

    5. Complications
- Uterine tachysystole (rare)
- Uterine rupture (very rare)

    6. Contraindications
- Preterm labor or certain women at high risk for preterm labor
- Placenta previa
- Uterine surgery
  – Classical cesarean incision (not confined to the lower uterine segment)
  – Extensive previous surgery, for example myomectomy
- Cervical incompetence
- Preterm rupture of membranes

D. Biophysical Profile (BPP)

The BPP assesses fetal well-being by evaluating 5 different factors.
- NST
- Amniotic fluid volume
- Fetal movement
- Fetal muscle tone
- Fetal breathing movements

Because BPP measures multiple components of fetal health, it may provide stronger evidence of fetal well-being or stress than an NST or CST alone. It may be used in place of an NST or CST as the primary means of fetal assessment.

    1. Indications: Same as for NST. In high-risk pregnancies, weekly NST or BPP testing is often started at 28 weeks' gestation.

    2. Description
- Ultrasound examination is performed to evaluate
  – Amniotic fluid volume
  – Fetal body movements
  – Fetal muscle tone
  – Fetal respiratory motion

If these 4 components are all normal (score of 2 for each), the NST may be omitted without compromising the value of the test results.
- NST is performed.

    3. Interpretation
- The scoring system for a BPP is shown in Table 3.1.
- Add the points for each component of the test to determine the final score.
  Note: The final score should never be an odd number, because the point system gives only 0 or 2 (not 1) for each component.

Table 3.1. Biophysical Profile

Component	0 Points	2 Points
Nonstress test	Abnormal (nonreactive)	Normal (reactive)
Amniotic fluid volume	No fluid pockets or 1 pocket less than 2 cm in 2 planes perpendicular to each other	1 or more pockets of at least 2 cm in 2 planes perpendicular to each other
Body movement	1 or 2 separate body or limb movements in 30 minutes	3 or more separate body or limb movements in 30 minutes
Muscle tone	No movement, slow extension with return to partial flexion, or limb movement in full extension	1 or more episodes of extremity extension with return to flexion, or opening or closing of a hand
Respirations	No breathing movements or no episode lasting 30 seconds or longer in 30 minutes of observation	1 or more episodes of rhythmic breathing lasting 30 seconds or longer in 30 minutes of observation

4. Implications
   a. Score of 8 or 10: Generally, if the indication for testing persists, the BPP is repeated in 1 week. Scores of 8 or 10 are reassuring and generally indicate fetal well-being at the time of the test.
   If the score is 8 with oligohydramnios present, consult with maternal-fetal medicine specialists because delivery may be indicated.
   b. Score of 6: If the patient is at term, it generally should lead to delivery. If preterm, repeating the BPP in 12 to 24 hours is recommended. If the score remains 6, consider delivery, depending on the clinical situation. If oligohydramnios is present, delivery is usually indicated. Consult with maternal-fetal medicine specialists.
   c. Score of 4: Delivery is warranted, although if the patient is extremely premature, management should be individualized in consultation with maternal-fetal medicine and neonatology specialists.
   d. Score of less than 4: Delivery should be expedited.

A BPP score of 6 indicates the fetus is at risk or sick. A BPP score of 4 or lower indicates the fetus is sick.

Immediate delivery may be needed. Consultation with maternal-fetal medicine and neonatology specialists is recommended.

5. Complications: None.
6. Contraindications: None.

E. Modified Biophysical Profile

   1. Indications: Same as for BPP.

   2. Description

   Uses NST and amniotic fluid index (AFI) to assess fetal well-being. These tests may be simpler to obtain than a complete BPP and seem to be as useful in evaluating fetal health.

   The AFI is a 4-quadrant assessment of amniotic fluid depth. See Book II: Maternal and Fetal Care, Unit 4, Various High-Risk Conditions, for additional information about AFI.

   3. Interpretation

   Interpretation of the NST is the same as for any NST. An AFI value of 5 cm or less indicates significant oligohydramnios, which suggests impaired placental function over some length of time.

   4. Implications
   • Reactive NST with oligohydramnios present suggests the fetus is at risk and may be sick.
   • Nonreactive NST with oligohydramnios present is non-reassuring and suggests the fetus is sick. Immediate delivery may be needed.
     For either situation, further investigation and consultation with maternal-fetal medicine and neonatology specialists is recommended.

   5. Complications: None.

   6. Contraindications: None.

Self-test

Now answer these questions to test yourself on the information in the last section.

A1. A contraction stress test is normal (negative) when
   A. No late decelerations of fetal heart rate occur
   B. Three late decelerations of fetal heart rate occur

A2. Which of the following conditions are contraindications for a nonstress test?

Yes	No	
____	____	Woman with a placenta previa and on strict bed rest
____	____	Woman with severe diabetes mellitus
____	____	Woman with ruptured membranes at 34 weeks' gestation

	True	False	
A3.	True	False	Eight times during a nonstress test, fetal heart rate accelerations occurred with fetal movement. This response is a danger sign.
A4.	True	False	Fetal activity determinations require electronic monitoring equipment.
A5.	True	False	If a woman reports a significant decrease in fetal activity, she should be seen the same day for further evaluation.
A6.	True	False	A biophysical profile score of 10 is reassuring of fetal well-being.
A7.	True	False	Fetal activity determinations can be used as a cost-free screening test in all pregnancies.
A8.	True	False	If the 4 ultrasound assessments in a biophysical profile each receive 2 points, the nonstress test may be omitted from the biophysical profile.
A9.	True	False	Fetal heart rate acceleration in response to acoustic stimulation is a reassuring sign.
A10.	True	False	A finding of oligohydramnios should prompt further investigation of fetal well-being.

A11. Which of the following are included in a biophysical profile?

Yes	No	
____	____	Nonstress test
____	____	Amniotic fluid volume
____	____	Biparietal diameter
____	____	Fetal body movements
____	____	Fetal respiratory activity
____	____	Contraction stress test
____	____	Fetal muscle tone

A12. Variable fetal heart rate decelerations during a nonstress test are
  - **A.** Common and of no special significance
  - **B.** A danger sign
  - **C.** Indicative of a healthy fetus

Check your answers with the list that follows the Recommended Routines. Correct any incorrect answers and review the appropriate section in the unit.

---

3. What Is Intrapartum Fetal Monitoring?

Intrapartum fetal monitoring is used to determine fetal well-being during labor. Monitoring can be done in 2 ways.

- Intermittent auscultation of fetal heart rate with a fetoscope or Doppler monitor
- Continuous electronic monitoring of fetal heart rate and uterine contractions

Scalp stimulation and acoustic stimulation tests are also used to assess fetal well-being, particularly when fetal heart rate monitoring findings are worrisome or unclear.

4. Why Is the Fetus Monitored?

The goal of intrapartum monitoring is to identify whether the fetus is well, at-risk, or sick. Fetuses that are well can be monitored routinely and labor allowed to continue. Fetuses that are at risk may require heightened surveillance and/or other interventions, including delivery. Fetuses that are sick require interventions and delivery if not promptly responsive to interventions.

Continuous electronic fetal heart rate monitoring correctly identifies fetal well-being 99% of the time when the pattern is normal.

Indeterminate and abnormal tracings are not equally predictive of a sick fetus. Some fetuses with these patterns are fine at birth; others are not.

If a pattern that is not normal is detected, maternal hypotension and decreased uterine blood flow, if present, are corrected. Oxygen is given to the woman, IV fluid infusion is started or increased, and she is repositioned. Labor-stimulating agents are discontinued. If these measures fail and the worrisome fetal heart rate pattern continues, prompt delivery is generally indicated.

5. Who Is Monitored?

All labors should be monitored in some way. Fetuses of high-risk pregnancies and those that develop problems during labor require continuous monitoring. Studies have shown very little difference in perinatal outcome whether continuous electronic monitoring or intermittent auscultation is used in uncomplicated pregnancies and labors.

The frequency with which the fetal heart rate should be checked and recorded during intensive monitoring usually means that this monitoring can be provided more easily and efficiently with continuous electronic monitoring. Women and/or fetuses with any of the following conditions should have *intensive* monitoring during labor.

A. Fetuses of Known High-Risk Pregnancies
- Chronic or gestational hypertension in the woman
- Maternal diabetes mellitus
- Maternal congenital or rheumatic heart disease
- Chronic renal disease in the woman
- Rh and other isoimmunization
- Prematurity (<37 weeks)
- Postmaturity (>41 weeks)
- Multifetal gestation
- Breech presentation
- Suspected fetal growth restriction
- Health of woman and/or fetus is unknown or uncertain (no prenatal care)
- Maternal substance use

B. Fetuses Subject to Intrapartum Stress
- Meconium-stained amniotic fluid
- Placenta previa
- Abruptio placentae
- Rupture of membranes longer than 12 hours
- Amniotic infection
- Whenever a fetal heart rate abnormality is detected during routine monitoring
- Any fetus being delivered because of abnormal antenatal testing results

6. How Is the Fetus Monitored?

Pregnancies without risk factors may be monitored routinely. The fetal heart rate and uterine activity should be evaluated at least

- Every 30 minutes during the active phase of the first stage of labor
- Every 15 minutes during the second stage of labor

Pregnancies with risk factors identified before labor or that develop problems during labor should have intensive monitoring. The fetal heart rate and uterine activity should be evaluated at least

- Every 15 minutes during the active phase of the first stage of labor
- Every 5 minutes during the second stage of labor until delivery occurs

A. Intermittent Auscultation of Fetal Heart Tones
A fetoscope or Doppler ultrasound transducer is used to listen to the fetal heart rate. Uterine contractions are felt and timed by hand, with contraction intensity estimated. This method of monitoring should be reserved for women without pregnancy complications.

1. Technique
   - A fetoscope or Doppler monitor is used to listen to the fetal heart rate.
   - The fetal heart rate is auscultated during, and for 30 seconds following, a contraction.

2. Advantages
   - Procedure easily carried out, with no risk to the woman.
   - Allows greater mobility for the woman than continuous electronic monitoring.
   - May be used before and after rupture of membranes.
   - Requires minimal equipment.

3. Disadvantages
   - Does not provide a record of fetal heart rate changes in relation to uterine contractions.
   - Fetal heart rate changes may be missed since the assessment of the fetal heart rate is not continuous.
   - Does not allow assessment of fetal heart rate variability.
   - Accurate use of a fetoscope requires a skilled person.
   - Estimation of contraction duration, intensity, and uterine tonus between contractions may be inaccurate or inconsistent.

 If a concerning fetal heart rate or pattern is detected with auscultation, continuous electronic monitoring and/or other tests of fetal well-being are recommended.

B. Electronic Monitoring of Fetal Heart Rate and Uterine Contractions
   Continuous electronic fetal monitoring (EFM) can be performed by using either an external or an internal monitor (Figures 3.1 and 3.2). Sometimes, a combination of external uterine contraction and internal fetal heart rate monitoring is used. Whether internal or external monitoring or a combination is used depends on the clinical situation.

   1. External monitoring
      This noninvasive technique can determine uterine contractions and fetal heart rate in labor, with or without rupture of membranes and/or dilatation of the cervix. This is the same technique used to monitor the fetus during antenatal nonstress and contraction stress testing. This method of monitoring may be used for all women unless the tracing is uninterpretable or the clinical situation requires internal monitoring.

      a. Technique
         - A pressure transducer is placed on the maternal abdomen where there is the greatest displacement of the uterus during a contraction. It is secured with an elastic belt. During a contraction, the transducer converts the change in uterine shape to an electrical signal.
         - A Doppler ultrasonic transducer is used to detect the fetal heart rate. A second belt holds the fetal heart rate sensor in place.
         - The settings for the fetal heart rate and uterine contraction tracings are adjusted for each patient.

      b. Advantages
         - Is noninvasive
         - Allows monitoring of the fetus prior to rupture of the membranes and dilatation of the cervix
         - Provides a permanent record

Tocodynamometer for
Uterine Pressure
Fetal Heart Rate Sensor

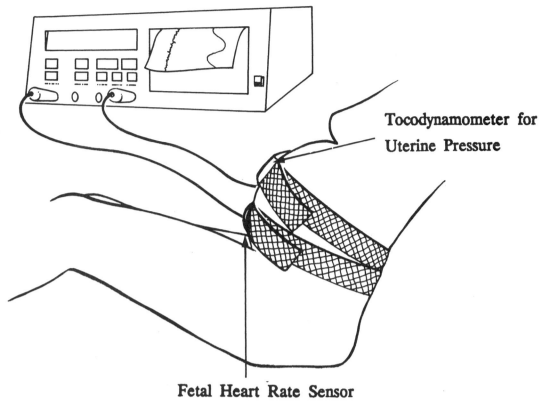

Figure 3.1. External Fetal Heart Rate Monitoring.

c. Disadvantages
- Correct placement and adjustment of the transducers requires a skilled person. Displacement or incorrect placement of the transducers resulting in inaccurate tracings can be a problem.
- May restrict maternal movement.
- Accurate monitoring may be difficult in obese women or with maternal and/or fetal movement.
- Although external monitoring indicates the timing of contractions, it cannot measure contraction intensity or uterine tonus between contractions as accurately as internal monitoring.

2. Internal monitoring

This technique requires that the membranes be ruptured and the cervix be sufficiently dilated to permit placement of instruments required for monitoring.

Note: Several types of intrauterine pressure transducers are available. Be sure you know how the ones in your hospital work.

a. Technique
- Under sterile conditions, an intrauterine pressure catheter is passed through the cervix and into the uterus. The transducer (sensor) measures intrauterine pressure, which is then transmitted to the monitor where it is displayed on the tracing.

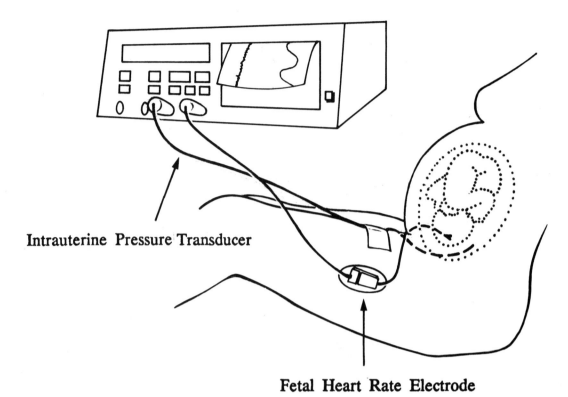

Intrauterine Pressure Transducer

Fetal Heart Rate Electrode

Figure 3.2. Internal Fetal Heart Rate Monitoring.

- The fetal heart rate is measured by an electrode that, under sterile conditions, is passed through the cervix and attached to the fetal presenting part. (The face, fontanels, and genitalia should be avoided.)
- Settings for the fetal heart rate and uterine contraction tracings are adjusted for each patient.

b. Advantages

- Allows quantitative measurement of contraction intensity and uterine tonus between contractions
- Provides continuous monitoring of the fetal heart rate and/or uterine activity when not achievable with external monitoring or when required by the clinical situation
- Allows for amnioinfusion
- Provides a permanent record

c. Disadvantages

- Is invasive.
- Rupture of membranes and some dilatation of the cervix are required.

d. Complications

- Placement of the intrauterine pressure catheter may cause bleeding and should not be forced because it can cause perforation of the uterus.
- Separation of a low-lying placenta.
- Fetal scalp laceration.
- Infection.

e. Possible contraindications

Internal monitoring should be avoided with certain obstetric conditions.

- Placenta previa. (This is an absolute contraindication.)
- Third trimester vaginal bleeding before the cause is identified.
- Suspected placental abruption. (Intrauterine pressure catheter is contraindicated, fetal electrode is not.)

Internal monitoring, particularly fetal heart rate scalp electrode, should be avoided when certain infectious organisms are known to be present.

- Human immunodeficiency virus
- Active genital herpes infection
- Hepatitis B or hepatitis C
- Inadequately treated gonorrhea or chlamydia

 Take care to rule out possible contraindications before beginning internal fetal heart rate and/or internal uterine pressure monitoring.

C. Other Tests of Fetal Well-being

1. Scalp stimulation test

   A healthy, sleeping, term fetus or a preterm fetus may have minimal fetal heart rate variability. If fetal heart rate accelerations are absent and/or variability is minimal, but there are no other concerning findings and the fetus is vertex, fetal response to mechanical stimulation of the scalp may help define whether the fetus is asleep or sick. This technique is an assessment technique and not a resuscitative technique.

   a. Technique
      - Woman is prepared as for a vaginal examination.
      - Fetal scalp is rubbed with the examiner's gloved finger.
      - Fetal heart rate response to scalp stimulation is monitored.

   b. Advantages: Can be performed easily without special equipment.

   c. Disadvantages: Requires vertex presentation. Results can be misleading. Not all fetuses without fetal heart rate response are sick. Clinical condition, gestational age, and other measures of fetal well-being should be taken into account.

2. Acoustic stimulation test

   This test is most often used when the cervix is closed or during an NST that is initially nonreactive.

   a. Technique: A device that produces a loud, short sound is placed against the woman's abdomen and triggered to give a brief (1-second) noise. The fetal heart rate response is monitored.

   b. Advantages: Does not require a vaginal examination or direct contact with the fetus.

   c. Disadvantages: Same as for scalp stimulation test.

Self-test

Now answer these questions to test yourself on the information in the last section.

B1. Name measures used to assess fetal well-being during labor.

_____

_____

_____

B2. Name 3 examples of *high-risk* pregnancies that require intensive monitoring during labor.

_____

_____

_____

B3. Name 3 examples of *intrapartum stress* that require intensive monitoring during labor.

_____

_____

_____

B4.	**True**	**False**	All high-risk pregnancies can be recognized before the onset of labor.
B5.	**True**	**False**	Continuous external monitoring can be done even if the membranes are intact.
B6.	**True**	**False**	Internal monitoring provides greater accuracy regarding contraction intensity and tonus between contractions than does external monitoring.
B7.	**True**	**False**	Third trimester vaginal bleeding of unknown origin is a reason to use internal fetal heart rate and uterine contraction monitoring.
B8.	**True**	**False**	Internal monitoring can only be done when rupture of membranes has occurred and the cervix is partially dilated.
B9.	**True**	**False**	Active genital herpes in the woman is a contraindication to the use of internal fetal heart rate monitoring.
B10.	**True**	**False**	Intensive intrapartum fetal heart rate and uterine contraction monitoring for high-risk women means assessment and documentation every 15 minutes during the second stage of labor.

B11. Possible complications of internal monitoring include which of the following?

Yes	No	
____	____	Scalp abscess in the baby
____	____	Perforation of the uterus
____	____	Bleeding
____	____	Uterine infection

Check your answers with the list that follows the Recommended Routines. Correct any incorrect answers and review the appropriate section in the unit.

7. How Are Electronic Fetal Monitoring Findings Interpreted?

An EFM tracing has 6 components that need consideration to interpret the pattern fully. These are

- Uterine activity
- Baseline rate
- Baseline fetal heart rate variability
- Presence of accelerations
- Presence of decelerations, and whether they are periodic (associated with uterine contraction[s]) or episodic (not associated with contraction[s])
- Trends over time in the pattern

Pattern interpretation must also take into account influencing factors, such as fetal gestational age, maternal medications and medical conditions, and results of other tests of fetal well-being, etc. The following table summarizes each of the characteristics, each of which will then be discussed in more detail.

Table 3.2. Interpretation of Fetal Heart Rate Tracings	

Baseline	• The mean fetal heart rate (FHR) rounded to increments of 5 beats per minute (bpm) during a 10-minute segment, excluding
	  – Periodic or episodic changes
	  – Periods of marked FHR variability
	  – Segments of baseline that differ by more than 25 bpm
	• The baseline must be for a minimum of 2 minutes in any 10-minute segment, or the baseline for that time period is indeterminate. In this case, one may refer to the prior 10-minute window for determination of baseline.
	• Normal FHR baseline: 110 to 160 bpm
	• Tachycardia: FHR baseline is greater than 160 bpm
	• Bradycardia: FHR baseline is below 110 bpm

Baseline variability	• Fluctuations in the baseline FHR that are irregular in amplitude and frequency
	• Variability is visually quantitated as the amplitude of peak to trough in beats per minute.
	  – Absent—amplitude range undetectable
	  – Minimal—amplitude range detectable but 5 bpm or fewer
	  – Moderate (normal)—amplitude range 6 to 25 bpm
	  – Marked—amplitude range greater than 25 bpm

Acceleration	• A visually apparent abrupt increase (onset to peak in less than 30 seconds) in the FHR. • At 32 weeks of gestation and beyond, an acceleration has a peak of 15 bpm or more above baseline, with a duration of 15 seconds or more but less than 2 minutes from onset to return. • Before 32 weeks of gestation, an acceleration has a peak of 10 **bpm** or more above baseline, with a duration of 10 seconds or more, but less than 2 minutes from onset to return. • Prolonged acceleration lasts 2 minutes or more but less than 10 minutes in duration. • If an acceleration lasts 10 minutes or longer, it is a baseline change.

Table 3.2. Interpretation of Fetal Heart Rate Tracings *(continued)*	
Early deceleration	• Visually apparent, usually symmetrical gradual decrease and return of the FHR associated with a uterine contraction. • A gradual FHR decrease is defined as from the onset to the FHR nadir of 30 seconds or more. • The decrease in FHR is calculated from the onset to the nadir of the deceleration. • The nadir (low point) of the deceleration occurs at the same time as the peak of the contraction. • In most cases, the onset, nadir, and recovery of the deceleration coincide with the beginning, peak, and ending of the contraction, respectively.
Late deceleration	• Visually apparent, usually symmetrical gradual decrease and return of the FHR associated with a uterine contraction. • A gradual FHR decrease is defined as from the onset to the FHR nadir of 30 seconds or more. • The decrease in FHR is calculated from the onset to the nadir of the deceleration. • The deceleration is delayed in timing, with the nadir of the deceleration occurring after the peak of the contraction. • In most cases, the onset, nadir, and recovery of the deceleration occur after the beginning, peak, and ending of the contraction, respectively.
Variable deceleration	• Visually apparent abrupt decrease in FHR. • An abrupt FHR decrease is defined as from the onset of the deceleration to the beginning of the FHR nadir of less than 30 seconds. • The decrease in FHR is calculated from the onset to the nadir of the deceleration. • The decrease in FHR is 15 beats per minute or greater, lasting 15 seconds or greater, and less than 2 minutes in duration. • When variable decelerations are associated with uterine contractions, their onset, depth, and duration commonly vary with successive uterine contractions.
Prolonged deceleration	• Visually apparent decrease in the FHR below the baseline. • Decrease in FHR from the baseline that is 15 bpm or more, lasting 2 minutes or more but less than 10 minutes in duration. • If a deceleration lasts 10 minutes or longer, it is a baseline change.
Sinusoidal pattern	• Visually apparent, smooth, sine wave-like undulating pattern in FHR baseline with a cycle frequency of 3 to 5 per minute that persists for 20 minutes or more.

Used with permission from Macones GA, Hankins GD, Spong CY, Hauth J, Moore T. The 2008 National Institute of Child Health and Human Development workshop report on electronic fetal monitoring: update on definitions, interpretation, and research guidelines. *Obstet Gynecol.* 2008;112:661-666.

A. Uterine Activity: Uterine contractions are measured as the number of contractions present in a 10-minute period, averaged over 30 minutes. Contraction duration, intensity, and uterine relaxation between contractions also must be assessed.

1. Normal: ≤5 contractions in 10 minutes, averaged over 30 minutes.

2. Tachysystole: >5 contractions in 10 minutes, averaged over 30 minutes.
   a. Significance
   Tachysystole may be due to the uterine response to labor stimulating agents.
   b. Treatment
   Decrease or discontinue any labor stimulating agents. If a more rapid response is required, a β₂-adrenergic drug, such as terbutaline, may be administered. The fetal heart rate response to uterine activity should always be evaluated.

B. Baseline Fetal Heart Rate: Usual rate 110 to 160 bpm
   This is the average fetal heart rate rounded to 5-beat increments during a 10-minute period. If periods of marked fetal heart rate variability, accelerations, or decelerations are present, the baseline is the rate between those changes. If segments of baseline differ by more than 25 beats, they represent 2 separate baselines.

   To be identified as a baseline heart rate, the rate must persist for a minimum of 2 minutes, not necessarily contiguous. If a 2-minute period of baseline fetal heart rate cannot be identified in the 10-minute segment being examined, review the previous 10-minute segment to determine the baseline.

1. Tachycardia: Baseline fetal heart rate greater than 160 bpm
   a. Significance
   Tachycardia alone may be due to
   • Maternal fever
   • Amniotic infection
   • Fetal anemia
   • Medications: Atropine, scopolamine, beta-agonists (eg, terbutaline)
   • Maternal hyperthyroidism
   • Fetal arrhythmia
   • Early fetal hypoxia

    Fetal compromise may be present if tachycardia is accompanied by
   • *Late decelerations*

   OR

   • *Lack of variability*

   OR

   • *Severe variable decelerations*

   b. Treatment
   Check for maternal fever and other signs of infection, clinical evidence of maternal hyperthyroidism, fetal arrhythmia, and medications listed previously. If fetal compromise cannot be ruled out, take the following actions:
   • Stop oxytocin, if used.
   • Position the woman in lateral decubitus to promote uterine blood flow. Avoid supine positioning.

- Give 100% oxygen by mask (not nasal cannula).
- Check maternal blood pressure, hydrate as necessary.
- Evaluate other indicators of fetal well-being.
- Determine whether prompt delivery is indicated.

2. Bradycardia: Baseline fetal heart rate below 110 bpm
   a. Significance

   Bradycardia alone may be due to
   - Fetal arrhythmia (heart block)
   - Local anesthesia given to the woman
   - Beta-adrenergic blocking agents
   - Prolapsed or compressed umbilical cord
   - Severe fetal hypoxia (acute or chronic)
   - Worsening acidosis
   - Impending fetal death (particularly if bradycardia is steadily worsening)

   Bradycardia, especially when accompanied by decelerations, indicates the fetus may be severely compromised.

   b. Treatment

    Begin assessment and possible intervention as soon as a consistent low heart rate is identified.

   - *Stop oxytocin, if used.*
   - *Position the woman in lateral decubitus or knee-chest position to promote uterine blood flow. Avoid supine positioning.*
   - *Give 100% oxygen by mask (not nasal cannula).*
   - *Check maternal blood pressure; hydrate as necessary.*
   - *Evaluate other indicators of fetal well-being.*
   - *Determine whether urgent delivery is indicated.*

    Sustained bradycardia is a concerning sign. Immediate delivery is usually indicated.

3. Variability (irregular fluctuations in fetal heart rate)
   There is normally some variation in fetal heart rate. The degree of fetal heart rate fluctuation can be evaluated reliably visually with either internal or external monitoring equipment.

   Variability is classified by the number of beats per minute between the peak and the trough of the fetal heart rate fluctuations around the baseline heart rate (Table 3.3). The precise number of peak-to-trough beats per minute is difficult to quantify visually, so ranges are used (Figure 3.3).

Table 3.3. Fetal Heart Rate Variability: Beats per Minute Ranges	
Baseline Fetal Heart Rate Variability	**Peak-to-Trough Beats per Minute (bpm) Range**
Absent	Undetectable
Minimal	Detectable, but ≤5 bpm
Moderate	6 to 25 bpm
Marked	>25 bpm

    a. Significance

- *Absent variability:* Amplitude range visually undetectable. Absent variability always required prompt evaluation. It may reflect a central nervous system impairment of the fetus and/or fetal acidemia.
- *Minimal variability:* Amplitude range visually detectable but ≤5 bpm. Minimal variability may be due to fetal sleep or, possibly, to low gestational age of the fetus. It also may be due to drugs given to the woman, including barbiturates, tranquilizers, certain narcotics, and magnesium sulfate. By itself, minimal variability may be a benign finding.

  Loss of variability may also be a warning sign for fetal acidosis or chronic fetal hypoxia. When it occurs with late or variable decelerations it is concerning, requiring prompt investigation and possible intervention.
- *Moderate variability:* Amplitude range of 6 to 25 bpm. It is the usual, and normal, finding. The presence of moderate variability is usually associated with a normal fetal acid-base status.
- *Marked variability:* Amplitude range >25 bpm. This pattern is very uncommon and the significance of marked variability is unclear.

  If findings are worrisome, be sure to assess all components of the fetal heart rate pattern, as well as other indicators of fetal well-being.

    b. Treatment: If minimal or absent variability occurs in association with recurrent late or variable decelerations, consider prompt cesarean delivery.

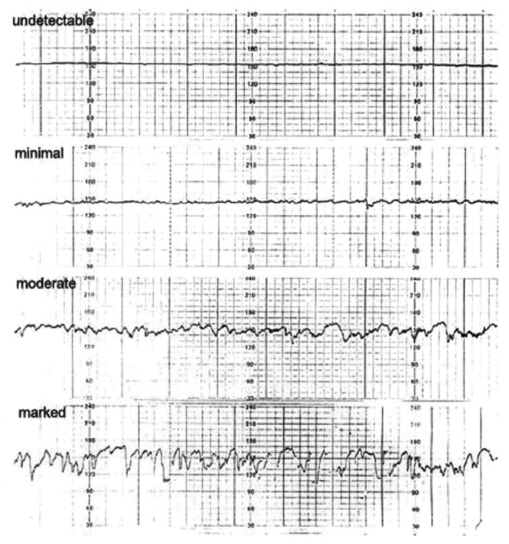

Figure 3.3. Baseline Fetal Heart Rate Variability: Electronic Fetal Monitoring Strip Images.
Reprinted with permission from National Institute of Child Health and Human Development Research Planning Workshop. 1997.

4. Sinusoidal pattern (Figure 3.4)
   a. Description
      • Regular, repeated increase and decrease of fetal heart rate in a sine wave pattern (uniform, smooth, rounded shape to peak and trough of waves).
      • *Not* a form of fetal heart rate variability.
      • Peak and trough of waves usually vary no more than 15 beats above and below baseline.
      • Waves occur at a frequency of at least 3 to 5 times per minute.
      • Waves do not change with contractions.

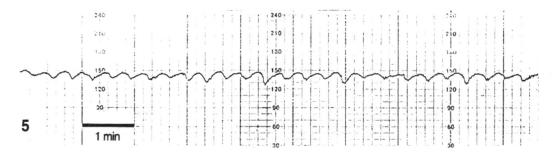

Figure 3.4. Sinusoidal Pattern.
Reprinted with permission from National Institute of Child Health and Human Development Research Planning Workshop. 1997.

   b. Significance
- Sometimes occurs as a transient pattern with no significance, or may be due to certain narcotics given to the laboring woman.
- Sinusoidal pattern also may be associated with
    - Severe fetal anemia
    - Fetal acidosis
    - Fetal hydrops

   c. Treatment
- Stop oxytocin, if used.
- Position the woman in lateral decubitus to promote uterine blood flow. Avoid supine positioning.
- Give 100% oxygen by mask (not nasal cannula).
- Hydrate the woman with normal saline or Ringer's lactate solution.
- If spontaneous contractions are present, consider using a beta-agonist to decrease uterine contractions.
- If the pattern continues after these measures, obtain a scalp or auditory stimulation test. Consider consultation with maternal-fetal medicine specialists.
- A Kleihauer-Betke test of fetal cells in maternal circulation may identify a feto-maternal transfusion. If that is the case, the fetus may be severely anemic.
- Determine if the woman is Rh-positive or Rh-negative and if she is sensitized to any other antigen.
- If the sinusoidal pattern still persists and cannot be attributed to maternal narcotic medication, consider prompt delivery. Cesarean delivery is usually performed. The longer the pattern goes on, the more likely there is to be fetal hypoxia and acidosis.

 Persistent sinusoidal fetal heart rate pattern requires prompt investigation and possible intervention.

C. Rate Changes
Fetal heart rate changes that are related to the timing of uterine contractions are called **periodic** heart rate changes. **Episodic** changes are not associated with uterine contractions.

1. Acceleration pattern
   a. Description
      - *32 weeks to term gestation*
         - Increase in fetal heart rate of 15 bpm or more above the baseline
         - Abrupt increase, with peak fetal heart rate reached in less than 30 seconds
         - Lasts 15 seconds to 2 minutes from onset to return to baseline
      - *Before 32 weeks' gestation*
         - Increase in fetal heart rate of 10 bpm or more above the baseline
         - Abrupt increase, with peak fetal heart rate reached in less than 30 seconds
         - Lasts 10 seconds to 2 minutes from onset to return to baseline
      - *Prolonged acceleration:* Acceleration that lasts longer than 2 minutes but less than 10 minutes before return to baseline (acceleration longer than 10 minutes constitutes a baseline change).
   b. Significance: Accelerations, either spontaneous or stimulated, reliably predict a normal fetal acid-base status. Accelerations occur normally with fetal movement (see Nonstress Test in Section 2). During labor, accelerations of 15 bpm and lasting 15 seconds or longer should be noted, just as decelerations (see following text) are noted.
   c. Treatment: None needed.

2. Deceleration patterns
   There are 3 types of fetal heart rate decelerations—early, late, and variable (Figures 3.5-3.7). The type of deceleration is determined by the shape of the pattern and the timing of the deceleration in relation to a uterine contraction.

   A *prolonged deceleration* is a decline in fetal heart rate of 15 bpm or more lasting 2 minutes or longer but less than 10 minutes. A deceleration lasting 10 minutes or longer constitutes a change in the baseline fetal heart rate.

   Recurrent decelerations are those that occur with 50% or more of contractions in any 20-minute period.

    A fetoscope or hand-held Doppler transducer cannot reliably detect fetal heart rate throughout a uterine contraction or changes in variability, and thus may miss subtle decelerations and/or loss of variability.

   Continuous electronic monitoring most accurately displays the relationship between fetal heart rate and uterine contractions.

   a. Early decelerations
   Description
      - Gradual decrease in fetal heart rate, beginning with the onset of a uterine contraction and returning to baseline heart rate by the end of the contraction.
      - Onset to lowest point takes 30 seconds or longer.
      - Uniform shape to pattern of fetal heart rate decline and recovery.
      - Lowest point of deceleration coincides with peak of contraction.

   Significance
      - Thought to result from vagus nerve response to fetal head compression.
      - Early decelerations are not associated with increased fetal mortality or morbidity.

   Treatment: None.

b. Late decelerations

Description

- Gradual decrease in fetal heart rate, beginning after the onset of a contraction, with the lowest point after contraction peak, and return to baseline after the contraction has ended.
- Onset to lowest point takes 30 seconds or longer.
- Uniform shape to pattern of fetal heart rate decrease and recovery.

Significance

- Thought to be associated with uteroplacental insufficiency due to decreased blood flow in the placenta or decreased oxygen levels in the blood.
- Seen particularly in patients with an increased risk for fetal intolerance of the transient hypoxemia associated with uterine contractions, such as diabetes mellitus, hypertension, Rh isoimmune disease, or post-term pregnancy.
- Other causes include maternal hypotension due to conduction anesthesia or uterine tachysystole due to excessive uterine activity.
- Recurrent late decelerations (occurring with ≥50% of the contractions) are concerning and may be associated with
  - Increasing risk for fetal compromise
  - Worsening fetal acidosis
  - Fetal central nervous system depression and/or direct myocardial hypoxia

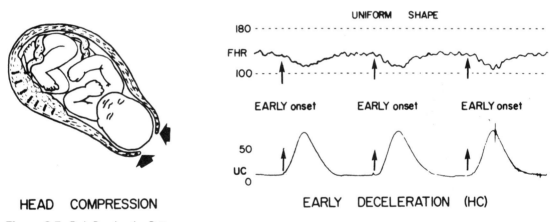

Figure 3.5. Early Deceleration Pattern.
Reprinted with permission from Hon EH. *An Introduction to Fetal Heart Rate Monitoring.* 2nd ed. 1975:29.

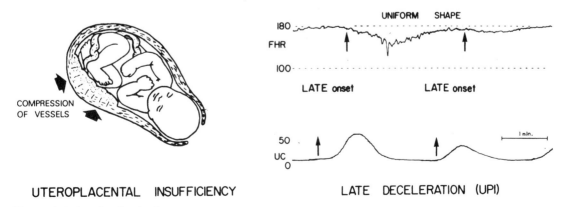

Figure 3.6. Late Deceleration Pattern.
Reprinted with permission from Hon EH. *An Introduction to Fetal Heart Rate Monitoring.* 2nd ed. 1975:29.

- Decelerations with minimal decline in beats per minute (often referred to informally as subtle late decelerations) may be as ominous as those with a much greater decrease in beats per minute.

 Regardless of the depth of the decelerations, recurrent late decelerations are a concerning finding that requires prompt investigation and treatment.

Treatment: Provide in utero resuscitation by improving fetal oxygenation and correcting factors that might restrict placental function.
- Give 100% oxygen by mask (not nasal cannula).
- Position the woman in lateral decubitus to promote uterine blood flow. Avoid supine positioning.
- Check maternal blood pressure; correct hypotension.
  - Hydrate with Ringer's lactate solution.
- Decrease uterine activity.
  - Stop oxytocin, if used.
  - Consider stopping contractions with a tocolytic drug. Tocolysis is sometimes used in preparation for an emergency cesarean delivery.
- Prepare for emergency delivery if
  - Variability is absent.
  - Resuscitation measures do not correct the late decelerations.

c. Variable decelerations

Description
- Abrupt decrease in fetal heart rate, with the lowest point of the deceleration reached in less than 30 seconds.
- Drop below baseline is at least 15 bpm and lasting at least 15 seconds but less than 2 minutes before returning to baseline.
- Shape of the fetal heart rate decrease and recovery pattern is frequently irregular.

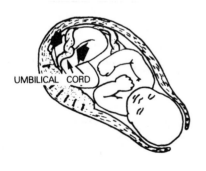

UMBILICAL CORD COMPRESSION

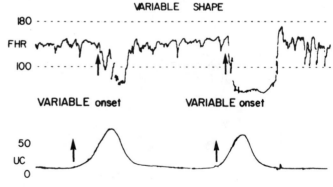

VARIABLE DECELERATION (CC)

Figure 3.7. Variable Deceleration Pattern.

Reprinted with permission from Hon EH. *An Introduction to Fetal Heart Rate Monitoring.* 2nd ed. 1975:29.

Significance
- Thought to be due to acute, intermittent compression of the umbilical cord between fetal parts and the contracting uterus or, possibly, to a nuchal cord (umbilical cord wrapped around the fetus's neck).
- Frequently seen in late labor.
- Variable decelerations may indicate fetal compromise if they are
  – Recurrent (ie, occur with more than half of contractions in a 20-minute period)
  – Accompanied by a decrease in variability
  – Not responsive to interventions

Treatment
- Check for prolapsed umbilical cord. If present, prepare for immediate operative delivery.
- Provide in utero resuscitation.
  – Stop oxytocin, if used.
  – Change maternal position.
  – Give 100% oxygen by mask (not nasal cannula).
  – Hydrate with Ringer's lactate solution.
  – Consider using a beta-agonist to decrease uterine contractions.
- If membranes are already ruptured, consider amnioinfusion (Book II: Maternal and Fetal Care, Unit 4, Various High-Risk Conditions, Oligohydramnios).
- Variable decelerations with moderate variability can usually be managed conservatively.
- Delivery may be indicated when
  – Variable decelerations are recurrent.
  and
  – There is a loss of variability.
- If bradycardia occurs, immediate delivery, usually by cesarean section, is generally indicated.

 Variable decelerations by themselves may be a benign finding. However, when they are recurrent, there also is often loss of variability or onset of bradycardia. Variable decelerations are concerning and nearly always require immediate intervention.

D. Other Tests of Fetal Well-being
These tests are most often used during labor when there is minimal or absent variability, but no other indications of fetal stress. Acoustic stimulation also may be used during nonstress antenatal testing. See Section 6C in this unit for a description of the tests and their use.

1. Scalp stimulation test
   a. Significance
   - Increase in fetal heart rate of at least 15 bpm and lasting 15 seconds or longer is associated with normal fetal blood pH.
   - While fetal heart rate acceleration in response to scalp stimulation is reassuring, lack of fetal heart rate response does not always indicate a sick fetus. Lack of response may indicate fetal acidosis, but also can occur in healthy fetuses.

   b. Treatment
   - If no accelerations in fetal heart rate occur with scalp stimulation, provide in utero resuscitative measures described earlier. Evaluate other indicators of fetal well-being.
   - If repeat stimulation test does not produce fetal heart rate accelerations, reevaluate the clinical situation and consider the need for delivery. Consider consultation with maternal-fetal medicine specialists.

 2. Acoustic stimulation test
   a. Significance: Same as scalp stimulation test.
   b. Treatment: Same as scalp stimulation test.

8. How Are Fetal Monitoring Tracings Classified?

Classification of fetal heart rate (FHR) tracing provides an evaluation of the fetus at the particular point in time the tracing was made. Tracing results can move back and forth between categories, depending on the clinical situation and response to intervention. Based on extensive review of available data, a 3-tiered classification system is now recommended.* It is recommended that tracings no longer be classified as reassuring or non-reassuring, but rather as normal, indeterminate, or abnormal, according to the following criteria:

CATEGORY I FHR Tracings (**Normal**) include *all* of the following:

- Baseline rate: 110 to 160 bpm
- Baseline variability: Moderate
- Late or variable decelerations: Absent
- Early Decelerations: Present or absent
- Accelerations: Present or absent

CATEGORY II FHR Tracings (**Indeterminate**) include tracings not meeting criteria for Categories I or III. Examples are tracings with any of the following:

- Bradycardia, not accompanied by absent variability
- Tachycardia
- Baseline variability
  - Absent, with no recurrent decelerations
  - Minimal
  - Marked
- Absence of accelerations following fetal stimulation (scalp or acoustic)
- Periodic or episodic decelerations
  - Recurrent variable decelerations accompanied by minimal or moderate baseline variability
  - Prolonged deceleration longer than 2 minutes but less than 10 minutes
  - Recurrent late decelerations with moderate variability
  - Variable decelerations with other characteristics, such as slow return to baseline, overshoots, or "shoulders"

A major thrust of the 2009 American College of Obstetricians and Gynecologists recommendations for classifying FHR patterns is to separate Category II patterns, which have less correlation with fetal acidosis, from Category III FHR patterns, which are associated with fetal acidosis.

---

*American College of Obstetricians and Gynecologists. ACOG Practice Bulletin No. 106: intrapartum fetal heart rate monitoring: nomenclature, interpretation, and general management principles. *Obstet Gynecol.* 2009;114:192-202.

CATEGORY III FHR Tracings (Abnormal)

Include either

- Absent FHR baseline variability with any of the following:
  - Recurrent Late Decelerations
  - Recurrent Variable Decelerations
  - Bradycardia

or

- Sinusoidal pattern

9. What Is an Appropriate Response to Each Fetal Heart Rate Tracing Category?

Category I tracings are strongly predictive of normal fetal acid-base status at the time the tracing was made. Continued routine monitoring is indicated, with no specific action needed, as long as the tracing remains in Category I.

Category II tracings occur frequently and are not predictive of abnormal fetal acid-base status at the time the tracing was made. Continued surveillance and frequent reevaluation are recommended, including the evolution of the pattern. Review the woman's medication list for medications that could contribute to reduced variability. Depending on the clinical situation, additional tests of fetal well-being or in utero resuscitative measures may be indicated. Clinical interventions vary depending on the circumstances, and may range from heightened surveillance to other ancillary tests to intrauterine resuscitation techniques to decisions regarding birth.

Category III tracings are associated with abnormal fetal acid-base status at the time the tracing was made. Category III tracings require prompt evaluation and probable intervention. In utero resuscitative efforts, including maternal oxygen, change in maternal position, efforts to decrease uterine activity, and correction of maternal hypotension by volume expansion or intravenous ephedrine (if caused by regional anesthesia), may each be indicated. If a Category III tracing does not resolve with these measures, delivery should be undertaken promptly.

Self-test

Fetal monitoring patterns in this quiz are from Paul RH, Petrie RH. *Fetal Intensive Care Current Concepts: Monitoring Records With Self Instruction.* **University of Southern California; 1973. Now answer these questions to test yourself on the information in the last section.**

C1. **True** **False** Lack of fetal heart rate acceleration in response to auditory stimulation occurs only in fetuses with abnormal acid-base status.

C2. **True** **False** Internal and external monitoring provide accurate information about fetal heart rate variability.

C3. **True** **False** Fetal heart rate acceleration in response to a scalp stimulation test is associated with normal fetal blood pH.

C4. **True** **False** Fetal tachycardia is a benign finding that can safely be ignored.

C5 **True** **False** Category II tracings usually require immediate delivery.

C6. Fluctuation of the fetal heart rate is

_____ Abnormal

_____ Normal

C7. You are monitoring a fetus and note early fetal heart rate decelerations. You would

   A. Continue to monitor the fetus.

   B. Rush the woman to the operating room for emergency cesarean delivery.

   C. Give the woman 100% oxygen by mask.

   D. Prepare for a fetal scalp stimulation test.

C8. You are monitoring the fetus of a woman with severe hypertension. Late fetal heart rate decelerations are noted. What would you do?

Yes	No	
____	____	Give the woman 100% oxygen.
____	____	Turn the woman onto her side.
____	____	Start an oxytocin infusion.
____	____	Check the woman's blood pressure.
____	____	Check for fetal heart rate variability.
____	____	Prepare for immediate cesarean section.

C9. Which of the following conditions or situations are most likely to produce variable decelerations?

Yes	No	
____	____	Uteroplacental insufficiency
____	____	Head compression
____	____	Gestational hypertension
____	____	Umbilical cord compression
____	____	Fetal arrhythmia
____	____	Fetal bradycardia

C10. A scalp stimulation test that does not produce accelerations in fetal heart rate can occur in which of the following?

_____ A non-acidotic fetus

_____ An acidotic fetus

C11. Which of the following is a concerning finding?

   A. Recurrent late decelerations

   B. Fetal heart rate variability of 6 to 10 beats per minute

   C. Recurrent fetal heart rate accelerations

   D. Early decelerations

C12. Which of the following auditory stimulation test results is reassuring that the fetus is not acidotic?

_____ Fetal heart rate remains constant throughout the test.

_____ Fetal heart rate increases 15 bpm for 15 seconds.

C13. Which of the following are included in a Category III tracing?

A. Early decelerations

B. Recurrent late decelerations with minimal variability

C. Recurrent variable decelerations with absent variability

D. Absence of acceleratory response to scalp stimulation

C14. **A.** What deceleration pattern is shown in the fetal heart rate tracing below?

_____

* 8:32:00 2/15/2006 3 cm/min   * 8:35:20

B. What would you suspect might be the cause of this fetal heart rate pattern?

_____ Umbilical cord compression

_____ Fetal head compression

_____ Uteroplacental insufficiency

C. What would you do to correct this fetal heart rate pattern? (Choose as many as appropriate.)

_____ Turn off oxytocin infusion (if there is one).

_____ Change the woman's position.

_____ Check maternal blood pressure.

_____ Give oxygen to the woman.

D. How would you categorize this tracing? _____

_____

C15. **A.** What deceleration pattern is shown in the fetal heart rate tracing below?

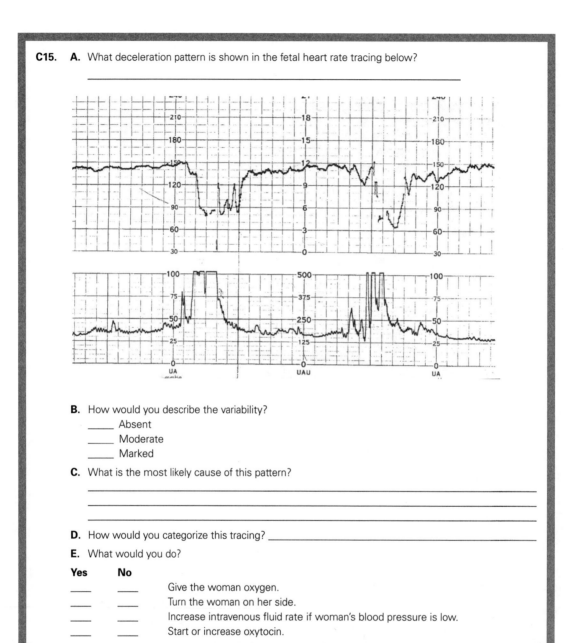

B. How would you describe the variability?
_____ Absent
_____ Moderate
_____ Marked

C. What is the most likely cause of this pattern?

D. How would you categorize this tracing? _____

E. What would you do?

Yes	No	
____	____	Give the woman oxygen.
____	____	Turn the woman on her side.
____	____	Increase intravenous fluid rate if woman's blood pressure is low.
____	____	Start or increase oxytocin.

C16. **A.** How would you describe the baseline fetal heart rate in the tracing below?

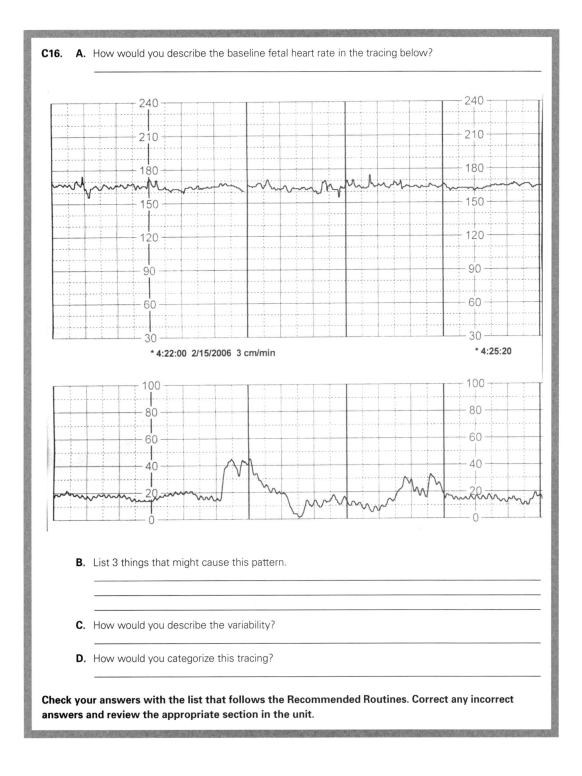

* 4:22:00 2/15/2006 3 cm/min   * 4:25:20

B. List 3 things that might cause this pattern.

C. How would you describe the variability?

D. How would you categorize this tracing?

Check your answers with the list that follows the Recommended Routines. Correct any incorrect answers and review the appropriate section in the unit.

Fetal Well-being

Recommended Routines

All the routines listed below are based on the principles of perinatal care presented in the unit you have just finished. They are recommended as part of routine perinatal care.

Read each routine carefully and decide whether it is standard operating procedure in your hospital. Check the appropriate blank next to each routine.

Procedure Standard in My Hospital   **Needs Discussion by Our Staff**

_____   _____   1. Establish a system so that each high-risk pregnancy has access to
   - Continuous electronic fetal monitoring for nonstress testing and contraction stress testing
   - Ultrasound evaluation for biophysical profile
   - Prompt consultation with maternal-fetal medicine specialists

_____   _____   2. Establish a system to ensure the availability of continuous electronic fetal monitoring for
   - All high-risk pregnancies during labor
   - All low-risk pregnancies that develop problems during labor

_____   _____   3. Develop a system for obtaining fetal scalp or acoustic stimulation tests whenever indicated for assessment of fetal well-being.

_____   _____   4. Develop training sessions and adjust staffing patterns to ensure that at least one individual skilled in recognizing abnormal fetal heart rate patterns is in attendance during all electronically monitored labors.

_____   _____   5. Establish a protocol and/or develop a checklist to ensure that each woman with an electronically monitored labor has the following evaluated systematically and frequently:
   - Uterine activity
     - Contraction strength
     - Contraction frequency
     - Contraction duration
     - Baseline uterine tonus (internal monitoring) or relative increase or decrease in tone (external monitoring)
   - Fetal heart rate pattern
     - Baseline fetal heart rate
     - Fetal heart rate variability
     - Periodic or episodic rate changes
   - Categorization of electronic fetal monitoring tracing

89

Self-test Answers

These are the answers to the self-test questions. Please check them with the answers you gave and review the information in the unit wherever necessary.

A1. A. No late decelerations of fetal heart rate occur.

A2.
Yes	No	
____	X	Woman with a placenta previa and on strict bed rest
____	X	Woman with severe diabetes mellitus
____	X	Woman with ruptured membranes at 34 weeks' gestation

A3. False. Fetal heart rate accelerations normally occur with fetal movement.

A4. False. Fetal activity determinations require only that the woman count the number of times she feels the fetus move.

A5. True

A6. True

A7. True

A8. True

A9. True

A10. True

A11.
Yes	No	
X	____	Nonstress test
X	____	Amniotic fluid volume
____	X	Biparietal diameter
X	____	Fetal body movements
X	____	Fetal respiratory activity
____	X	Contraction stress test
X	____	Fetal muscle tone

A12. B. A danger sign

B1. • Intermittent auscultation of fetal heart rate
 • Continuous electronic monitoring of fetal heart rate and uterine contractions
 • Fetal scalp stimulation or auditory stimulation

B2. Any 3 of the following:
 • Chronic or gestational hypertension in the woman
 • Maternal diabetes mellitus
 • Maternal congenital or rheumatic heart disease
 • Chronic renal disease in the woman
 • Rh and other isoimmunization
 • Prematurity (<37 weeks)
 • Postmaturity (>41 weeks)
 • Multifetal gestation
 • Breech presentation
 • Suspected fetal growth restriction
 • Health of woman and/or fetus is unknown or uncertain (no prenatal care)
 • Maternal substance use

B3. Any 3 of the following:
 • Meconium-stained amniotic fluid (particularly if presentation is vertex)
 • Placenta previa
 • Abruptio placentae
 • Rupture of membranes longer than 12 hours
 • Amniotic infection
 • Whenever a fetal heart rate abnormality is detected during routine monitoring
 • Any fetus being delivered because of abnormal antenatal testing results

B4. False.   Previously uncomplicated, low-risk pregnancies may develop problems during labor or delivery.

B5. True

B6. True

B7. False.   Internal fetal heart rate and uterine contraction monitoring should not be used until the source of the bleeding is identified.

B8. True

B9. True

B10. False.   Intensive monitoring for women who have or develop risk factors means fetal heart rate and uterine contraction assessment and documentation at least every 15 minutes during the active phase of the first stage of labor and at least every 5 minutes during the second stage of labor until delivery occurs.

B11.
Yes	No	
X	____	Scalp abscess in the baby
X	____	Perforation of the uterus
X	____	Bleeding
X	____	Uterine infection

C1. False.   Lack of fetal heart rate acceleration in response to auditory stimulation can occur in healthy fetuses and those who are acidotic. Fetal heart rate acceleration in response to either acoustic or scalp stimulation, however, is associated with normal fetal blood pH.

C2. True

C3. True

C4. False.   Fetal tachycardia may indicate fetal compromise and should be investigated.

C5. False.   Category II tracings require evaluation of possible causes, and usually require evaluation and treatment.

C6. Normal

C7. A. Continue to monitor the fetus.

C8.
Yes	No	
X	____	Give the woman 100% oxygen.
X	____	Turn the woman onto her side.
____	X	Start an oxytocin infusion.
X	____	Check maternal blood pressure.
X	____	Check for fetal heart rate variability.
____	X	Prepare for immediate cesarean section.

C9.
Yes	No	
____	X	Uteroplacental insufficiency
____	X	Head compression
____	X	Gestational hypertension
X	____	Umbilical cord compression
____	X	Fetal arrhythmia
____	X	Fetal bradycardia

C10. Non-acidotic fetus and an acidotic fetus

C11. A. Recurrent late decelerations

C12. Fetal heart rate increases 15 beats per minute for 15 seconds

C13. C. Recurrent variable decelerations with absent variability

C14. A. Late decelerations.
    B. Uteroplacental insufficiency.
    C. All the actions listed should be taken.
    D. This is a Category II tracing.

C15. A. Variable decelerations.

    B. Moderate.

    C. Umbilical cord compression.

    D. This is a Category II tracing.

    E.

Yes	No	
X	____	Give the woman oxygen.
X	____	Turn the woman on her side.
X	____	Increase intravenous fluid rate if woman's blood pressure is low.
____	X	Start or increase oxytocin.

C16. A. Tachycardia

    B. Any 3 of the following:
- Maternal fever
- Amniotic infection
- Fetal anemia
- Certain medications
- Maternal hyperthyroidism
- Fetal arrhythmia
- Early fetal hypoxia

    C. Moderate variability.

    D. This is a Category II tracing.

Unit 3 Posttest

If you are applying for continuing education credits, a posttest for this unit is available online. Completion of unit posttests and the book evaluation form are required to achieve continuing education credit. For more details, go to www.cmevillage.com.

SKILL UNIT

Electronic Fetal Monitoring

This skill unit will teach you about the application of continuous electronic monitoring and about the interpretation of monitor tracings. You will learn a systematic method for analyzing uterine activity and fetal heart rate patterns.

To master the skill, you will need to demonstrate each of the following steps correctly:

1. Determine uterine activity.
   - Frequency of contractions
   - Duration of contractions
   - Intensity of contractions
   - Baseline tonus

2. Determine fetal heart rate pattern.
   - Baseline heart rate
   - Variability
   - Periodic or episodic rate changes

3. Classify the electronic fetal monitor tracings.

In addition, you may be asked to learn to assemble, calibrate, apply, and troubleshoot the specific uterine contraction and fetal heart rate monitoring devices used in your hospital, as well as learn the specific requirements for documentation of your findings. More detailed training sessions for the evaluation of uterine contraction and fetal heart rate monitoring strips also may be scheduled. You may be asked to interpret and categorize patterns, in context with clinical findings, and outline an appropriate response to each sample situation.

PERINATAL PERFORMANCE GUIDE

Electronic Fetal Monitoring Pattern Interpretation

 Fetal heart rate and uterine contraction patterns cannot be interpreted correctly just by looking at a monitoring strip. Each of the individual components of the patterns needs to be analyzed separately. This requires a systematic method of evaluating uterine contractions, then fetal heart rate pattern.

It is common to analyze the fetal heart rate pattern first, and the uterine contraction pattern second. When this is done, because of the importance placed on the fetal heart rate pattern, the pattern of uterine contractions may not be analyzed in as much detail. This may result in overlooking subtle contraction abnormalities that may, in turn, influence the fetal heart rate pattern. Therefore, we recommend that, when you review a monitoring strip, you evaluate the uterine contractions first, and then analyze the fetal heart rate pattern.

ACTIONS	REMARKS
Analyzing the Components of the Uterine Activity Pattern	
1. What is the frequency of the contractions? _____ minutes	Contraction frequency is the time between the beginning of one contraction and the beginning of the next contraction. Excessive frequency of contractions (tachysystole) is commonly defined as more than 5 contractions within a 10-minute period.
2. What is the duration of the contractions? _____ seconds	Contraction duration is the time between the onset and the end of a contraction. Prolonged contractions are commonly defined as contractions lasting 90 seconds or longer.
3. What is the baseline tonus of the uterus? _____ mm Hg	Baseline tonus is the uterine tone between contractions. • Normal = Soft to palpation or 5 to 15 mm Hg • Increased = Firm to palpation or greater than 20 mm Hg
4. What is the intensity of the contractions? _____ mm Hg Note: Baseline tonus and contraction intensity can be measured accurately only with an *internal* monitor. Relative increase or decrease in uterine tone can be seen with an *external* monitor. Palpation of the maternal abdomen can help support these findings.	Contraction intensity is the increase in pressure, above the baseline tonus, during a contraction. Note: Various methods exist for describing contraction intensity. It is imperative that all members of the team are using the same method. Adequacy of labor is defined as cervical dilatation with fetal descent and will vary among laboring women.

ACTIONS

REMARKS

Analyzing the Components of the Fetal Heart Rate Pattern

5. What is the baseline fetal heart rate?
   _____ beats per minute (bpm)

This is the average fetal heart rate during any 10-minute period. It should be rounded to the nearest 5 bpm and reported as one value, rather than a range. For example, a tracing that fluctuates between 130 and 140 bpm would be recorded as 135 bpm baseline.

If periods of marked fetal heart rate variability, accelerations, or decelerations are present, the baseline is the rate between those changes. To be identified as a baseline heart rate, the rate must persist for a minimum of 2 minutes (not necessarily contiguous) in a 10-minute period. *Normal* fetal heart rate is between 110 and 160 bpm.

Does the fetal heart rate in the monitoring strip being analyzed represent fetal *tachycardia*?

Tachycardia is a fetal heart rate greater than 160 bpm for 10 minutes or longer. If 160 bpm or more lasts longer than 2 minutes but less than 10 minutes, it is considered a prolonged acceleration.

Does the fetal heart rate in the monitoring strip being analyzed represent fetal *bradycardia*?

Bradycardia is a fetal heart rate less than 110 bpm for 10 minutes or longer. If 110 bpm or less lasts longer than 2 minutes but less than 10 minutes, it is considered a prolonged deceleration.

Assessment and possible intervention should begin as soon as a consistent low heart rate is detected.

Do NOT wait for 2 or 10 minutes to go by before working to correct the bradycardia.

6. What is the variability?
   ___ Absent (undetectable)
   ___ Minimal (≤5 bpm)
   ___ Moderate (6-25 bpm)
   ___ Marked (>25 bpm)

Variability is classified by the number of beats per minute between the peak and the trough of the fetal heart rate fluctuations around the baseline heart rate.

7. Is there a sinusoidal pattern?
   _____ Yes _____ No

8. Are there periodic rate changes?
   • Accelerations?   ____ Yes ____ No
   • Decelerations—early?   ____ Yes ____ No
   • Decelerations—late?   ____ Yes ____ No
   • Decelerations—variable? ____ Yes ____ No

ACTIONS

REMARKS

Analyzing the Components of the Fetal Heart Rate Pattern (continued)

9. Evaluate systematically and frequently each electronically monitored labor for

- Uterine activity
  - Contraction frequency
  - Contraction duration
  - Contraction intensity
  - Baseline tonus
- Fetal heart rate pattern
  - Baseline fetal heart rate
  - Fetal heart rate variability
  - Periodic rate changes

In addition to consistent evaluation of uterine contractions and fetal heart rate, check the woman's vital signs; presence or absence of bleeding, pain, hydration, psychological adaptation to labor; and other measures of the woman's well-being according to protocols established for practice in your hospital.

Evaluating the Fetal Heart Rate and Uterine Contraction Pattern

10. Is the uterine activity and tone
    ___ Normal
    ___ Decreased
    ___ Increased

Keep in mind that, while it is important to analyze the components of uterine activity and fetal heart rate separately, your judgment of the pattern needs to consider all of the separate components together, as well as the stage of labor. For example, intermittent variable decelerations usually do not, by themselves, represent a threat to the fetus, but may become ominous if they become recurrent and there is loss of fetal heart rate variability.

11. What is the trend of the fetal heart rate pattern over time?

Changes during any period may be subtle. Over time, however, the sum of these changes may be quite dramatic. It is important not to focus exclusively on the segment of monitoring strip being analyzed but also to look at what has happened to the fetal heart rate and uterine contraction pattern over time.

12. What is the classification of the fetal heart rate tracing?
    ___ Category I
    ___ Category II
    ___ Category III

ACTIONS

Responding to the Evaluation Results

A. Normal Uterine Activity and Category I Fetal Heart Rate Pattern.

_____ Continue monitoring, no intervention needed at this time.

B. Category II Fetal Heart Rate Pattern. Ask The Following Questions:

_____ If external monitoring is being used, should internal monitoring be started?

_____ Is there excessive uterine activity or tonus that should be reduced?

_____ Are there factors that may influence the pattern, such as fetal sleep, maternal fever, maternal medical conditions, drugs given to the woman, etc?

_____ Is a vaginal examination indicated (check for prolapsed cord, etc)?

_____ Is in utero resuscitation indicated?

     _____ Give woman 100% oxygen by mask (8 to 10 L/min flow rate).

     _____ Check maternal blood pressure, correct hypotension.

          _____ Position the woman to promote uterine blood flow. Avoid supine positioning.

          _____ Hydrate with Ringer's lactate or normal saline.

     _____ Decrease uterine activity.

          _____ Turn off oxytocin, if used.

          _____ Consider use of tocolytic drug.

_____ Is fetal scalp stimulation test or acoustic stimulation test indicated?

_____ What is the evolution of the fetal heart tracing and clinical situation?

     _____ Is preparation for an emergency delivery indicated?

     _____ Surgical and anesthesia preparation for woman

     _____ Extra personnel and resuscitation equipment preparation for baby

C. Category III Fetal Heart Rate Pattern.

_____ In utero resuscitation is indicated

     _____ Give woman 100% oxygen by mask (8 to 10 L/min flow rate).

     _____ Check maternal blood pressure, correct hypotension.

     _____ Position the woman to promote uterine blood flow. Avoid supine positioning.

     _____ Hydrate with Ringer's lactate or normal saline.

     _____ Turn off oxytocin, if used.

     _____ Consider use of tocolytic drug.

_____ If the tracing does not resolve quickly with these measures, delivery should be undertaken immediately.

_____ Preparation for an emergency delivery is indicated, including

     _____ Surgical and anesthesia preparation for woman

     _____ Extra personnel and resuscitation equipment preparation for baby

Unit 4: Is the Baby Sick?

Objectives

In this unit you will learn

A. To classify all babies as being well, at risk, or sick

B. That these classifications may change from moment to moment and a baby must be *constantly* reassessed

C. The basic evaluation and management of each type of baby, which is used as the foundation for neonatal material presented throughout this program

Note: There is no pretest for this unit; there is only a brief quiz at the end of the unit. The concepts presented in the unit, however, are important to understanding all high-risk neonatal care.

Up to this point, you have learned how to identify women with high-risk pregnancies; assess fetal gestational age, well-being, and maturity; and recognize conditions that indicate that a newborn may experience problems at the time of delivery or soon after birth. In this unit, you will learn how to identify which babies are well, which are at risk, and which are sick. At-risk and sick fetuses may or may not be at-risk or sick newborns. Neonatal status needs to be assessed independently of fetal status, although it is important to know the fetal history.

1. What Is a Useful Way to Think About Babies?

When you see a baby, you should decide if the baby is

- Well
- At risk
- Sick

If a baby is well: You *observe* the baby at regular times.

If a baby is at risk: You *anticipate* the baby may have problems, and you test the baby frequently.

If a baby is sick: You *treat* the baby immediately.

2. Who Is a Well Baby?

A well baby has

- Normal vital signs, activity, color, and feeding

Note: Babies' respiratory rates and heart rates are extremely variable, and should be counted for 1 full minute.

- Normal
  - Maternal history
  - Labor and delivery history
  - Birth history

A well baby is

- Term gestational age
- An appropriate size for term

 You cannot assume a baby is well.
You must prove that a baby is well.

3. Who Is an At-Risk Baby?

An at-risk baby has

- Normal vital signs, color, and activity.
- Feedings, whether by tube or nipple, that are appropriate to the baby's gestational age and are tolerated well. (Some at-risk babies may not be feeding, but will be receiving intravenous fluids.)

An at-risk baby has *one or more* of the following conditions:

- Abnormal history
  - Maternal history (eg, diabetes mellitus)
  - Labor and delivery history (eg, bleeding)
  - Birth history (eg, low Apgar scores)

- Preterm or post-term gestation
- Large or small for gestational age
- Previously sick

 An at-risk baby does not need immediate treatment of any problems.

The baby's prognosis depends on continued, careful assessment of vital signs, anticipation of problems that are likely to occur, and either prevention of these problems or immediate treatment of them should they occur.

4. Who Is a Sick Baby?

A sick baby has

- Abnormal vital signs, activity, color, or feeding

A previously well baby or an at-risk baby may become sick by developing abnormal vital signs, color, activity, or feeding.

 A sick baby demonstrates an abnormality that requires immediate action.

Supportive care is begun and, when a cause for the abnormality is found, the abnormality is treated.

When a sick baby's vital signs become normal, the baby is then an at-risk baby.

The flow diagram on the next page is included to illustrate the previous points. It is presented to show what makes a baby at risk for certain problems and how a well or an at-risk baby may become sick.

Study the flow diagram (Figure 4.1). It shows the signs that help you classify babies as sick, at risk, or well. Read the sample cases and see how the babies are classified.

PCEP

Perinatal Continuing Education Program

WELL ←——————→ AT-RISK ←——————→ SICK BABIES

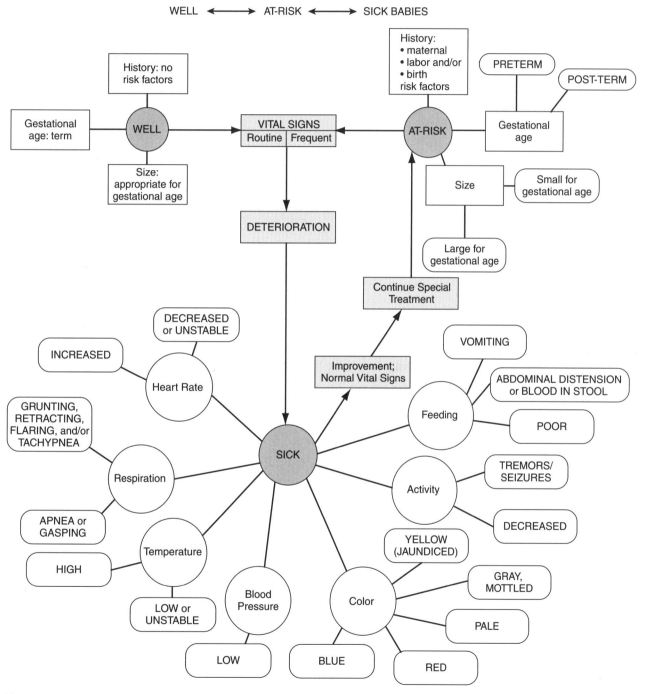

Figure 4.1. Well, At-Risk, and Sick Babies.

Case Examples

Sample Case 1
A term baby has normal maternal history, normal labor and delivery and birth histories, and normal vital signs.

> The baby *is well*.
> You should *observe the baby at regular intervals*.

The same baby develops jaundice, poor feeding, and temperature instability.

> The baby is now *sick*.
> You should *treat the baby immediately* and search for a cause of the illness.

Sample Case 2
A preterm baby is admitted to your nursery.

> She is *at risk*.
> You should *anticipate problems and monitor the baby* for them.

She develops increased respiratory rate and abnormal respiratory pattern.

> She is now *sick*.
> You should *treat the baby immediately* and search for a cause of the illness.

Sample Case 3
A baby requires resuscitation and has abnormal vital signs.

> He is *sick*.
> You should *treat the baby immediately* and search for a cause of the illness.

You stabilize his vital signs.

> He is now *at risk*.
> You should *anticipate problems and monitor the baby* for them.

In Book III: Neonatal Care, you will learn many individual techniques for treating sick and at-risk babies. In Book III: Neonatal Care, Unit 9, Review: Is the Baby Sick? the concepts introduced in this unit will be repeated and all the individual treatments will be combined in considering the total care of a sick or at-risk baby.

Is the Baby Sick?

Recommended Routines

All the routines listed below are based on the principles of perinatal care presented in the unit you have just finished. They are recommended as part of routine perinatal care.

Read each routine carefully and decide whether it is standard operating procedure in your hospital. Check the appropriate blank next to each routine.

Procedure Standard in My Hospital   **Needs Discussion by Our Staff**

_____ _____ 1. Establish a system for classifying all babies as well, at risk, or sick, with periodic reassessment and reclassification as indicated by the baby's condition.

_____ _____ 2. Provide continuous electronic cardiorespiratory monitoring for all sick babies and for all babies at risk for developing apnea.

_____ _____ 3. Provide continuous pulse oximetry monitoring for all babies receiving supplemental oxygen or positive-pressure ventilation, and have oximetry immediately available for all babies thought to be at risk for requiring supplemental oxygen.

_____ _____ 4. Obtain preductal oximetery screening for all newborns, whether sick, at risk, or well, to rule out cyanotic congenital heart disease.

Unit 4 Posttest

If you are applying for continuing education credits, a posttest for this unit is available online. Completion of unit posttests and the book evaluation form are required to achieve continuing education credit. For more details, go to www.cmevillage.com.

SKILL UNIT

Electronic Cardiorespiratory Monitoring

This skill unit will teach you how to electronically monitor a baby's heart rate and respirations.

Study this skill unit, then attend a skill practice and demonstration session.

To master the skill, you will need to demonstrate each of the following steps correctly:

1. Identify the features of the monitor(s) used in your hospital: oscilloscope, sensitivity adjustment (if present), audible signal, heart rate alarms, etc.
2. Apply monitoring electrode leads to a baby.
3. Connect electrodes, lead wires, monitor cable, and monitor.
4. Turn monitor on, adjust sensitivity (as appropriate), and set alarms correctly.
5. Make adjustments as necessary to maintain a clear, consistent heartbeat signal on the monitor.

PERINATAL PERFORMANCE GUIDE

Continuous Electronic Cardiorespiratory Monitoring

In this skill unit, you will learn *when* and *how* to use continuous electronic monitoring, and *why* electronic monitoring is important. You may not be familiar with some of the illnesses or conditions mentioned in this unit. All these conditions will be discussed in detail in the following units.

This skill unit will focus on electronic cardiac monitors. Cardiac monitors are also useful for monitoring preterm babies at risk for apneic episodes because they detect the bradycardia that will result from any significant apneic episode. Devices that detect both disturbances in heart rate and in respiratory pauses are most effective. Oximeters also will register heart rate and can provide another check on cardiac activity. Oximeters will be discussed in the skill unit that follows this one, and further in Unit 5, Resuscitating the Newborn, in this book, and again in Book III: Neonatal Care, Unit 1, Oxygen.

ACTIONS	REMARKS

Deciding to Use Continuous Electronic Monitoring

1. Use continuous electronic monitoring for a
• Baby who is sick
• Preterm newborn whose
   – Weight is 1,800 g (4 lb) or less
     and/or
   – Gestational age is less than 35 weeks
	All sick babies should have continuous electronic monitoring.
	
	Monitor a baby, even if you are providing care for only a few hours during stabilization, prior to transport of the baby to a regional intensive care nursery.
	
	Other babies who should be monitored include
	• Sick or at-risk babies born and cared for continuously in your hospital
	• Babies transported to an intensive care nursery but returned to your nursery for continuing care and still at risk

Choosing a Monitor

2. Use a monitor with the following features: waveform display, adjustable audio signal, and high/low alarms. These are the basic components of most cardiac monitors. • **Waveform display** (a panel that displays the image of each heartbeat, also called the screen).	Observing the heartbeat pattern and comparing it to the baby's pulse is useful in deciding between true bradycardia or tachycardia and false alarms. Visualizing each heartbeat also makes it possible to recognize *gross* abnormalities in the heart rhythm. Many monitors also display a tracing of the respirations.

ACTIONS	REMARKS

Choosing a Monitor (continued)

- **Audible signal** (beeps with each heartbeat), with an adjustment from silence to loud.

It is not necessary to have the monitor beep continuously, but it should have the capability to be heard during periods of instability in the baby's condition or during special procedures (endotracheal intubation, etc).

- **High and low heart rate alarms** (audible signal that sounds when the heart rate goes above or below the limits set).

Although tachycardia generally is not an immediately life-threatening condition, it should be investigated. Bradycardia, however, can be life-threatening and needs to be detected within seconds of its onset.

Cardio*respiratory* monitors also display chest movement and often are called "impedance" monitors. These monitors can be set to alarm when there has been no chest movement for a set number of seconds (eg, 15 or 20 seconds) and also to sound a different alarm when the heart rate falls below a certain level (eg, 80 or 100 beats per minute [bpm]).

The most effective monitor is one that displays several minutes of heart rate and chest movements simultaneously. Then, when an alarm goes off, you can look at the monitor and see what event triggered the alarm (eg, apnea or bradycardia).

Connecting the Monitor to the Baby

3. Apply monitoring electrode leads to the baby.

Many varieties are commercially available. You may want to test several types to see which you prefer and which work best with your monitor(s).

Generally, there are 3 leads—one on each side of the chest, and one on either the right leg or lower right quadrant of the abdomen.

Instructions regarding placement of the electrodes will accompany your monitor. As with any piece of machinery, be sure your sales representative provides a thorough in-service program for your entire staff.

111

ACTIONS   **REMARKS**

Connecting the Monitor to the Baby (continued)

A slight difference(s) in electrode placement can make a big difference in the clarity of the heart rate pattern and respiratory waveform (if so equipped) displayed on the monitor. For some babies, you may need to change the lead placement several times until a clear and consistent pattern is obtained. Placement of the leads widely separated on each side of the chest is important to achieve a good respiratory waveform.

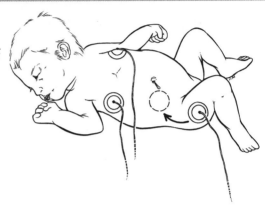

For accurate assessment of apnea, the respiration waveform needs to be clear. This requires the chest leads to move apart from each other with respirations—not on the anterior chest moving up and down without changing the distance between each other. Place the leads on the lateral chest wall.

4. Attach the thin lead wires to the electrodes, if they are separate from each other.

Most lead wires and electrodes are manufactured as one unit and are disposable. If the lead wires are separate from the electrodes, they are not disposable and should be reused. Follow the manufacturer's recommendations for cleaning wires between patients. Lead wires may be broken if, for example, an incubator door is accidentally closed on them. Therefore, be sure to keep extra leads available at all times.

5. Attach the lead wires to the cable, which connects to the monitor. The cable connector may have 4 markings, but only 3 (indicated by an asterisk [*]) may need to be used.
   *RA = right arm (or chest)
   *LA = left arm (or chest)
   *RL = right leg (or lower abdomen)
   LL = left leg (or lower abdomen)
   The monitor will not work properly unless the leads are attached to the electrodes that correspond to the positions indicated on the cable.

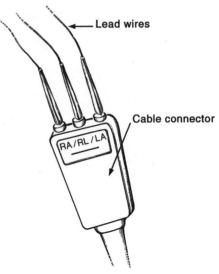

Lead wires

Cable connector

RA/RL/LA

ACTIONS   REMARKS

Connecting the Monitor to the Baby (continued)

6. Turn the monitor power "ON."

7. Wait for the electrocardiogram tracing to appear on the monitor screen.

8. If necessary, adjust the sensitivity control (if present), or lead placement, so that the frequency of the QRS complexes displayed on the oscilloscope corresponds to the digital display of the baby's heart rate.

The monitor should not skip beats, or pick up more than the peak of each QRS signal.

9. Test the audible signal by turning up the volume to be sure it beeps with each QRS peak.

After testing the signal, the monitor may be operated in silent mode.

10. Set the high and low alarms.
    - **Low heart rate:**   100 bpm
    - **High heart rate:**   180 bpm
    - **Respiratory pause (apnea):**   15 or 20 seconds

An undetected apnea and bradycardia spell can be fatal. Monitor alarms should ALWAYS be set.

The low alarm may be set at 80 or 90 bpm if the baby is a term newborn who normally has a low resting heart rate. Babies' respiratory rates are highly variable. Therefore, it usually is not necessary to set alarms for a high or low respiratory rate. However, most cardio-respiratory monitors will permit you to set an alarm for cessation of respirations (apnea).

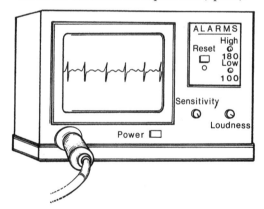

ACTIONS   REMARKS

Evaluating a Baby's Heart Rate

11. Determine the baby's heart rate.

    - **Normal** newborn heart rate is 120 to 160 bpm.
    - **Bradycardia** is a heart rate falling below 100 bpm.

Bradycardia generally means there is low blood oxygen; it may follow an apneic episode (stoppage of breathing) (see Book III: Neonatal Care, Unit 2, Respiratory Distress) and can be life-threatening unless proper attention is given immediately.

Well, term babies may normally have brief heart rate dips to below 100 bpm or demonstrate longer episodes during sleep. The following problems, however, should be ruled out before considering episodes of bradycardia to be normal:
- Hypoxia (low blood oxygen)
- Acidosis (low blood pH)
- Sepsis (blood infection)
- Hypothermia (low body temperature)
- Arrhythmia (congenital heart block)

- **Tachycardia** is a heart rate that is consistently faster than 180 bpm, while the baby is *quiet and at rest.*

Tachycardia should be investigated because it may be due to any of the following:
- Hypovolemia (low blood volume)
- Anemia (low hematocrit)
- Hyperthermia (high body temperature)
- Acidosis (excess acid in the blood)
- Sepsis (blood infection)
- Congestive heart failure
- Arrhythmia (supraventricular tachycardia)

Evaluating a Baby's Respiratory Pattern

12. If your monitor is equipped with a respiratory waveform, when an apnea alarm occurs, first look at the baby for signs of distress. Respond as described in Book III: Neonatal Care, Unit 2, Respiratory Distress. Then look at the monitor to see what led up to the event.

    - Was the baby apneic and, if so, for how long?
    - Was there bradycardia and, if so, did it occur before or after the apnea?

If the monitor does not have a respiratory waveform, you still will need to evaluate the baby and respond appropriately. Your characterization of the event will need to be developed from clinical observations alone.

ACTIONS   REMARKS

Evaluating a Baby's Respiratory Pattern (continued)

13. Record the characteristics of each alarm event.
    - Was the baby breathing?
    - Duration of apnea.
    - Presence of cyanosis.
    - Lowest heart rate and timing of onset.
    - Intervention required.

An accurate description of each event will be important for making decisions about possible medications, and when it may be safe to discharge the baby.

When Can You Stop Cardiorespiratory Monitoring?

Continuous electronic heart rate monitoring may be stopped when a baby
- Is no longer sick
- Weighs approximately 1,800 g (4 lb) or more and/or is 35 weeks' postmenstrual age or older

and
- Has been free of apnea episodes for an acceptable period (see Book III: Neonatal Care, Unit 2, Respiratory Distress, and Book IV: Specialized Newborn Care, Unit 5, Continuing Care).

Different hospitals and practitioners have different criteria for which babies should be monitored and for how long.

What Can Go Wrong?

1. The monitoring leads need to be repositioned.

The most common reason for monitor malfunction is that the position of the electrodes is not quite correct. As noted earlier, several trials at lead position may be needed. After repositioning the leads, it may be necessary to change the sensitivity adjustment, if present.

2. The paste in the electrodes dries.

The leads should be changed according to the manufacturer's recommendations and repositioned slightly with each change.

3. A monitoring electrode becomes loose.

This happens sometimes, especially if a baby is still covered with a thin layer of vernix caseosa or is very active. Clean the baby's skin and reapply the electrode according to the manufacturer's recommendations, or use a new lead.

4. The lead wires from the pad are incorrectly attached to the cable.

Make sure the lead attached to the baby's right arm or chest is the one connected to the RA slot in the cable, and so on for the other leads.

ACTIONS	REMARKS

What Can Go Wrong? (continued)

5. The leads are loose.

Be sure the ends are inserted completely into the cable slots.

6. A lead wire is broken.

It may not be easy to see a break in one of the wires, but the characteristic EKG or waveform pattern may not be present or will look like "noise." You will need to try another electrode and/or lead wire.

7. The cable connecting the lead wires to the monitor is broken.

After a great deal of use, a cable also may become broken or worn out. This is uncommon, but, if you have tried everything else, you may need to try another cable.

PERINATAL PERFORMANCE GUIDE
SKILL UNIT

Pulse Oximetry

A pulse oximeter consists of 2 parts—a light that shines through the baby's skin and a light detector that measures the color of light coming through the skin. The color of the light coming through the skin is determined by the amount of oxygen carried by the hemoglobin in the red blood cells. The oximeter also detects the heart rate by sensing the pulsing of blood in the arteries.

Some oximeters are designed to connect to a cardiac monitor so that the heart rate as determined by the pulse detector can be electronically checked against the heart rate as determined by the cardiac monitor. This comparison is made to determine the reliability of the oximeter reading.

Check the specifications of your oximeter.

- Is it supposed to be connected to a cardiac monitor?
- Is the sensor intended for use on babies? (Those made for adults generally do not work well when used on babies.)

This skill unit will teach you how to monitor a baby's oxygenation using a pulse oximeter. Study this skill unit, then attend a skill practice and demonstration session.

To master the skill, you will need to demonstrate each of the following steps correctly:

1. Identify the features of an oximeter (sensor, patient cable, pulse indicator, pulse and saturation displays, alarms, etc).
2. Connect the sensor to a patient before connecting it to the oximeter and turning it on.
3. Adjust the sensor to obtain an accurate reading.
4. Set the alarms.

ACTIONS   REMARKS

Deciding to Use a Pulse Oximeter

1. Will you be caring for a baby who may
   need assisted ventilation or supplemental
   oxygen?

   a. A newborn in the delivery room

   Yes: Collect the equipment and be sure
        someone is assigned whose primary
        job will be to set up the oximeter and
        connect the probe to the baby.

   No: Be sure the equipment for blending
       oxygen and air and monitoring pulse
       oximetry is quickly available in the
       delivery area.

   b. A baby in the nursery who requires
      oxygen therapy

   Yes: Plug in the oximeter, connect it to a
        cardiac monitor (if indicated), and at-
        tach the sensor cord to the monitor.

   No: Be sure the monitor and sensors are
       well maintained and ready for use.

As you will learn in Unit 5, Resuscitating
the Newborn, in this book, a pulse oximeter
should be available in every delivery area
and to be used for any birth in which

- Positive-pressure ventilation is needed.
- Supplemental oxygen is used or anticipated to be needed.
- Preterm birth at a gestation of less than
  35 weeks.
- Cyanosis persists beyond the first few
  minutes following birth.

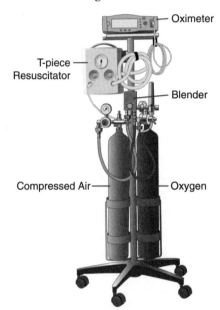

Portable blended oxygen and associated
equipment, for facilities without installed
compressed air source, such as in a delivery
area. However, be careful with small portable tanks that can empty quickly.

Reproduced with permission from photograph courtesy
of Swedish Medical Center, Seattle, WA.

An oximeter can be extremely valuable
when caring for any baby who requires
oxygen therapy. Although arterial blood gas
determinations are still necessary, use of an
oximeter will decrease the number of blood
gases needed. Pulse oximetry also allows
you to recognize very quickly the need for
change in the inspired oxygen concentration
(FIO_2) a baby is receiving.

ACTIONS	REMARKS

Preparing to Monitor a Baby

2. Examine the sensor.

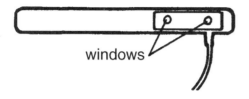

windows

Look at the sensor head. There are 2 dot-like "windows"—one is a light emitter, the other a light detector. For the sensor to work properly, the detector must be able to "see" light coming from the emitter.

3. Select an appropriate site for monitoring by considering
   • If the baby is a newborn

Newborn babies requiring resuscitation or supplemental oxygen should have the oximeter probe attached to the right upper extremity (right hand or wrist) so that the blood being sensed is "pre-ductal." (See Unit 5, Resuscitating the Newborn, in this book.)

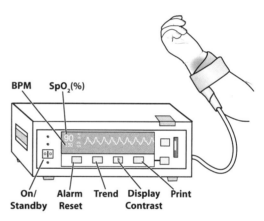

Figure from American Academy of Pediatrics, American Heart Association. Textbook of Neonatal Resuscitation. Kattwinkel J, ed. 6th ed. Elk Grove Village, IL: American Academy of Pediatrics; 2011.

   • If the baby is being cared for in the nursery.

By several hours after birth, and presumably after the ductus arteriosus has spontaneously closed, the oximeter probe may be placed on any extremity. (See figure on next page.)

ACTIONS   **REMARKS**

Preparing to Monitor a Baby (continued)

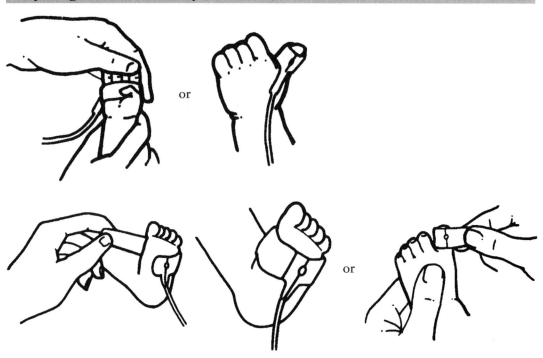

or

• Size and age of patient

Select a thin portion of the body where the emitter light can shine through the tissue and be detected on the other side. A finger or toe usually works best, but, in a small baby, a foot or hand generally works.

• State of perfusion

The sensor must be able to detect a pulse of blood within the tissue. If your patient is extremely ill and has poor peripheral perfusion, select a site with relatively good perfusion.

If the baby is very sick, you may want to use 2 oximeters—one attached pre-ductal (right arm) and the other post-ductal (one of the legs).

4. Before attaching the sensor to the monitor, wrap the sensor around the selected site, so the sensors are in contact with the baby's skin.

The 2 windows—light emitter and light detector—should be opposite each other to help the detector "see" the light.

Hold the sensor in place with Velcro, Coban, or tape. (See manufacturer's recommendations.)

 The wrap should be neither loose nor tight. Either may result in the sensor not being able to detect the pulse in the capillaries.

ACTIONS   **REMARKS**

Monitoring a Baby With Oximetry

NOTE: The following description is for use of an oximeter for a baby who has completed transition following birth. Use of oximetry in a newly born baby will be covered in a separate skill, presented in Unit 5, Resuscitating the Newborn, in this book.

5. Turn on the monitor.

The monitor will "search" for a pulse. If a pulse is detected, the monitor will indicate so with a flashing light-dot, a vertically stacked series of horizontal light-bars, and/or a tone that is activated with each heartbeat. Attaching the probe to the baby before plugging the lead into the monitor will permit the instrument to find the pulse faster.

6. Adjust the sensor, if necessary, until the baby's pulse is displayed and is coincident with the heartbeat signal displayed on the cardiac monitor.

Although a baby can be monitored with a pulse oximeter alone, simultaneous use of a cardiac monitor will help in determining the reliability of the oximeter readings. In addition, any baby sick enough to require oximetry probably also should have continuous electronic cardiorespiratory monitoring.

7. When the heart rate displayed on the cardiac monitor and on the oximeter agree (within approximately 5 beats per minute), note the % saturation displayed by the oximeter.

Be careful. Occasionally, an oximeter will display a % saturation reading even though the pulse is not being detected reliably. In such cases, the % saturation reading is inaccurate.

Oxygen saturation displayed by a pulse oximeter is accurate only when the oximeter is correctly detecting the pulse.

8. If the baby is under a bright light, shield the sensor by covering it lightly with opaque material.

The detector in the sensor is supposed to "see" only light from the emitter. If the baby is under phototherapy or bright procedure light and the sensor is not shielded, the sensor may not work or a false reading may be obtained.

9. When the oximeter reading is relatively stable, obtain an arterial blood sample for determination of Pao_2. Note the oximeter reading at the time the sample is drawn.

Oximetry is valuable for following trends and changes in a baby's oxygenation, but does not replace the need for precise measurement of arterial Pao_2 (as well as $Paco_2$ and pH).

10. Set the low and high alarms.
    Low: 85% saturation
    High: 95% saturation

The alarm limits should be set above and below the respective high and low thresholds of the target range you want.

ACTIONS	REMARKS

What Can Go Wrong?

1. The oximeter continues to "search" but cannot find a pulse, or there is a pulse displayed but no % saturation displayed.

Try readjusting the sensor or applying it to a new site that has better perfusion. Slight readjustments in the position of the light emitter and/or light detector can make the difference between a nonfunctional and a functional sensor. Also be sure that the "windows" are clean. Tiny bits of debris can interfere with the sensor. The sensor may not be plugged in securely to the monitor, or the sensor may be damaged.

2. The heart rate and % saturation readings fluctuate rapidly.

This is usually motion artifact caused by an active baby, although some of the fluctuations may be real.

3. The % saturation readings are misinterpreted to be the PaO_2, as determined from an arterial blood sample.

Remember that PaO_2 measures the oxygen dissolved in plasma, which is reported as "mm Hg." An oximeter measures oxygen bound to hemoglobin, which is reported as "SpO_2." Although the 2 values should correlate, the exact numbers will not be the same. (See figure below.) This concept is described in more detail in Book III: Neonatal Care, Unit 1, Oxygen.

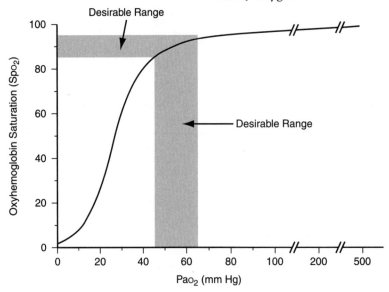

ACTIONS	REMARKS
What Can Go Wrong? (continued)	
4. The oximeter reading seems to be inaccurate.	Check to be sure that the pulse oximeter pulse rate is the same as the heart rate as determined by a cardiac monitor. If they are different, the sensor may need to be adjusted. Also, check to be sure the sensor is shielded from bright light.
5. The wrap holding the sensor in place may be too tight.	Check that the hand or foot beyond the wrap is pink with good perfusion.

Unit 5: Resuscitating the Newborn

Tables and Figures

Recommended Routines

Skill Units

Objectives

In this unit you will learn to

A. Anticipate and recognize newborns who need resuscitation.

B. Prepare adequately for resuscitation.

C. Resuscitate newborns effectively.

D. Anticipate and recognize complications that may arise in a baby who required resuscitation.

 Material in this unit is consistent with the Guidelines for Neonatal Resuscitation developed by the American Academy of Pediatrics and the American Heart Association.

These guidelines were published in

- *Circulation. 2010;122:S909-919*
- *Pediatrics. 2010;126:e1400-1413*

The Neonatal Resuscitation Program (NRP) flow diagrams, as well as segments of those diagrams within the unit, are reproduced, with permission, from American Academy of Pediatrics, American Heart Association. Textbook of Neonatal Resuscitation. *Kattwinkel J, ed. 6th ed. Elk Grove Village, IL: American Academy of Pediatrics; 2011.*

Unit 5 Pretest

Before reading the unit, please answer the following questions. Select the *one best* answer to each question (unless otherwise instructed). Record your answers on the test and check them against the answers at the end of the book.

1. Which of these babies needs resuscitation?
   A. A baby with meconium-stained amniotic fluid, normal breathing, and good tone
   B. A baby who is cyanotic but breathing regularly
   C. A term baby with gasping respirations and poor tone
   D. A preterm baby who has marked acrocyanosis

2. If epinephrine is given during a delivery room resuscitation, which of the following routes is preferred?
   A. Umbilical artery
   B. Extremity vein
   C. Umbilical vein
   D. Endotracheal tube

3. Which of the following is the *most* appropriate rate to provide assisted ventilation to a newborn (who does not need chest compressions)?
   A. 20 breaths per minute
   B. 40 breaths per minute
   C. 80 breaths per minute
   D. 120 breaths per minute

4. If a baby does not begin breathing spontaneously following delivery, which of the following would you do first?
   A. Stimulate by drying the baby.
   B. Start chest compressions.
   C. Administer epinephrine.
   D. Insert an umbilical venous catheter.

Match the following actions with the appropriate medication from the list on the right.

5. _____ Counteracts narcotic drugs   A. Epinephrine
6. _____ Improves heart rate   B. Normal saline
7. _____ Treats low blood volume   C. Sodium bicarbonate
                                               D. None of the above

8. Which of the following babies must be intubated immediately in the delivery room if resuscitation is required?
   A. A baby born to a mother whose membranes ruptured 30 hours before delivery
   B. A baby suspected of having a diaphragmatic hernia
   C. A baby with a 1-minute Apgar score of 6
   D. A baby with Turner syndrome

9. Which of the following concentrations of epinephrine is appropriate to use for newborns?
   A. 1:100
   B. 1:1,000
   C. 1:10,000
   D. 1:100,000

10. A newborn has been quickly rubbed dry following delivery but remains blue and limp, with gasping respirations and a heart rate of 80 beats per minute. Which of the following actions is recommended?
   A. Give free-flow oxygen.
   B. Administer naloxone HCl.
   C. Insert an umbilical arterial catheter.
   D. Begin assisted ventilation.

11. Which of the following concentrations of oxygen for resuscitation does the American Academy of Pediatrics recommend for a baby born at term who requires positive-pressure ventilation?
   A. 21%
   B. 40%
   C. 60%
   D. 100%

12. Which of the following problems is *least* likely to happen to a baby who required prolonged resuscitation at birth?
   A. Hypercalcemia
   B. Low urine output
   C. Seizures
   D. Low blood pH

13. Bag-and-mask ventilation is appropriate for all of the following babies, *except those*
   A. Who do not breathe after stimulation
   B. With an Apgar score of 2 and a respiratory rate of 10
   C. With a cleft lip who are not breathing
   D. With a sunken abdomen at birth

14. A baby will soon be delivered at term by emergency cesarean section because of a bleeding placenta previa. Which medication would you anticipate the baby is most likely to need?
   A. Naloxone HCl
   B. Normal saline
   C. Sodium bicarbonate 0.5 mEq/mL
   D. Vitamin K

15. **True** **False** Meconium aspiration may occur in utero minutes, hours, or days before delivery.

16. **True** **False** Initial positive-pressure inflation pressure of 40 to 45 cm H_2O is preferred.

17. **True** **False** Babies requiring resuscitation for as long as 20 minutes may have normal mental and physical development.

18. True   False   To avoid confusion, it is best if one person carries out all resuscitative procedures.

19. True   False   A CO_2 detector is the recommended way to confirm endotracheal tube placement.

20. True   False   A limp, meconium-stained baby with weak respiratory efforts and a heart rate of 120 beats per minute should be intubated, and the trachea should be suctioned directly.

21. True   False   Nearly all babies who require assisted ventilation should also receive chest compressions.

22. True   False   Overheating a compromised baby may worsen the extent of hypoxic brain injury.

1. What Is Resuscitation?

Resuscitation is the series of actions taken to revive a baby and restore to normal

- Respiratory rate and pattern
- Heart rate
- Oxygenation
- Blood pressure
- General activity level

There are 4 basic steps to resuscitation. They follow the first 4 letters of the alphabet.

A. Establish *Airway.* You will need to position a baby's head to open the airway. You also may need to suction amniotic fluid or secretions from the airway. If meconium is present and the baby is not vigorous, direct suctioning of the trachea will be indicated.

B. Assist *Breathing.* If a baby is not breathing spontaneously, you will need to administer positive-pressure ventilation (PPV) with a bag and mask or bag and endotracheal tube. If a baby is working hard to breathe, has grunting respirations or intercostal retractions, or has central cyanosis or hypoxemia, you may decide to support breathing with continuous positive airway pressure (CPAP).

C. Assist *Circulation.* If the heart rate is absent or low, you should assist cardiac output by rhythmically compressing the chest while PPV is continued.

D. Administer *Drugs.* Although seldom required, epinephrine and/or a blood volume expander may be indicated in certain clinical situations, after ventilation is established.

In this unit, you will learn to evaluate a baby to determine when each of these steps is needed and how each step should be carried out.

2. Which Babies Need to Be Resuscitated?

Babies *at birth* who make little respiratory effort, who are limp, or who have a heart rate less than 100 beats per minute (bpm) need resuscitation.

Babies *after birth,* whether in the nursery or mother's room, who experience deterioration in vital signs need resuscitation.

3. Who Should Perform Resuscitation?

At *every delivery,* there should be at least one person whose primary responsibility is the baby. This person should be capable of initiating resuscitation. An additional skilled person possessing the skills to perform a complete resuscitation, including endotracheal intubation and administration of medications, should be immediately available.

The concept of *resuscitation teams,* with specified leaders, identified roles for each team member, and 24-hour in-hospital presence, should be a goal of every delivery service.

If a pregnancy and/or labor is or becomes **high risk,** and thus need for neonatal resuscitation can be anticipated, at least 2 people should be present solely to manage the baby. One person should possess complete resuscitation skills and one, or more, other person should be present and skilled to assist with resuscitation. For multiple births, there should be a separate team for each baby.

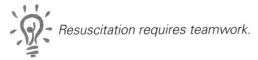 *Resuscitation requires teamwork.*

4. How Should You and Your Neonatal Team Prepare for Resuscitation?

Adequate preparation for resuscitation requires that each team member has studied the principles, learned and practiced the individual tasks they will need to perform, and, most importantly, be able to work together efficiently, with each team member having confidence that the other team members can be relied upon to perform his or her assigned tasks without requiring instruction to do so. This can only be accomplished if the team practices the sequences beforehand. Also, after there has been an actual resuscitation, the team should reconvene to discuss what went well and what could be improved.

You will need to practice each skill and the resuscitation sequence many times to have them become second nature, so you can use the information and skills to the fullest extent next time a baby in your hospital needs resuscitation.

Although 90% of babies are born without complications, you always need to be prepared for the 10% who need help at birth. For particularly complicated births, such as a baby unexpectedly born extremely preterm, you need to mobilize team members quickly, with the following assigned tasks:

- A leader, who has all of the resuscitation skills, including establishment of an airway and assisting ventilation.
- A second team member to help with the initial steps, listen for the heart rate, and be able to administer chest compressions, if required.
- Another nurse to prepare medications and help establish an umbilical venous line to deliver epinephrine, if required.
- An assistant to attach an oximeter and record all events.

Each team member should study the evaluation-decision-action sequences in the resuscitation flow diagram in Figure 5.1. In your mind, establish the content, sequence, and timing of each step. During neonatal resuscitation, evaluation and action are often carried out simultaneously. For the purpose of teaching and learning the process, each facet of the sequence is taught as a distinct segment in the Skill Units. In practice, however, components of each assessment are integrated into a total evaluation of the baby, with corresponding instantaneous intervention(s).

5. Can You Anticipate Before Delivery if a Baby Will Need Resuscitation?

In many situations, the need for resuscitation can be anticipated. In previous units, you learned conditions that place a fetus at risk. If any of these conditions are present at the time of delivery, at least one resuscitation team leader and one skilled assistant should attend the delivery and be prepared to resuscitate the baby.

The following conditions may jeopardize a fetus and necessitate newborn resuscitation:

A. Problems Identified During Pregnancy
- Maternal diabetes mellitus
- Hypertension
  - Gestational
  - Preeclampsia
  - Chronic
- Chronic maternal illness (neurologic, cardiovascular, thyroid, pulmonary, or renal)
- Anemia or isoimmunization

Newborn Resuscitation

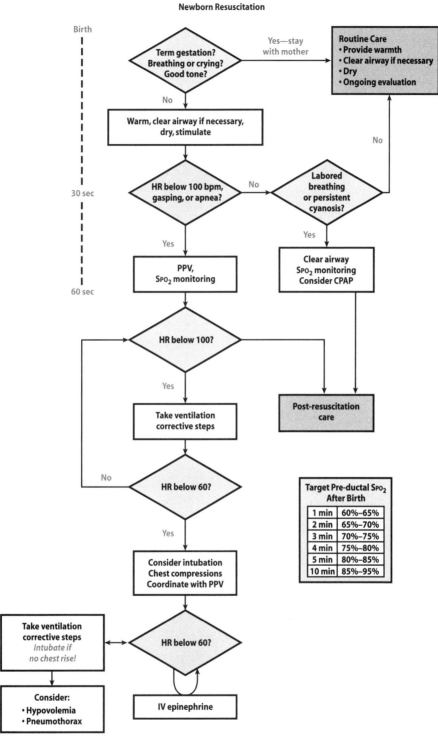

Figure 5.1. Resuscitation Flow Diagram.
Reprinted with permission from American Academy of Pediatrics, American Heart Association. *Textbook of Neonatal Resuscitation.* Kattwinkel J, ed. 6th ed. Elk Grove Village, IL: American Academy of Pediatrics; 2011.

- Previous fetal or neonatal death
- Bleeding in second or third trimester
- Maternal infection
- Hydramnios
- Oligohydramnios
- Premature rupture of membranes
- Post-term gestation
- Multifetal gestation
- Size-date discrepancy
- Drug therapy
  - Lithium carbonate
  - Magnesium
  - Adrenergic-blocking drugs
- Maternal substance use
- Fetal malformation
- Diminished fetal activity
- No prenatal care
- Age younger than 16 or older than 35 years

B. Problems Identified During Labor
- Emergency cesarean section
- Forceps or vacuum-assisted delivery
- Breech or other abnormal presentation
- Preterm labor
- Precipitous labor
- Chorioamnionitis
- Prolonged rupture of membranes (>18 hours before delivery)
- Prolonged labor (>24 hours)
- Prolonged second stage of labor (>2 hours)
- Fetal bradycardia
- Non-reassuring fetal heart rate pattern(s)
- Use of general anesthesia
- Uterine tetany
- Narcotics administered to woman within 4 hours of delivery
- Meconium-stained amniotic fluid
- Prolapsed umbilical cord
- Abruptio placentae
- Placenta previa (if undetected earlier)

No matter how carefully you screen for risk factors, some babies requiring resuscitation cannot be identified prior to delivery.

You must always be prepared to resuscitate.

6. Do Some Babies Require Resuscitation After Initial Stabilization?

Yes. Some babies may require resuscitation in the nursery, or in their mother's room, if their vital signs deteriorate. These babies require the same resuscitative measures as sick babies in the delivery room.

Resuscitate if a baby develops

- Heart rate below 100 bpm*
- Deep gasping respirations or apnea
- Low blood pressure

Resuscitate if a baby becomes

- Blue, gray, very pale, or mottled in color
- Limp with little or no response to stimulation

Self-test

Now answer these questions to test yourself on the information in the last section. Refer to the graphs or charts in the unit, as necessary, to answer these questions.

A1. **True** **False** It is possible to predict all babies who will require resuscitation at birth by evaluating their risk status.

A2. List the 4 basic steps of resuscitation.

A. _____

B. _____

C. _____

D. _____

A3. Name at least 4 conditions during *pregnancy* that would warn you to get ready to resuscitate a baby at birth.

A. _____   C. _____

B. _____   D. _____

A4. Name at least 4 conditions during *labor* that would warn you to get ready to resuscitate a baby at birth.

A. _____   C. _____

B. _____   D. _____

A5. You may have to resuscitate babies

A. At birth in the delivery room

B. Later in the nursery

C. Both A and B

A6. **True** **False** Only one skilled person is needed to perform the 4 basic steps of resuscitation.

A7. Describe the vital signs and appearance of a baby in the nursery who needs to be resuscitated.

Breathing: _____

Color: _____

Heart rate: _____

Activity: _____

Blood pressure: _____

Check your answers with the list that follows the Recommended Routines. Correct any incorrect answers and review the appropriate section in the unit.

---

*Some babies born at term may normally have a resting heart rate slightly below 100 bpm when in deep sleep.

7. How Should You Prepare for Every Delivery?

A. Provide or Obtain Pregnancy History

Close communication between obstetric and neonatal care providers is essential. Information should include all relevant history regarding maternal and fetal condition and the course of labor. Even if time is extremely limited, note the key points, such as if the woman has a serious medical illness or if there has been significant maternal blood loss, etc.

Knowing maternal and fetal history will help you anticipate the care a baby might need at delivery and understand the baby's risk factors to help you plan care following delivery.

B. Plan to Prevent Neonatal Heat Loss

Do not overlook general support measures that are needed for every baby. In particular, it is important to keep the baby warm. Cold stress can severely compromise a preterm or sick baby. Even healthy term newborns can lose a tremendous amount of body heat and may have difficulty maintaining normal body temperature as they move from the warm, wet intrauterine environment to the relatively cold, dry extrauterine environment.

Heat loss and the danger of hypothermia should be minimized for *all* babies (preterm, term, post-term, healthy, at risk, or sick) by using the following procedures:
- Maintain a relatively warm, draft-free delivery environment.
- Before each delivery, turn on the radiant warmer and preheat the bed.
- Use warm, dry towels to dry the baby immediately after delivery. (If possible, keep extra blankets and towels in a warmer immediately available to each room where deliveries occur.)
- Promptly remove any wet linen and replace with warm, dry linen.
- Be sure the baby's hair is dried and put a cap on the baby. (If the baby needs resuscitative measures, this step may need to be delayed.)

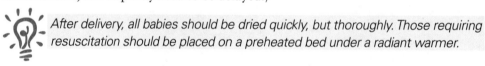

After delivery, all babies should be dried quickly, but thoroughly. Those requiring resuscitation should be placed on a preheated bed under a radiant warmer.

However, take care not to *over*heat a baby, particularly if the baby requires resuscitation. *Hyper*thermia should be avoided because it may provoke apnea, and may worsen the extent of hypoxic brain injury. The general goal is to maintain a normal body temperature.*

8. What Supplies Should Be Available for Every Delivery?

Resuscitation equipment should be kept well organized and immediately available at all times. This equipment should be in each room where deliveries take place, and in each nursery and postpartum unit. Essential neonatal resuscitation equipment kept only in a central location or on a hallway cart is not considered sufficient.

Check all equipment routinely and after every use to ensure proper functioning. Even the most skilled clinicians cannot perform a successful resuscitation without proper equipment in good working order. Be certain all essential resuscitation items are present and functioning properly.

---

*Intentionally induced hypothermia instituted after resuscitation of a severely compromised newborn may reduce the extent of brain injury following hypoxia in term babies. This newly recommended treatment will be discussed later in this unit.

Use of the neonatal resuscitation equipment in the following list is described in the skill units.

Essential Resuscitation Equipment

Suction Equipment

- Bulb syringe
- Mechanical suction with tubing and pressure regulator
- Suction catheters, 5F or 6F, 8F, and 10F or 12F
- 8F feeding tube and 20-mL syringe
- Meconium aspiration device

Bag-and-Mask Equipment

- Neonatal resuscitation bag with a pressure-release valve or flow-control valve and pressure manometer (bag must be able to deliver 90% to 100% oxygen) and/or T-piece resuscitator (mechanical device to control flow and pressures during ventilation)
- Face masks, newborn and preterm sizes (cushioned-rim masks preferred)

Oxygen equipment

- Oxygen blender with flowmeter (flow rate up to 10 L/min) and tubing
- Pulse oximeter with patient cable and neonatal sensor

Endotracheal Intubation Equipment

- Laryngoscope with straight blades, No. 0 (preterm) and No. 1 (term)
  No. 00 for extremely preterm babies (optional)
- Extra bulbs and batteries for laryngoscope
- Endotracheal tubes, 2.5-, 3.0-, 3.5-, and 4.0-mm internal diameter
- Stylet (optional)
- Scissors
- Stethoscope
- Tape or securing device for endotracheal tube
- Alcohol sponges
- Carbon dioxide (CO_2) detector
- Laryngeal mask airway

Medications

- Epinephrine in 1:10,000 concentration (0.1 mg/mL)
- Isotonic crystalloid (normal saline or Ringer's lactate) for volume expansion
- Dextrose 10%
- Normal saline for flushes
- Syringes, 1, 3, 5, 10, 20, 50 mL
- Needles, 25, 21, 18 gauge, or puncture device for needleless system

Umbilical Vessel Catheterization Supplies

- Sterile gloves
- Scalpel or scissors
- Mosquito or Kelly clamps (2)
- Iris forceps and toothed forceps (optional)
- Antiseptic prep solution
- Umbilical tape
- Umbilical catheters, 3.5F, 5F
- Three-way stopcock

Miscellaneous

- Gloves and appropriate personal protection
- Oropharyngeal airways (0, 00, and 000 sizes)
- Radiant warmer or other heat source
- Firm, padded resuscitation surface
- Clock with second hand (timer optional)
- Warmed linens
- Tape in 1/2- or 3/4-inch size

Thermal protection for preterm babies

- Reclosable, food-grade plastic bag (1-gallon size) or plastic wrap
- Chemically activated warming pad (optional)
- Transport incubator to maintain baby's temperature during move to the nursery

9. What Should You Do as Soon as a Baby Is Born?

A. Ask Yourself 3 Questions
   1. Was the baby born at term?
   2. Is the baby breathing or crying?
   3. Is there good muscle tone?

B. If the Answer to All 3 Questions Is "Yes"

   The *baby does not require resuscitation* (Figure 5.2) and usually can be placed on the mother's abdomen or chest to allow immediate maternal-newborn contact.

   You still will need to provide warmth and be sure that the baby has a clear airway and becomes pink, but these goals can generally be achieved by
   - Drying the baby well
   - Clearing secretions from the nose and mouth, if necessary
   - Placing the baby skin-to-skin with the mother, then covering with a warm blanket
   - Observing the baby frequently for breathing, heart rate, and adequate oxygenation (color and/or oxygen saturation from oximetry). If the baby does not require resuscitation, clamping the umbilical cord can be delayed 1 minute from the time the baby's head and body are completely delivered.

C. If the Answer to Any of the 3 Questions Is "No"
   The *baby requires resuscitation.* How you proceed will depend on whether meconium is present (Figure 5.3).

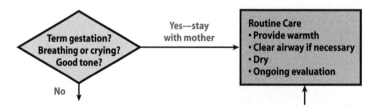

Figure 5.2. Identifying Babies *Not* Needing Resuscitation at Birth.
Reprinted with permission from American Academy of Pediatrics, American Heart Association. *Textbook of Neonatal Resuscitation.* Kattwinkel J, ed. 6th ed. Elk Grove Village, IL: American Academy of Pediatrics; 2011.

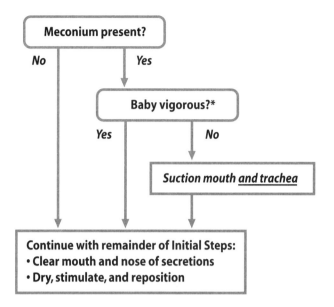

* Vigorous is defined as strong respiratory efforts, good muscle tone, and a heart rate greater than 100 bpm.

Figure 5.3. Decision Tree for Management of Meconium.
Reprinted with permission from American Academy of Pediatrics, American Heart Association. *Textbook of Neonatal Resuscitation.* Kattwinkel J, ed. 6th ed. Elk Grove Village, IL: America Academy of Pediatrics; 2011.

10. What Should You Do if Meconium Is Present?

A. Before Delivery of the Shoulders

A large, multicenter study revealed that the previously recommended practice of suctioning the mouth, posterior pharynx, and nose at the time a baby's head appears on the perineum, before delivery of the shoulders, does not make a difference in the incidence of meconium aspiration. Many occurrences of meconium aspiration are now thought to occur *in utero*, minutes, hours, or possibly days before birth.

For this reason, intrapartum suctioning of all meconium-stained babies, after delivery of the head and before delivery of the shoulders, is no longer recommended as a routine procedure. However, suctioning of the nasopharynx may be carried out in certain circumstances, such as thick meconium visible in the nares.

Repeated suctioning should not be performed on the perineum or at the incision because this may delay the resuscitation.

B. After Complete Delivery of the Baby

The next step depends on whether the baby is vigorous. Vigorous is defined as strong respiratory efforts, good muscle tone, and a heart rate greater than 100 bpm.

- *If the baby is vigorous,* proceed with routine care.
- *If the baby is not vigorous,* the trachea should be intubated with an endotracheal tube and suctioned directly prior to drying and stimulation. A suction adapter is attached to the endotracheal tube and the tube itself is used as a suction catheter. After suctioning the trachea, proceed with Resuscitation Step A: Airway.

Self-test

Now answer these questions to test yourself on the information in the last section. Refer to the graphs or charts in the unit, as necessary, to answer these questions.

B1. What 2 general measures should you do before every delivery?

_____

_____

B2.	**True**	**False**	Vigorous meconium-stained babies can be provided routine care.
B3.	**True**	**False**	All meconium-stained babies need endotracheal suctioning to help prevent meconium aspiration.
B4.	**True**	**False**	Neonatal resuscitation equipment should be kept in every room where deliveries occur.
B5.	**True**	**False**	Heat loss in the delivery room is dangerous only for preterm and sick babies.
B6.	**True**	**False**	When suctioning a baby's trachea to clear it of meconium, an endotracheal tube is used in place of a suction catheter.
B7.	**True**	**False**	A meconium-stained baby with a heart rate of 110 beats per minute who is pale and has weak, irregular respiratory efforts and poor muscle tone should be intubated and have direct tracheal suctioning.

B8. List 3 ways to minimize heat loss for any baby at the time of delivery.

_____

_____

_____

Check your answers with the list that follows the Recommended Routines. Correct any incorrect answers and review the appropriate section in the unit.

11. What Should You Do After Initial Assessment and Management of Meconium (if Present)?

Step A: Establish an Airway

The initial steps of resuscitation should take about 30 seconds and include

- Providing warmth
- Positioning and clearing residual meconium or secretions from the airway
- Stimulating the baby to breathe, which often can be accomplished by drying the skin, and then repositioning to ensure an open airway

These steps can be accomplished with the following actions:

Provide warmth by placing the baby under a pre-warmed radiant warmer or comparable heat source.

Place the baby supine on a flat, firm, but padded, surface. Do not tilt the bed. Extreme tilting of a radiant warmer bed in either direction increases the risk of aspiration of stomach contents, may abnormally increase or decrease cerebral blood flow, and may inhibit drainage of secretions from the lungs.

Put the baby in the "sniffing" position, with the nose as far anterior as possible and the neck slightly extended. This position provides maximum opening of a newborn's airway. Hyperextension or flexion of the head and neck can easily obstruct the airway of a newborn and should be avoided. A small cloth roll (0.5- to 1-inch thick) under a baby's shoulders may be helpful in maintaining proper head position.

Clear the airway of secretions or residual meconium by suctioning first the mouth and then the nose with a bulb syringe or large-bore suction catheter.

Avoid deep or excessively vigorous suctioning of a baby's mouth or nose, because this can stimulate the vagus nerve and cause bradycardia.

Dry and stimulate the baby to breathe. When babies are not breathing, they may begin breathing spontaneously, if stimulated. The most effective form of stimulation is to *rub a baby dry with a towel.* Rubbing the back or flicking the soles of the feet also may be used to stimulate a baby. More vigorous or prolonged stimulation should be avoided because it is likely to be ineffective and wastes time.

Reposition the baby in the sniffing position to ensure an open airway.

If a baby does not begin breathing adequately after several seconds of stimulation, start PPV (described in the next section).

12. What Should You Do After Initial Resuscitation Measures?

Reassess the baby's condition. After you have carried out Step A by providing warmth, positioning and clearing the airway, and stimulating the baby to breathe, you should reevaluate the baby's condition to determine if further resuscitation measures are necessary (Figure 5.5).

Evaluate respirations and heart rate to decide if it is necessary to move to the next step in resuscitation. These 2 physical signs provide the most rapid, effective assessment of a baby's well-being and an indication of whether PPV is needed.

Respirations
Look for good, spontaneous chest movement with each breath; however, gasping respirations are not a good sign and generally indicate the baby has been severely compromised and has a very low blood pH.

Heart Rate
The quickest way to determine the heart rate is to feel for pulsation at the base of the umbilical cord. Sometimes the umbilical arteries will be constricted, and, therefore, will not pulsate despite the presence of a good heart rate. If you cannot feel pulsation, listen to the chest with a stethoscope.

State of oxygenation. (See also Book III: Neonatal Care, Unit 1, Oxygen.)
Adequate oxygenation historically has been assessed by evaluating skin color for cyanosis. However, recent studies have shown that clinical assessment of skin color is very unreliable. Furthermore, fetuses normally have quite low blood oxygen levels, and uncompromised newly born babies may take as long as 10 minutes from birth to increase their levels to those expected of a healthy newborn. Current recommendations call for assessment of the state of oxygenation with a pulse oximeter during resuscitation and adjustment of the concentration of oxygen administered to match the increase in oxyhemoglobin saturation (SpO_2) demonstrated by a healthy newborn at term (Figure 5.4).

 If the need for resuscitation is anticipated before birth, or if a baby needs supplemental oxygen or assisted ventilation after birth, attach a pulse oximeter to measure pre-ductal arterial oxygen saturation and administer supplemental oxygen as indicated to achieve target saturations appropriate for the time after birth.

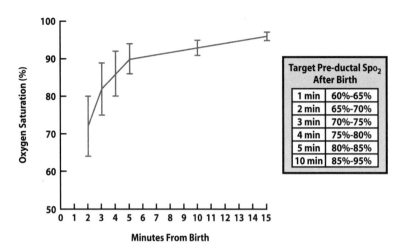

Figure 5.4. Pre-ductal Oxygen Saturation Changes Following Birth (Median and Inter-quartile Range).

Graph reprinted with permission from Mariani G, Dik PB, Ezquer A, et al. Pre-ductal and post-ductal O$_2$ saturation in healthy term neonates after birth. *J Pediatr.* 2007;150:418-421.

Table reprinted with permission from American Academy of Pediatrics, American Heart Association. *Textbook of Neonatal Resuscitation.* Kattwinkel J, ed. 6th ed. Elk Grove Village, IL: American Academy of Pediatrics; 2011.

"Pre-ductal" means that the saturation should be measured from tissue that is perfused with blood that comes from a vessel that leaves the aorta before the ductus arteriosus. Therefore, the oximeter probe always should be placed on the right arm (wrist or hand) to assess oxygenation immediately following delivery. Free-flow oxygen may be given by a flow-inflating bag-and-mask apparatus, a separate mask connected to oxygen tubing, a T-piece resuscitator, or oxygen tubing and your cupped hand to concentrate the oxygen around the baby's face. (See Book III: Neonatal Care, Unit 1, Oxygen.)

Acrocyanosis is a condition where a baby's hands and feet are blue, but the baby's body and mucous membranes are pink. **Acrocyanosis does *not* require oxygen** administration, but may indicate cold stress.

Clearing the airway may require endotracheal intubation, if meconium is present and baby is not vigorous.

- *If respirations, heart rate, and oxygenation are all normal,* the baby likely will not require further resuscitation. Because of the need for the initial resuscitation steps, this baby is still at risk for developing problems associated with transition from the intrauterine to extrauterine environment and should be monitored closely. However, this frequent assessment, perhaps even including continued pulse oximetry, often can be provided while the baby stays with the mother.

- *If respiratory distress and/or the need for supplemental oxygen to maintain target SpO$_2$* persists after appropriate clearing of the airway, application of CPAP may be helpful.

- **If a baby remains apneic, continues to have a heart rate <100 bpm, or cannot be adequately oxygenated with up to 100% supplemental oxygen,** despite drying, clearing the airway, and stimulation to breathe, PPV should be initiated.

 The most important part of resuscitation is ensuring adequate ventilation. Nearly all babies will improve if given adequate assisted ventilation.

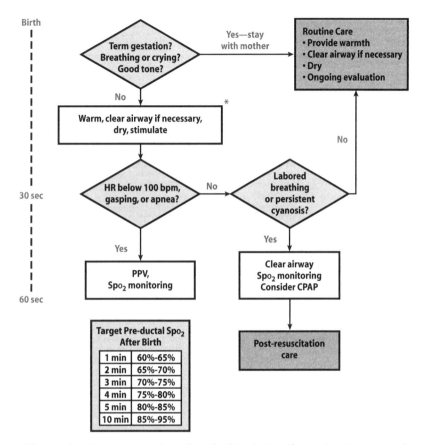

*Clearing the airway may require endotracheal intubation, if meconium is present and baby is not vigorous.

Figure 5.5. Resuscitation Sequence Through Step B: Breathing

Reprinted with permission from American Academy of Pediatrics, American Heart Association. *Textbook of Neonatal Resuscitation.* Kattwinkel J, ed. 6th ed. Elk Grove Village, IL: American Academy of Pediatrics; 2011.

13. How Do You Assist Ventilation?

Step B: Breathe for the Baby

Positive-pressure ventilation can be provided 2 ways.

- Face mask and ventilation bag or T-piece resuscitator
- Endotracheal tube and ventilation bag or T-piece resuscitator

 Do NOT use mask ventilation with babies who

- *Are meconium stained and have not been suctioned*
- *Have sunken abdomens (intestines may be in chest from a congenital diaphragmatic hernia)*

If these babies require assisted ventilation, their tracheas should be intubated.

What Should You Do?

- **Call for help.** If you are unsuccessful ventilating the baby adequately with mask ventilation, you will need to intubate the trachea. If intubation does not result in improvement, you will need to progress to further steps that will require extra personnel.

143

- **Use the appropriate amount of supplemental oxygen.** In term newborns, begin ventilation with room air (21% oxygen), unless you have already attached an oximeter and documented that supplemental oxygen is necessary to achieve the oximetry targets. Although sufficient oxygen is essential for life, tissues that have been deprived of oxygen can be injured further by abrupt exposure to excessive oxygen. Inflation of the lungs with air is often sufficient to restore spontaneous breathing. Onset of spontaneous respirations may occur more rapidly with 21% oxygen than with 100%. Preterm newborns (<32 weeks' gestation) often need moderate concentrations of supplemental oxygen (30% to 50%) to achieve the targeted rise in saturations after birth. Supplemental oxygen given in the delivery room should be guided by pulse oximetry.
- **Breathe for the baby at a rate of 40 to 60 breaths per minute.** This rate will be different if a baby also needs chest compressions. (See Section 14.) Prompt increase in heart rate and chest movement with audible breath sounds are the most rapid indications of effective ventilation. If the baby is not improving and there is no chest movement with each breath, take steps to improve ventilation. Consider the acronym, "**MR SOPA**":
  – Be sure the face **mask (M)** seals tightly over a baby's mouth and nose.
  – **Reposition (R)** the baby's head with the neck slightly extended.
  – Remove any **secretions (S)** from the airway.
  – Ventilate with the mouth slightly **open (O)**.
  – Squeeze harder on the bag to create more **pressure (P)** to deliver a larger breath. Although initial inflation pressures of about 20 cm H_2O are generally adequate, pressures up to 40 cm H_2O may be necessary in some babies with severe lung disease. However, excessive pressure will injure the lungs, particularly if the lungs are immature, and should be avoided. Use sufficient pressure to create slight movement of the chest with each inflation.
  – Consider establishing an **alternative (A)** airway. Endotracheal intubation is most effective. Placement of a laryngeal mask airway also may be effective.

14. What if There Is Little or No Improvement Despite Achieving Adequate Ventilation?

Reassess the baby's condition (Figure 5.6). If the heart rate remains less than 100 bpm, but above 60 bpm, continue to work to improve ventilation further. This likely will require intubation of the trachea, if not already done. If a baby's heart rate remains below 60 bpm after 30 to 60 seconds of PPV producing adequate chest rise, and oxygen has been increased to 100%, proceed to

Step C: Assisting *Circulation* With Chest Compressions

Encircle the baby's chest with your hands and use both thumbs, placed either side-by-side or on top of one another (depending on the baby's size) on the lower third of the sternum, to provide chest compressions. Compressions should be strong enough to depress the chest one-third the anterior-posterior diameter and result in a palpable pulse.

Because simultaneous chest compression and lung inflation may impede effective ventilation, coordinate compressions with assisted ventilations in a 3:1 ratio (3 compressions followed by a brief pause

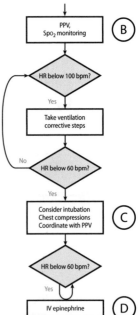

Figure 5.6. Resuscitation Sequence: Steps B Through D. Reprinted with permission from American Academy of Pediatrics, American Heart Association. *Textbook of Neonatal Resuscitation.* Kattwinkel J, ed. 6th ed. Elk Grove Village, IL: American Academy of Pediatrics; 2011.

144

for one ventilation). This cycle should be repeated every 2 seconds, so that 90 compressions and 30 breaths, or 120 events, occur each minute. Pause after 45 to 60 seconds of compressions to count the baby's heart rate. Discontinue chest compressions when the heart rate is above 60 bpm.

It is rare for a baby to need resuscitation beyond the actions taken in Steps A, B, and C; however, if a baby's heart rate remains below 60 bpm after approximately another 45 to 60 seconds of assisted ventilation with 100% oxygen and chest compressions, proceed to Step D: Drugs.

15. What Should You Do if There Is Minimal Improvement With Assisted Ventilation and Chest Compressions?

Reassess the baby's condition. Be sure all resuscitation techniques are being done correctly. Quickly review the baby's risk factors. Based on the baby's history and condition, consider the indications for administration of epinephrine and/or volume expander.

Step D: Administer *Drugs* to Assist Resuscitative Efforts

The most important resuscitation intervention is ventilation.

A baby being adequately ventilated and receiving adequate chest compressions rarely requires additional medications.

Use of the drugs listed below, however, may be indicated in certain circumstances.

- **Epinephrine:** This drug stimulates the heart and causes vasoconstriction. Epinephrine is used if a baby's spontaneous heart rate is less than 60 bpm despite a minimum of 45 to 60 seconds of adequate ventilation with 100% oxygen and chest compressions.

  Epinephrine is administered intravenously by infusing the drug through an umbilical venous catheter. Do *not* infuse epinephrine through an arterial catheter. Use only a 1:10,000 concentration of epinephrine. The intravenous dose is 0.1 to 0.3 mL/kg and may be repeated every 3 to 5 minutes. The drug also may be given into an endotracheal tube while intravenous (IV) access is being established, but higher doses may be required (0.5 to 1 mL/kg), and even they may be ineffective. Do *not* give these higher doses intravenously.

- **Blood volume expander:** An isotonic crystalloid solution is the fluid of choice for volume expansion. Normal saline or Ringer's lactate is generally the most readily available appropriate solution. O Rh-negative emergency-release blood also may be used when acute blood loss or profound anemia is suspected.

  A volume expander is indicated if a baby is responding poorly to other measures or blood loss is suspected. (See also Book III: Neonatal Care, Unit 4, Low Blood Pressure.) Signs of hypovolemia include bradycardia or tachycardia, pallor, poor perfusion, and gasping respirations or apnea.

  Administration of volume expansion is by steady, *slow* intravenous (IV) push, over 5 to 10 minutes, through an umbilical venous catheter. The dose is 10 mL/kg, which may be repeated if needed.

Self-test

Now answer these questions to test yourself on the information in the last section. Refer to the graphs or charts in the unit, as necessary, to answer these questions.

C1. **True** **False** Following delivery, a baby's head and neck should be in full extension to allow maximum opening of the airway.

C2. **True** **False** When suctioning secretions from a baby, clear the mouth first and then the nose.

C3. **True** **False** If a baby born at term needs assisted ventilation following delivery, 21% oxygen should be used.

C4. **True** **False** Both acrocyanosis and central cyanosis should be treated with oxygen.

C5. What 3 physical signs provide the most rapid, effective way to evaluate a baby's response to resuscitation?

_____, _____, and _____

C6. **True** **False** Heart rate less than 100 beats per minute despite stimulation, a clear airway, and proper head position indicate positive-pressure assisted ventilation should be started.

C7. **True** **False** Deep, slow, gasping respirations are a good sign that a baby will not need assisted ventilation.

C8. **True** **False** When giving positive-pressure ventilation to a baby who does not need chest compressions, 50 breaths per minute is an appropriate rate.

C9. **True** **False** All babies who require chest compressions should also receive epinephrine.

C10. **True** **False** You should anticipate the possible need for blood volume expansion for any baby born to a woman who experienced abruptio placentae or had a bleeding placenta previa.

C11. When a baby needs assisted ventilation and chest compressions, which ventilation-compression sequence is correct?
A. _breathe_-compress, compress, compress-_breathe_-compress, compress, compress-_breathe_. . .
B. _breathe_-compress, compress-_breathe_-compress, compress-_breathe_-compress, compress. . .
C. _breathe, breathe, breathe_-compress-_breathe, breathe, breathe_-compress. . .

C12. Following delivery, which of the following is the _first_ thing you should do to get a baby to breathe?
A. Start chest compressions.
B. Rub the baby dry with a towel.
C. Begin bag-and-mask assisted ventilation.
D. Carry out endotracheal suctioning.

C13. Epinephrine may be
A. Instilled into an endotracheal tube
B. Infused through an umbilical arterial catheter
C. Infused through an umbilical venous catheter

C14. Which 2 groups of babies should not have ventilations assisted with bag-and-mask ventilation?

_____, _____

Check your answers with the list that follows the Recommended Routines. Correct any incorrect answers and review the appropriate section in the unit.

16. What Should You Do for a Baby Who Has Depressed Respirations Because of a Narcotic Drug(s) Given to the Mother?

If a woman was given narcotic medication within approximately 4 hours of delivery, the drug will have been transferred to the fetus via the placenta by the time delivery occurs. Depending on timing of administration and drug dosage, the baby's spontaneous respirations may be depressed at birth.

Provide PPV and supplemental oxygen as necessary to establish normal heart rate and oxygen saturations. The baby should respond well to PPV, even if spontaneous respirations have been depressed by maternal medication. First, resuscitate and stabilize the baby, and then consider giving a narcotic antagonist (naloxone HCl).

Naloxone is NOT a resuscitation drug.

It should not be given until normal heart rate and normal oxygen saturations have been established with other resuscitative measures.

If there is a history of a woman having recently received a narcotic drug and the baby's spontaneous respirations are depressed, naloxone HCl may be appropriate. Administration may be by intramuscular or subcutaneous routes, although response will not be as rapid as when the drug is given intravenously.

Naloxone can be dangerous for babies born to women with drug addiction(s). It will cause acute withdrawal in a baby with chronic fetal exposure to narcotics, and it may induce neonatal seizures.

Naloxone should NOT be given to a baby whose mother is suspected of being addicted to narcotics.

17. When Should You Insert an Endotracheal Tube?

There are several points in the resuscitation sequence where endotracheal intubation may be appropriate. The timing of intubation will be determined by many factors, including the following:

- **Skill of resuscitator:** People who are not skilled at intubation should focus on providing effective ventilation with bag and mask and call for help, rather than wasting valuable time trying to intubate.
- **Suctioning for meconium:** If meconium is present and the baby is not vigorous (see Section 10), intubation of the trachea is the first step that should be taken before any other resuscitation measures are started.
- **Poor response:** If PPV is not resulting in an increase in heart rate, adequate chest movement, and improving oxygen saturations, or if the need for PPV lasts beyond a few minutes, intubation may be used to improve the effectiveness and ease of assisted ventilation.
- **Chest compressions needed:** If chest compressions are necessary, intubation may facilitate coordination of chest compressions and ventilation and maximize the efficiency of each positive-pressure breath.
- **Epinephrine administration:** If epinephrine is required to stimulate the heart, IV administration is preferred. Administration directly into the trachea, through an endotracheal tube, is acceptable while venous access is being established, although the drug is not absorbed reliably and predictably by this route, and higher doses may be required.
- **Certain conditions:** Some uncommon conditions, such as diaphragmatic hernia, are indications for endotracheal intubation.

147

18. What Can Interfere With Resuscitative Efforts?

When a baby does not respond well to resuscitation, consider the following:

A. Mechanical Equipment Failure

Although all equipment should be checked routinely and always be ready for use, failures may still occur.

- Check to be sure all **oxygen and air connections are tight.**
- Make sure the **bag can deliver 21% to 100% oxygen** (some bags can deliver only 40% oxygen).
- Check to be sure the **flow rate** of oxygen can be adjusted between 5 and 10 L/min.

B. Incorrect Skill Techniques

Skill techniques may not be applied correctly, or application may shift from correct to incorrect during the course of resuscitation. You should repeatedly check to be certain that

- **Airway is fully open.** Check to see that the baby's head is in the sniffing position. You may find it helpful to place a small cloth roll under the baby's shoulders to maintain proper head and neck position.
- **Positive-pressure ventilation is effective.** Watch the baby's chest to see if it rises and falls with each squeeze and release of the bag. Assess for an increase in heart rate and improved oxygen saturations.
- **Endotracheal tube is in the trachea.** Use a CO_2 detector to confirm endotracheal tube position. Be certain the tube is not in the esophagus or inserted too far into the trachea. Listen over both lungs and the stomach. Be sure that air movement with each squeeze of the bag is heard over the lungs and not the stomach. If in doubt, check the tube position with a laryngoscope.
- **Chest compressions are adequate.** Be sure the compressions are of adequate depth and well synchronized with ventilations. *Briefly* interrupt compressions to feel the femoral or umbilical pulse.
- **Epinephrine has been given effectively.** Epinephrine given intratracheally is absorbed poorly and unpredictably. Establish an IV line early. While doing so, if endotracheal epinephrine is given, use a higher dose (0.5 to 1 mL/kg) and make sure that the dose enters the trachea and does not remain in the connector of the endotracheal tube.
- **Hypovolemia has been considered.** If blood loss is suspected, consider giving a volume expander.

If there is any doubt, recheck each of the resuscitation techniques and call for help.

19. How Much Time Should You Allow for Each of the Steps?

Although learning the techniques of resuscitation may take many hours, the knowledge and skills must be applied over just a few minutes and in a highly coordinated fashion.

It should take no longer than approximately 30 seconds from birth for your rapid assessment of the baby and provision of the initial steps. Evaluation of the baby again determines if PPV is necessary. Positive-pressure ventilation should be provided by 1 minute after birth if the baby is not breathing adequately. Likewise, approximately 30 to 60 seconds should be sufficient time for a baby to show signs of improvement from any one of the resuscitation actions.

These guidelines are meant to be somewhat flexible. For example, more than 30 seconds will be required to complete the initial steps if meconium must be suctioned from the trachea. Nevertheless, it is vitally important that your evaluation and actions be performed efficiently and effectively.

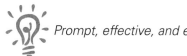 *Prompt, effective, and efficient resuscitation can prevent death or lifelong damage.*

20. What Else Should You Consider if There Is Minimal Improvement?

There are a few, relatively rare, conditions that may result in a baby showing only partial response to administration of optimal resuscitation techniques (Figure 5.7). A malformation of the airway (eg, choanal atresia or Robin syndrome) or mechanical compression of a lung (eg, pneumothorax or diaphragmatic hernia) may prevent adequate air movement. (See Book III: Neonatal Care, Unit 2, Respiratory Distress.)

Most forms of congenital heart disease do not cause severe problems at the time of delivery, although congenital heart block may cause a persistent bradycardia despite adequate ventilation and oxygenation.

After immediate stabilization of the baby, obtain consultation for all conditions listed below. See also Book III: Neonatal Care, Unit 2, Respiratory Distress, for additional care information. Continue respiratory and other support measures as needed.

- *Choanal atresia:* Insert oral airway or intubate trachea.

- *Robin syndrome:* Insert nasopharyngeal tube; position prone; consider nasal CPAP or insertion of laryngeal mask airway if there is persistent evidence of airway obstruction.

- *Pneumothorax:* Use transillumination and/or chest x-ray to diagnose; consider needle aspiration and/or chest tube insertion to evacuate pneumothorax and relieve lung compression.

- *Diaphragmatic hernia:* Intubate trachea; insert large bore orogastric tube to intermittent suction to evacuate air in stomach.

- *Congenital heart block:* Baby will probably be pink even with persistent bradycardia.

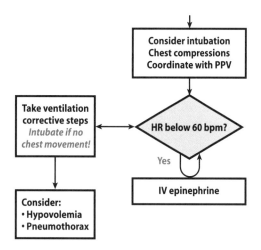

Figure 5.7. Expanded Resuscitation Flow Diagram.
Reprinted with permission from American Academy of Pediatrics, American Heart Association. *Textbook of Neonatal Resuscitation.* Kattwinkel J, ed. 6th ed. Elk Grove Village, IL: American Academy of Pediatrics; 2011.

21. How Long Should Resuscitation Efforts Be Continued?

There are very few viable babies who will not show some improvement after PPV, intubation, chest compressions, and epinephrine, assuming that these actions have been administered correctly.

Some people hesitate to conduct prolonged resuscitation efforts because of the possibility of saving a baby who has severe brain damage. Studies have shown, however, that withholding, or giving half-hearted, resuscitation efforts actually will result in more babies with brain damage than will aggressive resuscitation efforts. This is because some of these babies will live in spite of no or poor resuscitation efforts.

The possibility of brain damage increases the longer resuscitation is required. If a baby shows signs of improvement, even with a prolonged resuscitation of 15 to 20 minutes, the chances are favorable that the baby will survive and develop normally.

If there is no return of spontaneous circulation (ie, no spontaneous heart rate detected for 10 minutes or longer), the likelihood of intact survival is exceedingly small and it is reasonable to discontinue further resuscitative efforts.

 Avoid half-hearted resuscitations.

Optimum resuscitation technique should be employed until a baby's condition is stabilized or until the baby is pronounced dead.

Proper post-resuscitation care is also essential to a resuscitated baby's outcome. Information concerning monitoring and surveillance measures is given on the following pages.

 Resuscitation requires preparation, implementation, and follow-up.

- *Practice by all team members*
- *Smooth, coordinated teamwork*
- *Comprehensive post-resuscitation care*

Self-test

Now answer these questions to test yourself on the information in the last section. Refer to the graphs or charts in the unit, as necessary, to answer these questions.

D1. What serious complication can occur if naloxone HCl is given to a baby whose mother is addicted to narcotics?

_____

D2. **True** **False** Naloxone HCl should only be given intravenously.

D3. **True** **False** Naloxone HCl is the resuscitation drug used most often.

D4. **True** **False** The adequacy of chest compressions should be checked by feeling the femoral or umbilical pulse.

D5. **True** **False** Limited resuscitation has been shown to result in more babies with brain damage than vigorous resuscitation.

D6. List at least 3 indications for endotracheal intubation during a resuscitation.

_____
_____
_____

D7. You should allow approximately _____ seconds for the initial steps before going on to evaluation and the next step in the resuscitation sequence.

D8. List at least 3 things you should check if a baby is not responding well to resuscitation.

_____
_____
_____

D9. List at least 3 congenital malformations that could interfere with resuscitation efforts.

_____

D10. **True** **False** If a baby shows signs of improvement, even though resuscitation continues for 20 minutes, the chances are still favorable that the baby will survive and develop normally.

D11. If there is no documented spontaneous heart rate for _____ minutes of resuscitation measures, it is reasonable to discontinue further efforts.

Check your answers with the list that follows the Recommended Routines. Correct any incorrect answers and review the appropriate section in the unit.

22. What Care Should Be Provided to Babies Following Stabilization?

A. Routine Care

Approximately 90% of newborns require minimal assistance to make the transition from intrauterine to extrauterine environment. Most of these babies can remain with their mothers to facilitate maternal-newborn interaction, maintain warmth, and begin early breastfeeding. In vigorous newborns who do not require resuscitation, cord clamping should be delayed for at least 1 minute from the time the baby's head and body are delivered.

B. Post-resuscitation Care

Most of the remaining 10% of newborns respond well to the initial resuscitation measures described in Step A—drying and providing warmth, clearing the airway, and stimulating to breathe.

Some of these babies have significant risk factors, such as prematurity or having passed meconium in utero. Such risk factors increase the chance a baby will require supplemental oxygen or positive-pressure support of breathing and continue to have needs for special care. These babies should be monitored closely as they complete transition. Some can receive this monitoring while remaining with their mothers, while many will need to be admitted to a special care nursery for electronic, visual, and laboratory monitoring.

Less than 5% of newborns require PPV or more invasive measures to establish cardiorespiratory stability. These babies are at relatively high risk for developing complications from perinatal compromise and should be monitored very closely during the early neonatal period. Some of these babies will require IV therapy and/or cardiorespiratory support. Usually, this level of care requires consultation with neonatal teams and admission to a special care nursery for a time.

The term *perinatal compromise* is used to describe a wide spectrum of situations in which a baby might have experienced an episode of hypoxia or decreased blood flow to vital organs. These situations range from a baby who is quickly resuscitated, and demonstrates no further evidence of compromise, to a severely depressed baby who has documented hypoxia and severe metabolic acidosis with resulting abnormal cardiac, renal, gastrointestinal, and/or neurologic function.

The term *asphyxia* should be reserved for those severely affected babies in whom hypoxia and alterations in blood flow result in metabolic acidosis and organ injury. In general, asphyxia is best used to describe only the most extreme situations. Asphyxial injury to the brain is often referred to as hypoxic-ischemic encephalopathy.

23. How Should You Transfer a Resuscitated Baby to the Nursery?

Babies who continue to require assisted ventilation following resuscitation should have PPV or CPAP continued without interruption during transfer to the nursery. Similarly, any supplemental oxygen should be maintained as indicated by SpO$_2$. Babies use oxygen as they increase their metabolism to keep warm. Make certain the transport incubator is warm and the baby is on warm, dry linen. Just as it is important to prevent a baby from being chilled, it is important to avoid overheating a baby. Unless therapeutic hypothermia is being considered, the goal is to maintain a baby's normal body temperature. (See Unit 7, Thermal Environment, in this book.)

Babies greater than 36 weeks' gestation who have evidence of significant perinatal compromise and certain signs of neurologic injury should be considered for cooling according to a specific protocol (therapeutic hypothermia) to decrease the likelihood of hypoxic-ischemic encephalopathy. Consult your regional perinatal center rapidly to initiate therapy under their protocol, as hypothermia must be initiated within 4 to 6 hours of birth for maximum efficacy. A consistent approach to therapeutic cooling, using a recognized protocol, is essential to match the efficacy demonstrated in multicenter trials and for ongoing evaluation of this care.

24. What Care Should You Provide for Any Baby Who Required Extended Resuscitation?

Newborns who required extended resuscitation at birth need careful observation and monitoring for at least 48 hours following delivery. Even though their vital signs may be normal, these babies may develop problems that were caused by lack of oxygen and acidosis.

Anticipation of possible problems is helpful to

- Prevent some problems from occurring.
- Recognize and treat problems quickly should they develop.

Monitoring and care practices listed below should be considered to help you detect problems early and/or prevent abnormal findings from becoming serious problems.

- Attach an electronic cardiorespiratory monitor to the baby in addition to a pulse oximeter.
- Check all vital signs (heart rate, blood pressure, respiratory rate, body temperature, SpO_2), color, and activity frequently.
- Do not feed enterally (npo); administer IV fluids until bowel sounds are heard.
- Weigh at least once a day. Weighing twice a day may be appropriate for some babies.
- Obtain glucose screening test frequently.
- Check calcium levels in addition to glucose screening if baby is jittery or has seizures.
- Check serum electrolytes.
- Check arterial blood gases.
- Measure and record urine output.
- Check urine for blood and protein.
- Restrict fluids to 40 to 60 mL/kg per day until urine output is established.

A description of problems that may result from perinatal compromise is shown in Table 5.1. Study the table to learn what problems can be due to perinatal compromise and how to recognize them.

The table need not be memorized, but may serve as a useful guide in the management of a baby who was resuscitated. A copy should be kept near any baby who required vigorous resuscitation.

Table 5.1. Potential Complications Following Neonatal Resuscitation		
Recommended Monitoring	**Potential Problems**	**Reasons and Comments**
	Cardiovascular System	
Pulse oximetry and cardiac monitor	• Rapid heart rate	• Low blood volume • Compromised cardiac function
Pulse oximetry and cardiac monitor	• Low heart rate	• Hypoxia • Severely low blood volume or compromised cardiac function
Pulse oximetry and/or arterial blood gas	• Desaturation and/or • Low arterial oxygen	• Pulmonary blood vessels may constrict with hypoxia and acidosis. • There may be a shunt from right to left (ductus arteriosus or foramen ovale).
Check blood pressure.	• Low blood pressure	• Low blood volume and/or • Compromised cardiac function and/or • Acidosis

Table 5.1. Potential Complications Following Neonatal Resuscitation *(continued)*

Recommended Monitoring	Potential Problems	Reasons and Comments
	Respiratory System	
Observation and/or electronic monitor	• Rapid respiratory rate	• Respiratory distress syndrome in preterm newborn • Aspiration
	• Apnea	• Acidosis, hypoxia • Central nervous system depression
	• Sudden cyanosis	• Pneumothorax
	Gastrointestinal System	
Observation	• No stools passed • Blood in stools • Distended abdomen	• Hypoxia may affect the gastrointestinal system, causing decreased motility (ileus) and/or necrotizing enterocolitis.
	• Absent bowel sounds	• Many experts advise withholding feedings and providing intravenous fluids for 3 to 5 days following severe perinatal compromise.
	Genitourinary System	
Measure intake and output. Weigh daily. Obtain urinalysis. Check serum sodium.	• Low urine output • Excessive weight gain • Hematuria (blood in urine) • Hyponatremia (low blood sodium)	• Hypoxia may affect the kidneys. • Excessive weight gain and hyponatremia usually indicate kidneys are damaged and unable to handle a fluid load. Consider restricting fluids.
	Central Nervous System	

Observation	• Abnormal neurologic examination with documented severe metabolic acidosis
	
	• Seizures
		• Consult regional center promptly for possible initiation of therapeutic hypothermia following hypoxic-ischemic insult.
		• Seizures may be caused by brain hypoxia, ischemia, or hemorrhage, or by low blood glucose, sodium, or calcium.
		• If cause of seizures is unknown,
		  – Give phenobarbital 20 mg/kg (may give as many as two 10 mg/kg additional doses to achieve suppression of seizures, but be prepared to ventilate baby if respiratory depression occurs).
		  – Provide maintenance dose of 3.5 to 5 mg/kg per day and check blood levels.

Table 5.1. Potential Complications Following Neonatal Resuscitation (continued)		
Recommended Monitoring	**Potential Problems**	**Reasons and Comments**
	Metabolic System	
Screen blood glucose.	• Hypoglycemia • Seizures due to hypoglycemia	• Baby may have depleted glucose stores.
Check blood calcium.	• Seizures due to low calcium	• Cause of low calcium commonly seen post resuscitation is unknown.
Check blood pH and bicarbonate.	• Acidosis	• Babies may require several hours to clear the acidosis after resuscitation. Bicarbonate or increase in ventilation may be indicated.
Check blood pH and bicarbonate.	• Alkalosis	• Occasionally babies who required resuscitation will breathe very rapidly. If they have normal lungs, they will blow off carbon dioxide and become alkalotic.

Self-test

Now answer these questions to test yourself on the information in the last section. Refer to the graphs or charts in the unit, as necessary, to answer these questions.

E1. What precautions should you take when transferring a resuscitated baby from the delivery room to the nursery?

A. _____

B. _____

E2. List at least 4 monitoring and care activities that should be done for babies who required vigorous resuscitation.

_____

_____

_____

E3. List at least 2 potential problems that may affect the gastrointestinal system of a baby who required vigorous resuscitation.

_____

_____

E4. **True** **False** Fluid restriction until urine output is ensured is recommended for babies who required vigorous resuscitation.

E5. **True** **False** Metabolic acidosis is a potential complication that may develop in any baby who required vigorous resuscitation.

E6. **True** **False** If seizures occur in a baby who required vigorous resuscitation, the cause is always brain hypoxia.

E7. **True** **False** It is important to prevent hypothermia (low body temperature) and hyperthermia (high body temperature).

Check your answers with the list that follows the Recommended Routines. Correct any incorrect answers and review the appropriate section in the unit.

Resuscitating the Newborn

Recommended Routines

All the routines listed below are based on the principles of perinatal care presented in the unit you have just finished. They are recommended as part of routine perinatal care.

Read each routine carefully and decide whether it is standard operating procedure in your hospital. Check the appropriate blank next to each routine.

Procedure Standard in My Hospital	Needs Discussion by Our Staff	
_____	_____	1. Use a system of prenatal identification of high-risk pregnant women to recognize high-risk situations immediately on admission to the hospital and
_____	_____	• Allow for elective transfer of a woman and her fetus for delivery at a regional center, as appropriate.
_____	_____	• Mobilize extra personnel skilled in newborn resuscitation to the delivery room.
_____	_____	2. Establish a routine when meconium is present, and a baby is not vigorous, of direct endotracheal suctioning.
_____	_____	3. Ensure the immediate 24-hour-a-day availability of a resuscitation team, consisting of at least 2 people, including someone skilled in endotracheal intubation.
_____	_____	4. Conduct resuscitation practice sessions periodically to be sure team members work together and communicate effectively and efficiently.
_____	_____	5. Develop a system for periodically checking the presence and the operation of all resuscitation equipment in each delivery room, in the nursery, and in postpartum rooms.
_____	_____	6. Identify an independent person at each delivery to assign the Apgar score and record the points (0, 1, or 2) for each of the 5 components of the score.
_____	_____	7. Establish the capability for immediate availability of equipment for mixing oxygen and compressed air and for pulse oximetry monitoring in every delivery area.
_____	_____	8. Ensure continuous availability of equipment for transferring a resuscitated baby from the delivery room to the nursery (eg, warmed incubator, portable oxygen, pulse oximeter, etc).

_____ _____   9. Develop a checklist of things to observe and record in all babies who required resuscitation.

_____ _____ 10. Establish a protocol with obstetric providers to delay umbilical cord clamping for at least 1 minute, following complete delivery of the baby, for vigorous babies who do not require resuscitation.

Self-test Answers

These are the answers to the self-test questions. Please check them with the answers you gave and review the information in the unit wherever necessary.

A1. False.   Although determining risk status will identify many who will require resuscitation, many babies with no risk factors may require resuscitation following birth.

A2. A = Airway
    B = Breathing
    C = Circulation
    D = Drugs

A3. Any 4 of the following conditions:
- Maternal diabetes mellitus
- Hypertension
  - Gestational
  - Preeclampsia
  - Chronic
- Chronic maternal illness (neurologic, cardiovascular, thyroid, pulmonary, or renal)
- Anemia or isoimmunization
- Previous fetal or neonatal death
- Bleeding in second or third trimester
- Maternal infection
- Hydramnios
- Oligohydramnios
- Premature rupture of membranes
- Post-term gestation
- Multifetal gestation
- Size-date discrepancy
- Drug therapy
  - Lithium carbonate
  - Magnesium
  - Adrenergic-blocking drugs
- Maternal substance use
- Fetal malformation
- Diminished fetal activity
- No prenatal care
- Age younger than 16 or older than 35 years

A4. Any 4 of the following conditions:
- Emergency cesarean section
- Forceps or vacuum-assisted delivery
- Breech or other abnormal presentation
- Preterm labor
- Precipitous labor
- Chorioamnionitis
- Prolonged rupture of membranes (>18 hours before delivery)
- Prolonged labor (>24 hours)
- Prolonged second stage of labor (>2 hours)
- Fetal bradycardia
- Non-reassuring fetal heart rate pattern(s)
- Use of general anesthesia
- Uterine tetany
- Narcotics administered to mother within 4 hours of delivery
- Meconium-stained amniotic fluid

- Prolapsed umbilical cord
- Abruptio placentae
- Placenta previa (if undetected earlier)

A5. C. Both at birth and in the nursery

A6. False.   At least 2 people are required.

A7. Breathing: Stopped or gasping respirations
    Color: Blue, gray, very pale, or mottled
    Heart rate: Below 100 beats per minute
    Activity: Limp, little or no response to stimulation
    Blood pressure: Low

B1. Obtain at least the key points of maternal and fetal history.
    Prepare to prevent heat loss.

B2. True

B3. False.   Meconium-stained babies who are *not* vigorous should have endotracheal suctioning. Vigorous babies with meconium in the amniotic fluid can be treated as if no meconium was present.

B4. True

B5. False.   Heat loss is dangerous for all babies, whether they are preterm, term, post-term, well, or sick.

B6. True

B7. True

B8. Any 3 of the following:
- Maintain a relatively warm delivery room temperature.
- Before each delivery, turn on the radiant warmer and preheat the bed.
- Use warm, dry towels to dry baby immediately after delivery.
- Promptly remove any wet bed linen and replace with warm, dry linen.
- Dry the baby's hair and put on a cap (may need to be delayed if resuscitation is needed).

C1. False.   A baby should be in the sniffing position, with the nose and mouth as far anterior as possible and the neck in neutral position to allow maximal airway opening. Extension or flexion of the head/neck can obstruct a newborn's airway.

C2. True

C3. True.   Current national guidelines recommend using 21% oxygen if positive-pressure ventilation is required and the baby is born at term.

C4. False.   Acrocyanosis does not require oxygen therapy, but *may* indicate cold stress. Central cyanosis, however, is an indication for pulse oximetry monitoring and immediate oxygen administration and/or assisted ventilation as needed to achieve target oxygen saturations.

C5. Color, respirations, heart rate

C6. True

C7. False.   Gasping respiration is *not* a good sign. It generally means a baby has been severely compromised, has a low blood pH, and assisted ventilation is needed.

C8. True.   When chest compressions are not needed, a rate of 40 to 60 ventilations per minute is appropriate.

C9. False.   There is no indication to give epinephrine routinely whenever chest compressions are used.

C10. True   See Book III: Neonatal Care, Unit 4, Low Blood Pressure, for further details.

C11. A. *Breathe*-compress, compress, compress-*breathe*-compress, compress, compress-*breathe*. . .
    There should be 90 chest compressions and 30 ventilations per minute, with each ventilation given during a pause after 3 chest compressions.

C12. B

C13. A and C

160

C14. • Meconium-stained babies who are not vigorous at birth. (See Section 10 in this unit.)
   • Babies with sunken abdomens. (Intestines may be in the chest due to a diaphragmatic hernia; bag-and-mask ventilation would force air into the lungs and into the stomach so babies who need resuscitation and are suspected of having a diaphragmatic hernia should always have endotracheal intubation and assisted ventilation through an endotracheal tube.)

D1. Acute narcotic withdrawal, with possible seizures

D2. False.   Naloxone HCl may be given intravenously, intramuscularly, or subcutaneously.

D3. False.   Naloxone HCl is *not* a resuscitation drug. It should not be given until a baby has been resuscitated and stabilized with 100% oxygen and positive-pressure ventilation, as necessary.

D4. True

D5. True

D6. Any 3 of the following:
   • Meconium-stained, nonvigorous baby who needs endotracheal suctioning.
   • Poor response associated with inadequate chest movement with bag-and-mask ventilation that cannot be corrected with positioning, more forceful squeezing of the bag, etc.
   • Need for extended period of positive-pressure ventilation.
   • Chest compressions are necessary and endotracheal intubation and assisted ventilation allow more effective ventilation and easier coordination with chest compressions.
   • Epinephrine needs to be administered and an umbilical venous catheter is not yet in place.

   Note: The skill of the resuscitators also may influence the timing of intubation. Personnel who are not skilled at intubation should concentrate on providing effective positive-pressure ventilation and call for help.

D7. 30

D8. Any 3 of the following:
   • Oxygen connections are tight.
   • Bag can deliver 100% oxygen.
   • Flow rate of oxygen is strong.
   • Airway is fully open.
   • Chest moves perceptibly with each positive-pressure ventilation.
   • Endotracheal tube is in the trachea.
   • Chest compressions are adequate.
   • Epinephrine, if used, has truly reached the baby.
   • Hypovolemia, if present, has been corrected.

D9. Any 3 of the following:
   • Choanal atresia
   • Robin syndrome
   • Pneumothorax (not a congenital malformation, but can occur shortly after birth due to lung disease and/or positive-pressure ventilation)
   • Diaphragmatic hernia
   • Congenital heart block

D10. True.   If a baby shows signs of improvement within 20 minutes of birth, the chances are favorable that the baby will survive and develop normally.

D11. 10

E1. A. Provide the same oxygen and/or assisted ventilation support during the entire transfer as was used for the baby in the delivery room.

   B. Keep the baby warm and body temperature normal.

E2. Any 4 of the following:
- Attach an electronic cardiorespiratory monitor and pulse oximeter to the baby.
- Check all vital signs (heart rate, blood pressure, respiratory rate, body temperature), color, and activity frequently.
- Do not feed by mouth (npo); administer intravenous fluids until bowel sounds are heard.
- Weigh at least once a day. Weighing twice a day may be appropriate for some babies.
- Obtain glucose screening test frequently.
- Check calcium levels if baby is jittery or has seizures.
- Check serum electrolytes.
- Check arterial blood gases.
- Measure and record urine output.
- Check urine for blood and protein.
- Restrict fluids to 40 mL/kg per day until urine output is ensured.

E3. Any 2 of the following:
- No stools passed
- Blood in stools
- Distended abdomen
- Absent bowel sounds

E4. True

E5. True

E6. False. Seizures may be due to hypoxic-ischemic insult to the brain, or cerebral hemorrhage or low blood glucose, sodium, or calcium.

E7. True. Being chilled and being overheated are dangerous for newborns. Whole-body or head cooling will decrease the severity of brain injury for some asphyxiated babies *following* resuscitation, but this should generally be performed only under protocol conditions established with your regional perinatal center.

Unit 5 Posttest

If you are applying for continuing education credits, a posttest for this unit is available online. Completion of unit posttests and the book evaluation form are required to achieve continuing education credit. For more details, go to www.cmevillage.com.

SKILL UNIT

Suctioning

This skill unit will teach you how to suction a baby's airway. Not everyone will be required to learn all aspects of the suctioning techniques described here. However, everyone should read this unit and attend a skill session to learn the equipment and sequence of steps to perform the skill or to assist with suctioning.

Study this skill unit, then attend a skill practice and demonstration session. To master the skill, you will need to demonstrate each of the following steps correctly:

1. Use a bulb syringe to suction a baby's (manikin's) mouth and nose.
2. Assemble
   - Suction catheter, tubing, and suction source
   - Endotracheal tube, suction adapter for removal of meconium
3. Regulate the suction pressure.
4. Use a suction catheter to suction a baby's mouth, posterior pharynx, and nose.
5. Use an endotracheal tube to suction a baby's trachea.
6. Monitor the baby's heart rate throughout the procedure.

PERINATAL PERFORMANCE GUIDE

Suctioning

ACTIONS	REMARKS
Anticipating Suctioning, Clear Amniotic Fluid	
1. Before the baby is delivered, determine if the amniotic fluid is clear or meconium stained.	Your subsequent actions will be guided by whether there is meconium present and whether the baby requires resuscitation.
2. Prepare suction system for use.	**Resuscitation equipment should be prepared in advance.**
• Attach the catheter and tubing to a mechanical suction source, either a wall outlet or portable machine.	
• Regulate the suction strength so that it is strong and constant but does not exceed -100 mm Hg (-136 cm H_2O) when the catheter is occluded.	The suction source should be equipped with a pressure gauge and regulator.
Clear amniotic fluid; no resuscitation needed	
3. Wipe the baby's face and nose free of secretions with a cloth and place the baby on the mother's chest.	Most healthy newborns do not require suctioning.
Clear amniotic fluid; resuscitation needed	
4. Suction the baby's mouth and nose with a bulb syringe or suction catheter to clear secretions.	*Suction the mouth and pharynx first so that, if a baby gasps when the catheter is inserted in the nose, fluid in the mouth will not be inhaled into the lungs.*
Suctioning the back of a baby's throat or nose with a catheter may lead to severe bradycardia.	*Whenever a catheter is used for suctioning, the baby's heart rate should be monitored throughout the procedure.*
5. Continue with initial steps of resuscitation.	
Anticipating Suctioning, Meconium-Stained Amniotic Fluid	
1. Prepare equipment and personnel as if the baby's trachea may need to be intubated.	If there is meconium in the amniotic fluid, a person with endotracheal intubation skills should be present at the delivery. You should always be prepared to intubate because you cannot anticipate how vigorous a baby will be.
2. Consider clearing the airway after delivery of the head and before delivery of the shoulders.	Suctioning of the mouth, posterior pharynx, and nose before delivery of the shoulders in meconium-stained babies has been shown to be of no benefit in preventing meconium aspiration syndrome, and is no longer recommended as a routine procedure.

ACTIONS	REMARKS

Anticipating Suctioning, Meconium-Stained Amniotic Fluid (continued)

	However, a brief period of suctioning meconium from the mouth and nose before delivery of the shoulders may facilitate neonatal intubation after delivery. Intrapartum suctioning is reasonable when a depressed baby is anticipated, as long as it does not worsen bradycardia or delay handing the baby to the neonatal resuscitation team.
3. Quickly hand the baby to the neonatal team for placement on the resuscitation table, under a radiant warmer.	Do not spend valuable time excessively suctioning the baby at the mother's perineum or operative incision. This may stimulate the baby to breathe, which may lead to more aspiration of meconium and a delay in intubating the trachea.
4. Decide if the baby is *vigorous* or *nonvigorous*. Knowing this will determine what you do next.	
Vigorous (yes to all 3 questions) • Breathing or crying? • Good muscle tone? • Heart rate 100 beats per minute (bpm) or more?	*A vigorous* meconium-stained baby should be treated as if no meconium is present. See Step 3 under clear amniotic fluid section.
Nonvigorous (yes to any 1 question) • Respiratory effort poor? • Muscle tone poor? • Heart rate less than 100 bpm?	*A nonvigorous* meconium-stained baby should be intubated, and the trachea should be suctioned directly.

Suctioning a Nonvigorous Meconium-Stained Baby After Delivery

1. Attach a large-bore (10F or 12F) catheter and suction tubing to a mechanical suction source, either a wall outlet or portable machine, and regulate suction strength as described earlier.	
2. After the baby has been fully delivered, suction the mouth and posterior pharynx first, then the nose, with a bulb syringe or large-bore (10F or 12F) suction catheter.	The duration and extent of suctioning of the mouth, pharynx, and nose should be just sufficient to clear the airway for visualization needed for endotracheal intubation.
3. Visualize the larynx with a laryngoscope and insert an endotracheal tube into the trachea.	See Skill Unit: Endotracheal Intubation for a detailed description.

ACTIONS	REMARKS

Suctioning a Nonvigorous Meconium-Stained Baby After Delivery (continued)

4. Immediately attach an adapter and suction tubing to the endotracheal tube.	Use a specially designed adapter, with a suction control port, to connect to the endotracheal tube to the suction tubing (illustrated below).
5. Use an endotracheal tube as a suction catheter. The lumen of the endotracheal tube is large enough to remove even thick meconium.	Suction catheters small enough to fit through an endotracheal tube are too small for effective initial removal of meconium.

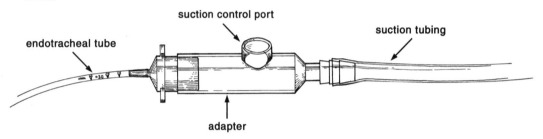

NOTE: A variety of meconium suctioning devices are commercially available. The device illustrated above is one example.

ACTIONS	REMARKS

Suctioning a Baby's Trachea Using an Endotracheal Tube

1. Place your thumb over the suction control port of the endotracheal tube adapter.	Be sure the suction pressure does not exceed −100 mm Hg (−136 cm H_2O).
2. Continue to apply suction as the endotracheal tube is slowly withdrawn. To minimize the duration of hypoxemia or the risk of bradycardia, avoid applying suction pressure continuously for longer than approximately 5 seconds at a time.	A plug of meconium may cling to the end of the endotracheal tube.
3. Repeat the procedure until no more meconium is recovered.	Judgment will be required to decide how many times to re-intubate and repeat suctioning with an endotracheal tube used as a suction catheter. Visualization of the larynx may be maintained to facilitate reintubation with a second endotracheal tube, if necessary. *Monitor the baby's heart rate throughout the procedure.*

ACTIONS	REMARKS

Suctioning a Baby's Trachea Using an Endotracheal Tube (continued)

ACTIONS	REMARKS
4. Assess the baby's condition and provide assisted ventilation, as necessary.	*Try to avoid giving assisted ventilation to a nonvigorous, meconium-stained baby until the mouth, nose, and trachea have been suctioned thoroughly and cleared of meconium.*
5. Attach an oximeter probe and adjust oxygen concentration to achieve time-specific oxygen target saturations (see next skill unit).	
6. In babies who are expected to need assisted ventilation, it may be more efficient to leave an endotracheal tube in place. Additional meconium can often be removed over the next several hours by passing a suction catheter through the endotracheal tube.	Although the initial meconium will often be too thick to pass through a suction catheter, once the large chunks are removed, a suction catheter passed through an endotracheal tube may be effective in removing additional meconium.
7. Continue with the resuscitation sequence.	

SKILL UNIT

Management of Oxygen in the Delivery Setting

This skill unit will summarize the equipment and skills required to manage oxygen delivery at the time of birth. For the complete Perinatal Performance Guide for Pulse Oximetry, refer to Unit 4, Is the Baby Sick?, in this book.

The required equipment includes the following:
- Compressed gas sources for both oxygen and air
- A blender to mix oxygen and air, adjustable from 21% to 100% oxygen, and an adjustable flowmeter to regulate the gas flow of the mixture
- Tubing, masks, and a positive-pressure delivery device (If you normally use a flow-inflating bag or T-piece resuscitator—either of which requires compressed gas to function, you also should have a self-inflating bag as backup.)
- A pulse oximeter and oximetry probes designed for use with neonates

Some hospitals will have all the necessary equipment available for every delivery, while others may mount the equipment on a moveable stand that can immediately be brought to the delivery. Some examples of the equipment are shown below.

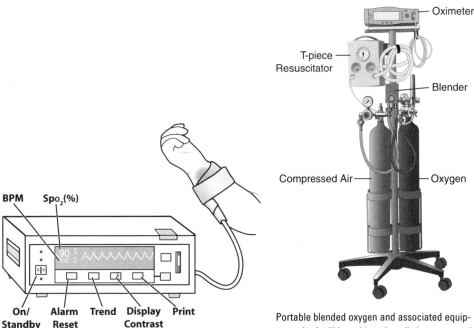

Pulse oximeter, with placement of probe on baby's right wrist or hand for use during newborn resuscitation.
Reprinted with permission from American Academy of Pediatrics, American Heart Association. *Textbook of Neonatal Resuscitation.* Kattwinkel J, ed. 6th ed. Elk Grove Village, IL: American Academy of Pediatrics; 2011.

Portable blended oxygen and associated equipment, for facilities without installed compressed air source, such as in a delivery area. However, be careful with small portable tanks that can empty quickly.
Reproduced with permission from photo courtesy of Swedish Medical Center, Seattle, WA.

The above equipment should be immediately available for use in the following situations:
- Anticipated need for supplemental oxygen or assisted ventilation.
- A preterm birth at a gestation of less than 35 weeks.

- If cyanosis is felt to persist beyond the first few minutes following birth.
- Whenever supplemental oxygen or assisted ventilation (positive-pressure ventilation or continuous positive airway pressure) is used.

Oxyhemoglobin saturation normally increases gradually in healthy babies born at term, according to the following graph. You should attach an oximeter as soon as any of the conditions listed above occur. Then adjust the inspired oxygen concentration to achieve an SpO_2 to match the values shown in the following table.

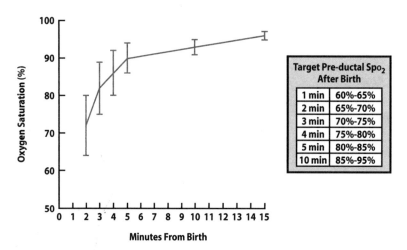

Target Pre-ductal Spo₂ After Birth	
1 min	60%-65%
2 min	65%-70%
3 min	70%-75%
4 min	75%-80%
5 min	80%-85%
10 min	85%-95%

Pre-ductal oxygen saturation changes following birth (median and interquartile range).
Graph reprinted with permission from Mariani G, Dik PB, Ezquer A, et al. Pre-ductal and post-ductal O₂ saturation in healthy term neonates after birth. *J Pediatr.* 2007; 150:418-421.
Table reprinted with permission from American Academy of Pediatrics, American Heart Association. *Textbook of Neonatal Resuscitation.* Kattwinkel J, ed. 6th ed. Elk Grove Village, IL: American Academy of Pediatrics; 2011.

 Apply the pulse oximeter probe to the right hand or wrist to measure pre-ductal saturations.

 Apply the probe to the baby's hand or wrist before connecting to the pulse oximeter to obtain the fastest reading.

SKILL UNIT

Free-Flow Oxygen and Positive-Pressure Ventilation

This skill unit will teach you how to give free-flow oxygen in the delivery room and how to assist a baby's ventilation with bag and mask or T-piece resuscitator.

Study this skill unit, then attend a skill practice and demonstration session.
To master the skills, you will need to demonstrate each of the following steps correctly:

Free-Flow Oxygen Administration
Assemble equipment which is attached to a blender.

- Oxygen tubing
- Oxygen mask
- Flow-inflating bag-and-mask
- T-piece resuscitator

Positive-Pressure Ventilation With Bag-and-Mask
1. Select appropriate-sized mask.
2. Assemble bag, mask, and tubing.
3. Adjust pressure valve.
4. Position baby.
5. Position mask on baby's face.
6. Squeeze-release cycle

- Force of assisted ventilation
- Rate of assisted ventilation

7. Check effectiveness of bag-and-mask ventilation.

- Baby's response (heart rate, color and oxygen saturation, activity, etc).
- Breath sounds.
- Chest movement. (Notice pressure reading on the manometer or pressure gauge with each breath and maintain consistency in inflation pressure and positive end-expiratory pressure [PEEP].)

Positive-Pressure Ventilation With T-piece Resuscitator and Mask

A T-piece resuscitator is a commercially available device designed to deliver controlled flow and preset pressures. This device may be used for resuscitation in the delivery room and transport to the nursery, but a bag-and-mask apparatus must also be available for backup and for resuscitation use outside of the delivery room.

1. Select appropriate-sized mask.
2. Assemble T-piece resuscitator and tubing (refer to manufacturer's instructions).
3. Obstruct the mask or mask connector, and adjust maximum pressure relief (safety feature). A typical limit is 40 cm H_2O.

4. Obstruct the mask or mask connector and adjust the inspiratory pressure and PEEP. Typical values are 20 to 25 cm H_2O and 5 cm H_2O, respectively.
5. Position the baby with the neck slightly extended.
6. Position mask on baby's face. When properly sealed, the manometer will register the PEEP pressure.
7. Deliver breaths of appropriate duration by occluding the aperture in the PEEP cap with your fingertip.
8. Check effectiveness of positive-pressure ventilation.

PERINATAL PERFORMANCE GUIDE

Delivering Free-Flow Oxygen to a Baby Who Is Breathing

A system to provide a variable amount of free-flow oxygen (from 21% to 100%) must be available in each delivery room. This is needed for babies who have adequate spontaneous respirations but need additional oxygen.

Free-flow oxygen can be given in several ways. It is most important that a method be used that will concentrate the oxygen around a baby's nose, where it will enter the lungs with each breath. When connected to compressed air and oxygen flow through a blender, any of the following is an acceptable method for delivering free-flow oxygen after birth:

- Oxygen tubing (held close to face)
- Oxygen mask and tubing held close to face
- Flow-inflating bag and mask
- T-piece resuscitator and mask

Deciding Which Type of Resuscitation Bag to Use

There are 2 types of bags that can be used to provide positive-pressure ventilation (PPV) to a baby. Each bag has its own advantages and disadvantages. Free-flow oxygen and PPV also can be provided with a commercially available device known as a T-piece resuscitator that will be described separately.

- A *self-inflating bag,* as the name implies, fills spontaneously with oxygen or air when released after being squeezed. It does not require a compressed gas source to fill.
- A *flow-inflating bag* (also called an anesthesia bag) fills only when it is connected to a compressed oxygen (or air) source and the outlet is being partially or completely occluded.

Both types of bags

- Can be connected either to a face mask for bag-and-mask ventilation or to an endotracheal tube for bag-and-tube ventilation
- Come in several sizes, from newborn to adult; but only smaller bags, with 750-mL capacity or less, should be used for newborns

Self-inflating Bag

A self-inflating bag is often thought to be easier to use than a flow-inflating bag because the self-inflating bag always refills. This easy refilling may be misleading because it does not require a tight seal with the patient. The connection between a mask and the baby's face or between an endotracheal tube and the bag may be loose, but a self-inflating bag would still reinflate. A tight seal is necessary to give effective assisted ventilation. Refilling of a self-inflating bag does not ensure that appropriate pressure is being delivered and the baby's lungs are being inflated.

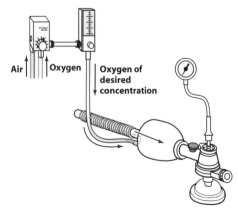

Reproduced with permission from American Academy of Pediatrics, American Heart Association. *Textbook of Neonatal Resuscitation.* Kattwinkel J, ed. 6th ed. Elk Grove Village, IL: American Academy of Pediatrics; 2011.

Self-inflating bags may be used alone to deliver room air, or can be connected to oxygen. When connected to 100% oxygen, most self-inflating bags deliver only 40% oxygen. This is because the bag draws in room air and dilutes the 100% oxygen. When connected to blended oxygen, the concentration delivered will be less than the concentration flowing into the self-inflating bag.

A reservoir or "tail" adapter can be attached to increase the amount of oxygen a self-inflating bag can deliver to a maximum of approximately 85% to 90% with 100% oxygen. A reservoir should always be attached when a self-inflating bag is used with a blender to deliver variable concentrations of oxygen.

Note: Oxygen will **not** reliably flow through many self-inflating bags unless someone is squeezing and releasing the bag. Placing the mask of a self-inflating bag over the face of a spontaneously breathing baby does **not** deliver a reliable flow of oxygen to the baby, even if a reservoir is attached. Detach the oxygen tubing from the self-inflating bag and hold the tubing near the baby's face, monitoring oxygen saturation.

A self-inflating bag has an automatic pressure pop-off valve. This means it may not be useful for ventilating babies with stiff lungs. Some bags have a button that allows override of a pop-off valve.

Advantages
- Always refills after being squeezed
- Will deliver room air without a compressed gas source
- Pressure-release valve makes over-inflation less likely

Disadvantages
- Bag always inflates even with inadequate seal, which may be misleading and lead to inadequate inflation of a baby's lungs
- Oxygen flow to the baby depends on resistance of internal valves, and thus cannot deliver free-flow oxygen reliably
- Requires override of pressure-release valve to inflate very stiff lungs
- If a manometer is not part of the device, it will need to be added to monitor the pressure being delivered.
- Cannot be used to deliver continuous positive airway pressure (CPAP), and delivers positive end-expiratory pressure (PEEP) unreliably even after having a special PEEP valve attached.

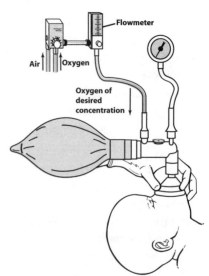

Flow-inflating Bag

Flow-inflating bags are sometimes considered difficult to use because there must be a tight connection with the patient for the bag to refill after each squeeze. Because there must be a tight connection for any type of bag to fulfill its function of ventilating the lungs, this filling characteristic can be used to help determine if you are using the bag correctly and effectively.

Reproduced with permission from American Academy of Pediatrics, American Heart Association. *Textbook of Neonatal Resuscitation.* Kattwinkel J, ed. 6th ed. Elk Grove Village, IL: American Academy of Pediatrics; 2011.

Slow or inadequate refilling of a flow-inflating bag may be due to inadequate mask-patient seal or inadequate oxygen flow into the bag. Usually a flow rate of 5 to 10 L/min is needed for brisk refilling of a flow-inflating bag between breaths given to a baby.

Flow-inflating bags will deliver supplemental oxygen when attached to an oxygen source and blender, even when the bag is not being squeezed. This can be used to provide free-flow oxygen of any concentration from 21% to 100% to a baby.

Note: Oxygen will flow through a flow-inflating bag and mask whether or not someone is squeezing and releasing the bag. The concentration of oxygen flowing out of the bag will be the same as that flowing into the bag. In the delivery room, a flow-inflating bag may be held next to the face of a baby who needs additional oxygen but does not need assisted ventilation.

Flow-inflating bags have an adjustable pressure valve. The valve may be located at the back, or tail, of the bag or be part of the connector between the bag and the mask.

The pressure valve is hand-regulated according to the amount of pressure needed to ventilate the baby. It can supply low pressure for babies with normal lungs or pressures high enough to ventilate babies with stiff lungs. The pressures generated by a flow-inflating bag vary with how hard the bag is squeezed, how many breaths are given per minute, the gas flow to the bag, and the setting of the valve. A second person may be needed to adjust the valve during ventilation.

The pressure valve also can allow too much pressure to be delivered, causing a pneumothorax (ruptured lung). For this reason, it is important to use an in-line pressure manometer with a flow-inflating bag. The manometer measures the pressure given with each breath as well as the pressure maintained between breaths.

Care must be taken to adjust the pressure valve so (1) the baby's chest moves appropriately and (2) consistent peak pressures are achieved with each breath, as registered on the manometer. Between breaths, the pressure should be permitted to drop to the desired PEEP.

Advantages
- Easy to determine if mask-patient seal is tight
- Delivers to the patient the same oxygen concentration that flows into the bag.
- Allows adjustable pressure, as well as sufficient pressure to inflate stiff lungs
- Can be used for delivering free-flow oxygen

Disadvantages
- Requires a gas source, adequate flow, and adequate seal with the patient to inflate, and to reinflate after each squeeze
- Usually does not have an automatic safety pop-off valve
- Can deliver pressures that are too high
- Requires an in-line pressure manometer for safe operation

T-piece Resuscitator

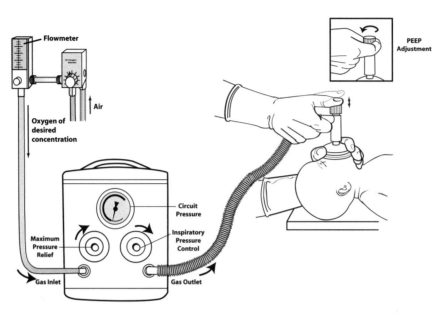

Reproduced with permission from American Academy of Pediatrics, American Heart Association. *Textbook of Neonatal Resuscitation.* Kattwinkel J, ed. 6th ed. Elk Grove Village, IL: American Academy of Pediatrics; 2011.

There are several brands of mechanical resuscitators for babies available commercially. T-piece resuscitators must be connected to a compressed gas source with a blender to mix oxygen and compressed air to deliver oxygen concentrations from 21% to 100%, similar to the 2 types of resuscitation bags. A flexible tubing from the device ends in a valve and connector which will fit either a mask or an endotracheal tube. A breath is delivered when the clinician alternately occludes and opens an aperture on the top of the valve. The valve can be adjusted to deliver a desired amount of CPAP or PEEP. The device must be pre-adjusted to deliver the desired level of inspiratory pressure, which can be viewed by a pressure gauge mounted on the device. One type of T-piece resuscitator is in the following drawing. Be sure to follow the specific manufacturer's directions included with the device used in your hospital.

Advantages
- Pressure delivered is consistent.
- There is a reliable control of peak pressure.
- Delivers to the patient the same oxygen concentration that flows into the device.
- Can be used for delivering free-flow oxygen.

Disadvantages
- Requires a gas source, adequate flow, and adequate seal with the patient to deliver a breath
- Requires pressure to be set prior to use and may be cumbersome to change during resuscitation
- Can deliver pressures that are too high
- Significant risk for delivering an excessive inflation time if operator leaves finger on the aperture too long

ACTIONS   **REMARKS**

Anticipating Positive-Pressure Ventilation

1. Newborns may require PPV in the delivery room and/or in the nursery.

   The following equipment is necessary:
   - Masks
     - Preterm size
     - Newborn size
   - Bag
     - That can deliver 21% to 90% or 100% oxygen
     - With pressure valve adjustment or pressure pop-off valve
     - With pressure manometer (if flow-inflating bag)
   - T-piece resuscitator (optional)
   - Stethoscope
   - Oxygen and compressed air source with flowmeter, blender, and tubing
   - Pulse oximeter

Check daily and after every delivery to make sure this equipment is always ready for immediate use in each
- *Delivery room*
- *Nursery*
- *Postpartum mother-baby unit*

Neonatal resuscitation guidelines released in 2010 recommend that all delivery settings have the capability to deliver oxygen concentrations from 21% to 100% and guide supplemental oxygen delivery with pulse oximetry.

2. Select an appropriate-sized mask. The mask should cover the baby's nose and mouth, with the top (pointed side) of the mask over the nose and the bottom just covering the tip of the chin.

The mask must fit over the nose and mouth, but not be so large that pressure is placed on the eyes or that an adequate seal cannot be made.

Face masks with cushioned rims are most effective in achieving a tight seal.

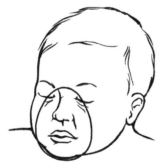

INCORRECT
too large, covers eyes

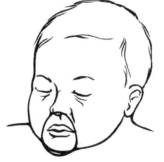

INCORRECT
does not cover
mouth and nose

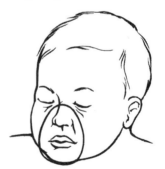

CORRECT
covers mouth and nose
but not eyes

ACTIONS   REMARKS

Deciding to Use Positive-Pressure Ventilation

3. Use PPV when the initial steps have failed to establish adequate respirations and heart rate.

4. Beyond the delivery room, PPV may be used when a baby has apnea or severe bradycardia and does not respond to tactile stimulation.

5. Do *not* use PPV with

   - Nonvigorous meconium-stained babies until their tracheas have been suctioned

   - Babies with suspected diaphragmatic hernia   If a baby with a diaphragmatic hernia requires assisted ventilation, an endotracheal tube should be inserted.

Note: A diaphragmatic hernia may be diagnosed by ultrasound before birth or be detected at birth in a baby with severe respiratory distress and a scaphoid (sunken) abdomen.

Deciding Which Oxygen Concentration to Use

6. The goal of supplemental oxygen administration is to help achieve the time-specific rise in saturations as occurs in healthy term newborns after birth.

Target Pre-ductal Spo$_2$ After Birth	
1 min	60%–65%
2 min	65%–70%
3 min	70%–75%
4 min	75%–80%
5 min	80%–85%
10 min	85%–95%

Reproduced with permission from American Academy of Pediatrics, American Heart Association. *Textbook of Neonatal Resuscitation.* Kattwinkel J, ed. 6th ed. Elk Grove Village, IL: American Academy of Pediatrics; 2011.

This will require awareness of the time-specific oxygen targets in the first 10 minutes after birth and the ability to deliver oxygen concentrations between 21% and 100%. A compressed air source, a means of mixing oxygen and compressed air, and a pulse oximeter to rapidly and objectively measure saturation are needed to deliver the concentration of oxygen required to keep the baby's blood oxygen saturation within an acceptable range. Use the table of normal saturations following birth as a goal. Details of oxygen delivery and pulse oximetry use after resuscitation are given in Book III: Neonatal Care, Unit 1, Oxygen.

- <u>Babies born at term and not anticipated to require resuscitation:</u> *Begin resuscitation with 21% oxygen, attach oximeter, and adjust upward as necessary to achieve time-specific saturation targets.*

ACTIONS   **REMARKS**

Deciding Which Oxygen Concentration to Use (continued)

- <u>Babies born preterm:</u> *Begin with an intermediate concentration of oxygen, attach oximeter, and adjust oxygen concentration upward or downward as necessary to achieve time-specific saturation targets.*

- <u>Any baby reaching the point of requiring PPV or given supplemental oxygen:</u> *Attach an oximeter and adjust oxygen concentration to achieve time-specific saturation targets.*

Several studies show that very preterm newborns consistently require oxygen concentrations above 21% to initiate the desired rise in saturations after birth. One recommendation is to start the resuscitation with 30% to 50% oxygen and then increase or decrease the concentration as guided by pulse oximetry targets. Once target saturations are achieved, oxygen concentrations can often be decreased nearly to room air. Administration of CPAP to the spontaneously breathing baby can aid in achieving target saturations more rapidly. (See Book IV: Specialized Newborn Care, Unit 3, Continuous Positive Airway Pressure.)

Preparing for Positive-Pressure Ventilation

7. **Be sure that the oxygen line is firmly connected to the bag and adjust the flow to 8 to 10 L/minute.** If you are using a self-inflating bag, be sure the oxygen reservoir is attached. If you are using a T-piece resuscitator, follow manufacturer's instructions.

Low flow may result in
- Insufficient filling of the bag, if a flow-inflating bag is being used.
- Low oxygen concentration, if a self-inflating bag is being used. (Room air drawn in with each squeeze-release dilutes low-flow oxygen more than high-flow oxygen.)

High flow may cool a baby from cold oxygen blowing on the baby.

8. **Attach mask to bag and adjust pressure.**

Placing your gloved thumb inside the mask to push the connection together with the ventilation bag helps prevent accidental leaks and disconnection.

If you are using a flow-inflating bag

Adjust pressure valve.
- Place your hand tightly over mask opening.
- Allow bag to fill with oxygen.
- Adjust pressure until some oxygen escapes and the bag is filled but no longer tense.

Pressure adjustment is generally made with a valve located between the bag and the mask. Consult manufacturers' instructions for your device.

The pressure manometer should read 3 to 5 cm H_2O when the bag is not being squeezed and 20 to 40 cm H_2O when it is squeezed.

It is important to have a constant leak at the pressure valve so a baby does not receive too much pressure when the mask is held tightly to the baby's face. Peak inspiratory pressures and positive end-expiratory pressures will vary with ventilation rate and how hard the bag is squeezed, even when flow rate is constant to the bag.

181

ACTIONS   REMARKS

Preparing for Positive-Pressure Ventilation (continued)

If you are using a self-inflating bag

Test the functioning of the pressure-release valve.

- Place your hand tightly over mask opening.
- Squeeze the bag firmly and be sure that gas escapes from the pressure-release valve.

The pressure-release valve should open at approximately 40 cm H_2O as registered on the manometer.

Be certain the various tubings are connected to the correct ports and that the pressure-release valve functions properly. Incorrect assembly of the apparatus has been associated with excessive pressure being delivered to a baby. Consult manufacturer's instructions for your specific ventilation device.

If you are using a T-piece resuscitator

Test the setting of the of the pressure settings previously set by

- Placing your hand tightly over mask opening.
- Noting the PEEP setting and adjusting the PEEP valve if not 3 to 5 cm H_2O.
- Occluding the aperture opening to test the peak pressure and adjusting the peak inspiratory pressure valve if not reading 20 cm H_2O.

Consult manufacturer's instructions for your specific ventilation device.

9. **Be sure the baby's airway is clear of secretions.**

10. **Place baby in the sniffing position.**

This position may be accomplished by lifting the baby's lower jaw forward from the back, just below each ear, and making sure the nose is the highest point of the baby's face.

Placing the baby in the sniffing position opens the airway, puts the neck in a neutral position, and displaces the tongue away from the posterior pharynx.

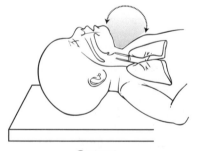

Correct

Reproduced with permission from American Academy of Pediatrics, American Heart Association. *Textbook of Neonatal Resuscitation.* Kattwinkel J, ed. 6th ed. Elk Grove Village, IL: American Academy of Pediatrics; 2011.

Correct Position for mask ventilation

ACTIONS   **REMARKS**

Preparing for Positive-Pressure Ventilation (continued)

A 0.5- to 1-inch cloth roll under the shoulders (not shown) may help to maintain the sniffing position.

If the chin is higher than the nose, the baby's neck is hyperextended.

Too large a cloth roll under the neck or hyperextending the baby's head will result in obstruction of the posterior pharynx.

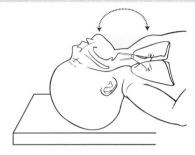

Incorrect
(hyperextension)

Reproduced with permission from American Academy of Pediatrics, American Heart Association. *Textbook of Neonatal Resuscitation*. Kattwinkel J, ed. 6th ed. Elk Grove Village, IL: American Academy of Pediatrics; 2011.

Incorrect Position: Too large a cloth roll under neck or allowing the baby's head to be hyperextended over the edge of the table will result in obstruction of the posterior pharynx.

If the forehead is higher than the nose, the baby's neck is flexed and the posterior pharynx will occlude the airway.

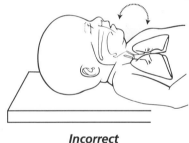

Incorrect
(flexion)

Reproduced with permission from American Academy of Pediatrics, American Heart Association. *Textbook of Neonatal Resuscitation*. Kattwinkel J, ed. 6th ed. Elk Grove Village, IL: American Academy of Pediatrics; 2011.

Incorrect Position: Flexed neck produces airway closure.

Ventilating a Baby Using a Mask

11. **Position mask on the baby's face.** Place your thumb and index finger over the mask to make a seal with the face and lift up under the chin with the middle finger to maintain slight extension of the neck.

Pressing downward on the mask and lifting upward on the chin help create a tight seal between the mask and the baby's face; Without a tight seal, a flow-inflating bag will not fill and a self-inflating bag or T-piece resuscitator will not deliver pressure to the baby.

ACTIONS   REMARKS

Ventilating a Baby Using a Mask (continued)

12. Squeeze the bag with your other hand or
    occlude the PEEP aperture of the T-piece
    with your finger until some of the gas is
    delivered to the baby. Enough gas should
    enter the baby's lungs so the chest rises
    slightly with each squeeze of the bag.

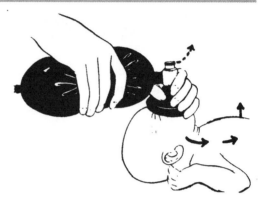

13. **Watch for slight chest movement** each time
    you squeeze the bag.

The chest should appear as if the baby is
taking a relatively normal breath—not too
deep and not too shallow. A manometer is
recommended on all positive-pressure devices to help you watch how much pressure
is required.

Because a newborn's lungs are initially filled
with fluid, it may take higher pressures to
move the chest with the first few breaths. You
also may choose to hold each inflation for a
slightly longer period during the first several
breaths than you will when providing PPV after the lungs have been filled with air.

Higher pressure and longer inflation time
may help establish lung volumes more
quickly; however, the ideal strategy for lung
inflation has not been determined.

Note: If you are using a self-inflating bag, you
may need to disable the automatic pop-off
valve to give adequate pressure to achieve
chest movement and an increase in heart rate.

Be sure you practice how to disable and re-
enable the pop-off valve of a self-inflating
bag. An emergency situation is not the time to
learn how to do this quickly and efficiently.

14. **Release your squeeze on the bag or remove
    your thumb from the PEEP cap** of the
    T-piece device, but keep the mask in place.
    Let the bag fill again with oxygen.

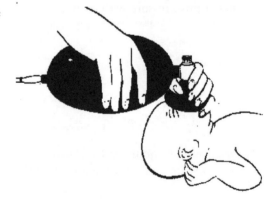

Release: The baby will exhale, even though
the mask is kept in place while oxygen refills the bag. Flow continues through the
T-piece device to provide PEEP.

ACTIONS   **REMARKS**

Ventilating a Baby Using a Mask (continued)

Continue this squeeze (occlude)-release breathing cycle at a rate of 40 to 60 breaths per minute. Initial pressures of about 20 cm H_2O, with a good seal at the mask, are generally sufficient; however, if the heart rate does not rise promptly and the chest does not move, take appropriate corrective steps. Higher pressures may be needed.

15. **Check for rise in heart rate on the pulse oximeter.** If heart rate is not being displayed reliably, feel the umbilical pulse or listen to the heart rate with a stethoscope.

A rise in heart rate is the first sign of effective ventilation. The pulse oximeter or feeling the umbilical cord pulse gives continuous feedback on heart rate while ventilation is provided. If the umbilical cord pulse is not palpable, listen for a heart rate over the chest. Sometimes you may need to pause ventilation to hear the heart rate.

16. **Listen for breath sounds.** Place a stethoscope on either side of the baby's chest in the axillary region, not on the front of the chest.

If you are adequately ventilating a baby, you should hear good breath sounds in both lungs.

17. **Observe baby's color and oxygen saturation and watch for breathing.**

If bag-and-mask ventilation is effective, a cyanotic baby should become pink quickly and saturations should rise to target range. Note when the baby begins to breathe spontaneously.

18. **Note the inflation pressure on the manometer that results in chest movement.** Try to match this pressure with each inflation, while periodically checking the chest rise.

Subsequent breaths may require less pressure than the first few breaths. The pressure manometer is helpful to maintain consistency, but chest movement is much more important than any specific number.

19. **If PPV is prolonged, an orogastric tube should be placed and the stomach decompressed.**

Positive-pressure ventilation may cause gastric distension because some oxygen will be forced into the stomach as well as into the lungs.

ACTIONS	REMARKS

What Can Go Wrong?

1. You could ventilate a baby inadequately.

If the chest is not moving well or there are no signs of improvement (rising heart rate, signs of spontaneous respirations, improved color and oxygen saturations), consider these corrective actions.

- Reapply the mask to the face to ensure an adequate seal; be sure mask size is correct.
- Reposition the baby's head.
- Suction the mouth, posterior pharynx, and nose to ensure a patent airway and ventilate with the mouth slightly open.
- Increase your squeeze on the bag.

OR

- Increase the gas flow to the bag.

OR

- Tighten the pressure valve to allow less oxygen to escape from a flow-inflating bag to increase the end-expiratory pressure.

OR

- Increase the peak inspiratory pressure and/or PEEP on the T-piece device.

OR

- Override the pop-off valve of a self-inflating bag.

If there is still no improvement, endotracheal intubation or insertion of a laryngeal mask airway is indicated.

2. You could push secretions or meconium into a baby's lungs.

3. The abdomen could become distended. Insert an orogastric tube for decompression.

Consider the following acronym to help remember the corrective steps:

	Corrective Steps	Actions
M	Mask adjustment.	Be sure there is a good seal of the mask on the face.
R	Reposition airway.	The head should be in the "sniffing" position.
S	Suction mouth and nose.	Check for secretions; suction if present.
O	Open mouth.	Ventilate with the baby's mouth slightly open and lift the jaw forward.
P	Pressure increase.	Gradually increase the pressure every few breaths, until there are bilateral breath sounds and visible chest movement with each breath.
A	Airway alternative.	Consider endotracheal intubation or laryngeal mask airway.

Reproduced with permission from American Academy of Pediatrics, American Heart Association. *Textbook of Neonatal Resuscitation.* Kattwinkel J, ed. 6th ed. Elk Grove Village, IL: American Academy of Pediatrics; 2011.

If you disable a safety pop-off valve, be sure to re-enable the valve after you no longer need the higher pressures.

Avoid using PPV until you have suctioned the baby. Avoid using it on nonvigorous, meconium-stained newborns until the trachea has been suctioned.

A distended stomach will push up on the diaphragm and make lung inflation more difficult.

ACTIONS   **REMARKS**

What Can Go Wrong? (continued)

4. **You could rupture a baby's lungs.**

Evacuation of air with needle thoracentesis may be necessary.

If you squeeze too hard or if the adjustable valve of your flow-inflating bag is closed too far or the peak inspiratory pressure of the T-piece is set too high, excess pressure may build up and cause a pneumothorax (rupture in the lung tissue). Use of a pressure manometer or T-piece device will help you be consistent in the amount of pressure you deliver with each breath. The chest should rise normally but not excessively, and the pressure between breaths should drop to 3 to 5 cm H_2O.

When Can You Stop Positive-Pressure Ventilation?

1. **When a baby has spontaneous respirations, has a heart rate above 100 bpm, and is pink with target saturations, there is no further reason for bag-and-mask ventilation.**

Many babies respond quickly to several breathing cycles given by bag and mask; however, a baby may still require additional oxygen.

2. **If a baby does not improve, the chest is not moving adequately despite corrective measures, or subsequent resuscitative steps are indicated (chest compressions or medications), you should perform endotracheal intubation.**

Although chest compressions can be given while a baby's ventilation is being assisted with bag and mask, ventilation through an endotracheal tube usually makes coordination of ventilation and compressions easier and more effective.

How to Withdraw Positive-Pressure Ventilation as a Baby Improves

1. **After the heart rate has risen above 100 bpm, look for the baby to begin taking spontaneous breaths.** Gradually decrease the rate of assisted ventilation as you stimulate the baby by rubbing the extremities and back.

If your assisted ventilation has been successful, the baby's carbon dioxide may be low, resulting in insufficient respiratory drive. Cutaneous stimulation will help increase the baby's spontaneous efforts.

2. **As the baby begins to breathe, continue to administer free-flow supplemental oxygen as indicated by pulse oximetry, and then gradually withdraw the oxygen as saturations permit.**

Abrupt withdrawal of supplemental oxygen from a baby who has undergone perinatal compromise may cause decreased blood flow to the lungs and possibly lead to the serious condition of pulmonary hypertension.

3. **Move the baby to an area where close monitoring and management can be provided.**

Continue to monitor saturations with a pulse oximeter to better gauge the appropriate concentration of oxygen (Book III: Neonatal Care, Unit 1, Oxygen).

SKILL UNIT

Endotracheal Intubation

This skill unit will teach you how to insert an endotracheal tube into a baby's airway. Not everyone will be required to learn and practice this skill. However, everyone should read this unit and attend a skill session to learn the equipment and sequence of steps to be able to assist with endotracheal intubation. Your perinatal education coordinators will contact the nurses and/or respiratory therapists who will be asked to master endotracheal intubation.

Study this skill unit, then attend a skill practice and demonstration session. A special, additional practice session for physicians, nurses, and other selected staff in your hospital may be arranged with regional center staff.

The staff members who will be asked to master all aspects of this skill will need to demonstrate each of the following steps correctly:
1. Assemble laryngoscope handle, blade, bulb, and batteries.
2. Insert stylet (if used) into endotracheal tube.
3. Position baby (manikin).
4. Hold laryngoscope correctly.
5. Insert laryngoscope blade into baby's mouth.
6. Visualize vocal cords.
7. Suction (as necessary).
8. Insert endotracheal tube within 30 seconds.
9. Adjust tube position by checking location of vocal cord line (printed on tube).
10. Remove laryngoscope.
11. Attach bag.
12. Check tube placement.
    - Baby's response (heart rate, color and oxygen saturation, activity, etc)
    - Color change of carbon dioxide (CO_2) detector from bluish-purple to yellow
    - Breath sounds (listen over both axillae and the stomach)
    - Chest movement
13. Secure tube in place.

 Endotracheal intubation may be a life-saving procedure. Someone skilled in neonatal intubation should be available in your hospital at all times.

PERINATAL PERFORMANCE GUIDE

ACTIONS	REMARKS
Anticipating Intubation	

1. The following equipment is necessary:

   - Oxygen, compressed air, and suction sources.
   - Oxygen/air blender.
   - Ventilation bag or T-piece device that can deliver variable oxygen concentrations from 21% to 100% oxygen. Ventilation bags must have an adjustable pressure valve and manometer or pressure-release valve.

Check daily or after every delivery to make sure this equipment is always ready for use in each

   - Delivery room
   - Nursery
   - Postpartum mother-baby unit

Laryngeal mask airway may provide an alternative route for ventilation if endotracheal intubation is not successful. (Refer to *Textbook of Neonatal Resuscitation, 6th Edition,* for details.)

   - Suction catheters
     - Size 5F to 6F
     - Size 8F
     - Size10F
     - Size 12F
   - Laryngoscope handle with extra batteries
   - Laryngoscope blades with extra bulbs
     - Size "0" and size "1" straight blade
     - Size "00" for extremely preterm newborn

Put laryngoscope blade and handle together and check light daily to make sure it is bright. Change the batteries as necessary to ensure a bright light. Also check to see that the bulb is screwed in tightly.

   - Endotracheal tubes
     - 2.5 mm
     - 3.0 mm
     - 3.5 mm
     - 4.0 mm
   - Stylet (optional)

Endotracheal tubes should be non-tapered (no shoulder), have a natural curve, and have a vocal cord line.

   - Carbon dioxide (CO_2) detector

A CO_2 detector is a disposable device that connects to an endotracheal tube after insertion. It changes color when CO_2 is present, thus indicating correct placement of the tube in the trachea, rather than in the esophagus.

   - Endotracheal tube stabilizing device or moisture-resistant tape

Endotracheal tube stabilizing devices are commercially available. Follow manufacturers' instructions for appropriate application.

   - Face masks
     - Preterm
     - Newborn

Clear masks with cushioned rims are recommended.

ACTIONS   **REMARKS**

Anticipating Intubation (continued)

2. There are several points in the resuscitation sequence where endotracheal intubation may be appropriate. Factors that influence the timing of intubation include

   • Skill of resuscitator

   • Presence of meconium in a baby who is not vigorous

   • Baby's response to positive-pressure ventilation (PPV)

   • Need for chest compressions

   • Need for epinephrine administration before intravenous access is established

   • Certain conditions, such as diaphragmatic hernia

These factors, and the consideration they should receive in making your decision whether to intubate, are discussed in the main unit.

Preparing for Intubation

3. Baby should be connected to pulse oximeter or one person should continuously take the baby's pulse and call or tap out the heart rate.

4. Select correct-size tube, blade, and suction catheter for baby's weight.

Positive-pressure ventilation with supplemental oxygen and chest compressions, if indicated, should continue while you prepare the equipment for intubation.

Use the information in the table as guidelines for equipment selection.

Weight of Baby (g)	Gestational Age (wks)	Tube Size (mm) (inner diameter)	Laryngoscope Blade	Insertion Depth (from upper lip) (cm)	Suction Catheter (F)
<1,000	<28	2.5	0 or 00	6.5-7	5, 6
1,000-2,000	28-34	3.0	0-1	7-8	5, 6, or 8
2,000-3,000	34-38	3.5	1	8-9	8
>3,000	>38	3.5-4.0	1	>9	8 or 10

ACTIONS	REMARKS

Preparing for Intubation (continued)

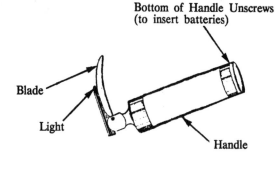

Bottom of Handle Unscrews
(to insert batteries)

Blade

Light

Handle

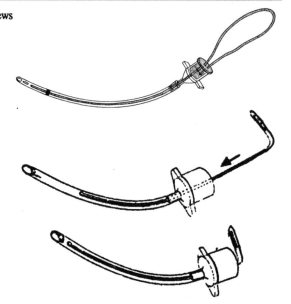

5. **Assemble equipment.**

   - Assemble laryngoscope handle and blade.

   - Check light.

   - Insert stylet into tube, as shown (optional). Two types of stylets are shown, but each serves the same purpose of making an endotracheal tube rigid.

   - If using a stylet, bend the tube slightly upward, as shown.

   Note: Intubations can often be carried out *without* a stylet. This may be preferable because a stylet can lacerate the trachea and/or esophagus if used incorrectly.

   Make sure the stylet does not extend beyond the end or side of the tube.

   - Keep the resuscitation bag connected to supplemental oxygen.

   The same bag used for bag-and-mask ventilation may be used with an endotracheal tube to ventilate a baby.

   - Ventilate the baby for a few seconds with PPV before starting the intubation procedure.

   The baby will not be ventilated while the tube is being inserted, so begin intubation with the baby stable and normally saturated, if possible. Use a pulse oximeter to monitor heart rate and oxygen saturation during intubation.

ACTIONS   **REMARKS**

Inserting an Endotracheal Tube Using a Laryngoscope

6. **Keep the baby positioned as for bag-and-mask ventilation, on a flat surface in the sniffing position.** A 0.5- to 1-inch cloth roll under the baby's shoulders may be helpful.

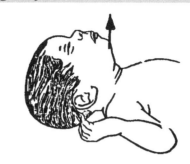

Correct Position

Hyperextension of the head over the edge of the table is *not* the proper position for intubating a baby. The head and shoulders should be on the same surface. The chin should be extended.

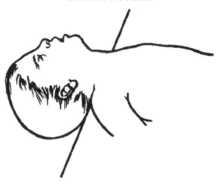

Incorrect Position

7. **Hold the laryngoscope in your left hand with thumb, index, and middle finger.** Leave the fourth and fifth fingers free to steady your hand on the baby's chin.

   If you are left-handed, you will need to learn to hold the laryngoscope in your left hand and use your right hand to insert the endotracheal tube.

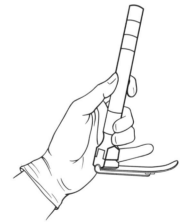

8. Steps 9 through 16 must be done very quickly because the baby is without oxygen during this time.

ACTIONS   REMARKS

Inserting an Endotracheal Tube Using a Laryngoscope (continued)

Some people use the technique of holding their breath as they insert the laryngoscope and tube. As soon as they can no longer hold their breath, it is assumed that the baby needs a breath too. The laryngoscope is removed and bag-and-mask ventilation, with supplemental oxygen as appropriate, is resumed.

If a baby's heart rate drops below 60 to 70 beats per minute for more than a few seconds, STOP and remove the laryngoscope. RESUME bag-and-mask ventilation.

When heart rate and saturation are normal, try inserting the tube again.

Intubation attempts generally should be limited to 30 seconds.

It may take more than one attempt to insert the tube. A second person should be monitoring the baby's heart rate continuously.

9. Insert the laryngoscope blade into the baby's mouth along the *right* side of the tongue, until about three-fourths of the blade is in the baby's mouth.

   The blade is designed to push the tongue to the left. It is important, therefore, to insert it down the right side of the mouth. Then, shift the blade to the center of the mouth, keeping the tongue to the left of the blade.

10. Lift the laryngoscope so the blade lifts the baby's chin and tongue away from you.

    Do *not* tilt the laryngoscope handle back toward you.

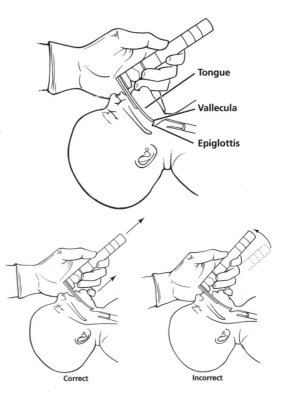

NEVER PRY up with a laryngoscope.

11. Are the vocal cords visible?

    Yes: Insert the tube between the vocal cords.

    The key to successful intubation is visualizing the vocal cords. You should be able to see the tip of the tube go between the cords and into the trachea.

194

ACTIONS   **REMARKS**

Inserting an Endotracheal Tube Using a Laryngoscope (continued)

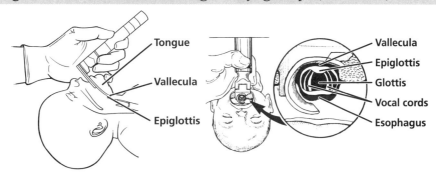

Correct View: Vocal cords are visible.

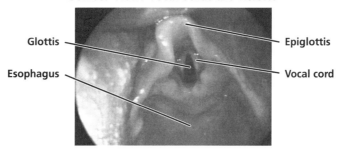

Reproduced with permission from Klaus M, Fanaroff A. *Care of the High Risk Neonate.* Philadelphia, PA: WB Saunders, 1996.

No: Do *not* attempt to insert the tube.

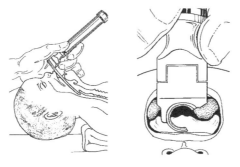

Incorrect View: Vocal cords are not visible.

- *If only the tongue is visible,* lower laryngoscope, insert blade farther, and lift again. If the vocal cords are still not visible, the blade is probably too deep. Pull back, just until you feel the epiglottis fall off the blade. Lift again and look for the vocal cords.

- *If the epiglottis obscures the larynx,* lower laryngoscope, insert blade farther, and lift again to pin the epiglottis under the blade and out of view.

ACTIONS   **REMARKS**

Inserting an Endotracheal Tube Using a Laryngoscope (continued)

> • *If mucus secretions block the view,* suction secretions with a suction catheter.
>
> **If you cannot see the cords, do not insert the tube. Unless the vocal cords can be seen, the tube almost certainly will go into the esophagus and not the trachea.**

12. **Insert the tube** (with the bend upward) along the right side of the mouth. **Watch the tip of the tube as it slides between the vocal cords and into the trachea.**

    Keep the laryngoscope in place and continue to observe the tube.

13. **Stop inserting the tube when the stripe on the tube reaches the vocal cords.**

Do *not* slide the tube down the groove of the blade. An endotracheal tube will fit in the groove, but putting it there will obstruct your view. The groove is designed for you to see to the end of the blade and observe the tube as it enters the line of sight from the right.

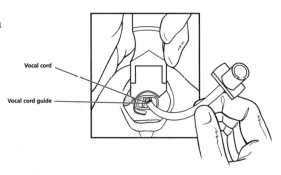

Reproduced with permission from American Academy of Pediatrics, American Heart Association. *Textbook of Neonatal Resuscitation.* Kattwinkel J, ed. 6th ed. Elk Grove Village, IL: American Academy of Pediatrics; 2011.

This will place the tip of the tube about 1.5 to 2 cm (one-half inch to three-fourths inch) below the vocal cords.

14. Remove the laryngoscope while holding the tube in place against the palate with your finger.

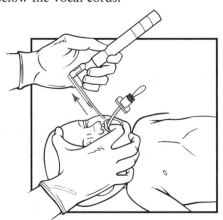

Reproduced with permission from American Academy of Pediatrics, American Heart Association. *Textbook of Neonatal Resuscitation.* Kattwinkel J, ed. 6th ed. Elk Grove Village, IL: American Academy of Pediatrics; 2011.

ACTIONS   **REMARKS**

Inserting an Endotracheal Tube Using a Laryngoscope (continued)

15. Remove the stylet (if used) while holding the tube in place with your other hand.

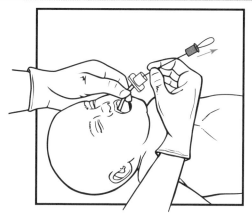

Reproduced with permission from American Academy of Pediatrics, American Heart Association. *Textbook of Neonatal Resuscitation.* Kattwinkel J, ed. 6th ed. Elk Grove Village, IL: American Academy of Pediatrics; 2011.

16. **Hold the tube in place by pressing it against the palate with your finger.**

17. **Connect the ventilation device to the tube and begin ventilation with supplemental oxygen** as indicated at a rate of 40 to 60 breaths per minute.

18. *Remember, steps 9 through 17 must be done quickly, with a goal of less than 30 seconds.*

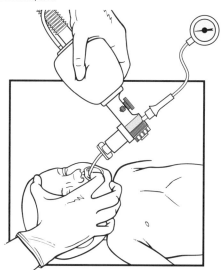

Reproduced with permission from American Academy of Pediatrics, American Heart Association. *Textbook of Neonatal Resuscitation.* Kattwinkel J, ed. 6th ed. Elk Grove Village, IL: American Academy of Pediatrics; 2011.

 The tube must be held securely, but be careful not to press so hard that you collapse the lumen.

ACTIONS **REMARKS**

Inserting an Endotracheal Tube Using a Laryngoscope (continued)

If you do not get the tube in place within 30 seconds, STOP. Remove the laryngoscope and tube. Provide assisted ventilation and oxygen as indicated until you and the baby are ready for another intubation attempt.

Do not persist with intubation at the expense of a baby's oxygenation. Likewise, do not insert a tube without adequate visualization. It may take several attempts to intubate the trachea. Between attempts, ensure adequate ventilation by providing PPV with a mask.

Checking Endotracheal Tube Placement

19. Check to make sure the tube is in the right place.

   • Connect a CO_2 detector between the bag and the endotracheal tube. Monitor for improvement in heart rate and saturation after PPV is resumed. If the baby's heart rate was low, it generally will rise rapidly after endotracheal intubation and ventilation.

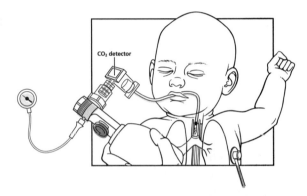

Reproduced with permission from American Academy of Pediatrics, American Heart Association. *Textbook of Neonatal Resuscitation.* Kattwinkel J, ed. 6th ed. Elk Grove Village, IL: American Academy of Pediatrics; 2011.

The CO_2 detector should change color within several positive-pressure breaths.

Note: Although not shown, the endotracheal tube should be held in place.

If the heart rate is not increasing and CO_2 is not detected after several positive-pressure breaths, consider removing the tube, resuming bag-and-mask ventilation, and repeating intubation steps 9 through 17.

Alternatively, confirm endotracheal tube placement through the vocal cords by visualizing with the laryngoscope.

ACTIONS   REMARKS

Checking Endotracheal Tube Placement (continued)

- *Look* for symmetrical chest movement with each PPV breath.

- *Listen* with a stethoscope over the baby's
  – **Left lung**
  – **Right lung**
  – **Stomach**

Listen over both sides of the chest, in the axillary region, not over the front of the chest.

Because of a baby's small chest size, assisted ventilation breaths forced down the esophagus may be heard in the chest, but will be loudest over the stomach. Listening over the stomach as well as both lungs is *essential* for accurate determination of tube placement.

A second team member should **give 3 quick, low-pressure puffs** with the bag so the first person can clearly hear which breath sounds are created by assisted ventilation. Unless you do this, you may hear the baby's own, slower breathing and think the tube is placed correctly.

When you hear the sounds described and illustrated below, take the actions indicated.

Sounds Heard   *Response Needed*

Loud over both lungs, soft over stomach (tube is in the trachea)   No action needed.

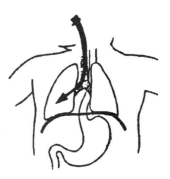

Sounds Heard   *Response Needed*

Loud over right lung, soft over left lung (tube is in the main bronchus leading to the right lung)   Check tube marking at lip.

Consider pulling tube back 1 cm (one-half) and listening again.

ACTIONS   **REMARKS**

Checking Endotracheal Tube Placement (continued)

Sounds Heard   *Response Needed*

*Loud over stomach, soft   *Remove tube immediately and*
over lungs* (tube is in the   *reintubate!*
esophagus)

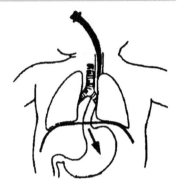

20. **Confirm tube distance inside the trachea by checking which mark on the endotracheal tube is at the baby's lip.**

    - <1,000 g = 6.5-7 cm
    - 1,000-2,000 g = 7-8 cm
    - 2,500-3,500 g = 8-9 cm
    - >3,500 g = >9 cm

    An easy-to-remember approximation is "6 cm plus the baby's weight in kilograms." For example, the 9-cm mark on an endotracheal tube would be approximately at the lip of a baby that weighs 3,000 g.

Once you have determined that the tube is in the trachea (not the esophagus), adjust the distance the tube has been inserted. Follow the guidelines given (at left). Listen again over the chest and stomach, then secure the tube in place. Confirm position with a chest x-ray.

Securing an Endotracheal Tube in Place

21. **Thoroughly dry the skin around the baby's mouth.**

Continue to ventilate the baby while someone else secures the tube in place. Hold the tube firmly against the palate with your finger until it is secured.

22. **Secure the tube in place with a stabilizer or tape.**

Some hospitals prefer to use a commercially available endotracheal tube stabilizer.

ACTIONS   **REMARKS**

Securing an Endotracheal Tube in Place (continued)

- Place a strip of clear adhesive dressing between the baby's nose and upper lip.

- Cut 2 pieces of one-half inch adhesive tape 4 inches (10 cm) long.

- Split each piece for half its length.

- Stick the unsplit section of the tape and one tab across the baby's upper lip (on top of the clear adhesive dressing).

- Wrap the other tab in a spiral around the endotracheal tube.

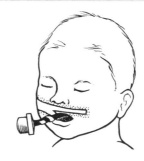

- Place second tape in reverse direction.

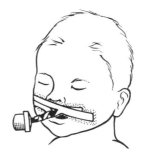

- Listen again after securing the tube, to be sure it has not been displaced.

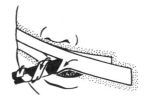

Removing an Endotracheal Tube

23. **Prepare to remove the tube** when the baby is breathing adequately without assistance and has good heart rate, saturations, and activity.

      Oximetry and arterial blood gas measurements can be helpful in deciding when to remove the tube.

24. **Disconnect the bag from the tube.**

25. **Suction any mucus from the tube. Reconnect the bag and ventilate the baby for a few breaths.**

26. **Suction any mucus from the back of the baby's throat.**

27. **Pull out the tube as the baby is exhaling.**

28. **Continue to give the baby supplemental oxygen, as necessary.**

      Be ready to assist ventilation using a mask and perhaps to re-intubate.

ACTIONS	REMARKS

What Can Go Wrong? Observing a Baby With an Endotracheal Tube

1. **If a baby turns blue or the heart rate drops, consider the following:**

Immediately increase the baby's oxygen, then promptly investigate the cause.

a. The tube may be in the esophagus instead of the trachea.

Even if a tube was originally in the trachea, it may slip out. If a baby becomes cyanotic or bradycardic, listen again for breath sounds over both lungs and the stomach and/or use a CO_2 detector. If breath sounds are heard over the stomach, but not in either lung and the CO_2 detector is negative for carbon dioxide, remove the tube and re-intubate.

b. The tube may become plugged with blood or mucus.

Using sterile technique, suction the tube. If secretions are thick, instill approximately 0.5 mL of saline into the tube prior to suctioning.

When suctioning an endotracheal tube, be careful not to insert the suction catheter too far or damage to the trachea may occur. The catheter should be inserted only 1 cm beyond the tip of the endotracheal tube. Many suction catheters are marked with numbers indicating the length of the catheter (in centimeters). The proper insertion distance can be determined by matching these numbers with corresponding numbers on an endotracheal tube. Some commercially available closed-system suctioning devices are designed to facilitate correct suctioning depth.

c. The posterior pharynx may bleed.

Trauma to the pharynx is generally a result of prying instead of lifting the laryngoscope.

d. Stylet may have been used incorrectly, resulting in puncture or tear of the esophagus and/or trachea.

If a stylet is used, be sure the stylet does not extend beyond the tip of the endotracheal tube.

e. The baby may develop a pneumothorax (ruptured lung).

Some babies who are intubated and require PPV develop a pneumothorax. If a baby's condition suddenly deteriorates and the tube is judged to be placed correctly, consider a pneumothorax. Transilluminate the baby's chest and/or obtain an emergency portable chest x-ray. (See Book III: Neonatal Care, Unit 2, Respiratory Distress, for detection and management of a pneumothorax.)

ACTIONS   **REMARKS**

What Can Go Wrong? Observing a Baby With an Endotracheal Tube (continued)

f. The tube may have slipped in too far.

Listen for breath sounds. They should be equally loud over the right and left lung. If you can hear the positive-pressure breaths louder over the right lung than the left lung, the tube probably has slipped down into the right mainstem bronchus. Carefully pull the tube back a tiny bit at a time until the positive-pressure breaths are equally loud over both lungs.

Checking with a laryngoscope for the position of the vocal cord line on the tube can also be helpful.

g. The pressure or rate used to ventilate a baby may be inadequate.

Pressure: Sometimes you may not give enough pressure to move sufficient oxygen into the baby's lungs for adequate ventilation.

1. If the ventilation bag is slow to refill from the oxygen source, increase the liter-per-minute flow rate.

2. If the ventilation bag fills rapidly, but you do not seem to hear good breath sounds in the baby's lungs and/or the baby's chest does not rise with each breath,

   - Squeeze harder on the bag.
   - Tighten the pressure valve to increase the PEEP if you are using a flow-inflating bag.
   - Check the actual pressure delivered to the baby with a pressure manometer. Sick babies may require 25 to 30 cm H_2O of pressure, or more, with each breath.
   - Increase the peak inspiratory pressure and/or PEEP on the T-piece device.

Rate: The recommended rate is 40 to 60 breaths per minute. Occasionally, a faster or a slower rate may be needed.

h. The lungs may be over-inflated.

Make certain the bag deflates after you squeeze it. If it does not, the liter-per-minute flow rate may be excessive.

ACTIONS   **REMARKS**

What Can Go Wrong? Observing a Baby With an Endotracheal Tube (continued)

i. CO_2 detector may read inaccurately.

CO_2 detectors are nearly always accurate for detecting misplaced endotracheal tubes, but they can occasionally give false readings.

- Circulation must be adequate and heart rate present for CO_2 to be delivered to exhaled air. Babies in cardiac arrest and/ or those not receiving effective chest compressions may not exhale sufficient CO_2 to change the detector's color.

- If a detector becomes wet with an acidic solution, such as epinephrine, it will change color, even if there is no CO_2.

- Extremely low birth weight babies may not produce sufficient CO_2 to change the detector's color, although CO_2 detectors are usually accurate even in very small babies if they are being adequately ventilated.

SKILL UNIT

Chest Compressions

This skill unit will teach you how to give chest compressions to a baby.

Study this skill unit, then attend a skill practice and demonstration session.

To master the skill, you will need to demonstrate each of the following steps correctly:

1. Position of baby
2. Position of your hands on baby's chest
3. Force of compressions
4. Rate of compressions
5. Coordination of compressions with ventilations
6. Checking effectiveness of chest compressions

PERINATAL PERFORMANCE GUIDE

ACTIONS	REMARKS
Deciding to Begin Chest Compressions	

ACTIONS	REMARKS
1. **Chest compressions should be started when the heart rate remains below 60 beats per minute (bpm) despite 30 seconds of effective positive-pressure ventilation (PPV).** Assess the heart rate by • Feeling the pulse by lightly grasping the base of the umbilical cord • Listening to the apical beat with a stethoscope • Monitoring heart rate with a pulse oximeter Assess the heart rate continuously with a pulse oximeter or every 45 to 60 seconds during PPV.	Beginning chest compressions too early is unwise because • The most common reason for brady-cardia is insufficient expansion of the lungs. • Administering chest compressions will diminish your ability to ventilate a baby.

Preparing to Begin Chest Compressions	

ACTIONS	REMARKS
2. **Is the airway secure?** **Yes: Endotracheal tube in place.** **No:** Endotracheal intubation should be performed if chest compressions are needed.	***Effective ventilation MUST be given in conjunction with chest compressions.*** Any resuscitation that requires chest compressions needs 2 people (one to manage the airway and one to give chest compressions). If medications are needed, a third person is required.
3. **Is the baby in the proper position?** **Yes: Supine on a flat surface.** **No:** Place the baby on his or her back on a firm surface.	The person giving chest compressions may be at the side or head of the baby's bed, with the person ventilating in the alternative position.
4. **Locate the lower third of the sternum.**	Run your finger along the lower edge of the baby's ribs until you find the xiphoid (a small protrusion where the ribs meet in the midline). Press on the lower third of the sternum, just above the xiphoid. Be careful not to press on the xiphoid itself.

ACTIONS	REMARKS

Giving Chest Compressions

5. **Wrap your hands around the baby's chest. Place both thumbs on the lower third of the sternum on a line just below the nipples and above the xiphoid.**

Note: The *thumb* chest-encircling technique is generally preferred; however the 2-*finger* technique may allow better access to the umbilicus during insertion of a catheter for medication administration.

Two-finger technique (not shown), with your index and middle fingers held next to each other, fingers straight, at a right angle to the chest, may be used if a baby is very large or your hands are small. Use your other hand to support the baby's back.

For a very small baby, your thumbs may be placed one on top of the other (not shown).

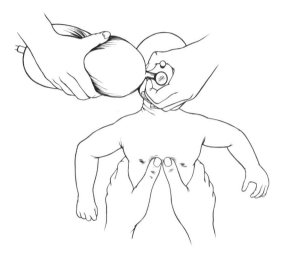

Experience has shown that the thumb technique can be performed at the head of the bed while the umbilical catheter is being inserted. This will require some coordinated positioning of the person giving PPV and the person performing the compressions.

6. **Compress the baby's chest with enough force to depress the sternum approximately one-third of the anterior-posterior diameter of the chest.** Then release the pressure.

Do *not* lift your thumbs (or fingers) off the sternum between compressions, but be sure to release the pressure completely.

When the chest is compressed, the entire thorax serves as a bellows pump, thus pumping blood through the circulatory system. The compressions should be smooth, not jerky, and equal or slightly shorter than the relaxation (release) phase.

7. **Give 3 compressions, then pause for delivery of one breath.** Continue this 3:1 cycle, so there are 2 "events" delivered per second and 120 "events" per minute (90 compressions plus 30 ventilations).

If a ventilation and a chest compression are delivered simultaneously, it is likely that chest inflation will be impaired. Effective coordination will require practice as a team.

Counting out loud may help keep the cadence: "1-and-2-and-3-and-breathe-and-1-and-2-and...."

207

ACTIONS	REMARKS

Giving Chest Compressions (continued)

8. Continue to provide coordinated chest compressions and ventilations until the baby has a spontaneous heart rate above 60 bpm.	Compressions should be interrupted briefly every 45 to 60 seconds to feel for the umbilical pulse or check the heart rate by pulse oximetry. If no pulse is detected, you will need to interrupt ventilation briefly to listen to the chest for heart sounds.

What Can Go Wrong?

1. You may not ventilate the baby adequately.	Positive-pressure ventilation will not be as effective while chest compressions are being given. Because of this, • Do not start compressions before they are indicated. • Intubate the trachea if compressions are indicated. • Stop compressions when no longer indicated. • Coordinate compressions and ventilations.
2. You may not give compressions effectively.	Be sure to compress the chest to a full one-third of the diameter of the chest. If done effectively, you should be able to create a palpable pulse.
3. You may injure the baby.	Fractured ribs and injured organs have occurred with aggressive or inappropriately administered chest compressions. Be sure to compress only one-third of the diameter of the chest and be careful to compress the sternum above the xiphoid.

SKILL UNIT

Emergency Medications

This skill unit will teach you how to prepare and administer emergency medications for newborn babies.

This unit should be completed only by personnel licensed to prepare/administer medications.

However, all perinatal health care providers should know where emergency medications are kept in each delivery room and nursery. A table of preparation instructions and dosages also should be kept wherever the drugs are stored.

Study this skill unit now. Sessions to practice and demonstrate administration of emergency medications may be scheduled later, at the same time as umbilical catheterization practice sessions. The educational unit for umbilical catheters is in Book III: Neonatal Care, Unit 3, Umbilical Catheters.

You do not need to memorize the dosage for each medication. You may use the table at the end of this skill unit when demonstrating how to prepare and administer emergency medications.

To master the skill, you will need to demonstrate each of the following steps correctly for each of the medications:

1. Prepare each medication (mock solutions may be used) in the desired concentration and in a dosage appropriate for babies described in examples presented by your coordinators.
2. Label each syringe with all necessary information.
3. Show the administration technique using the appropriate route(s) and speed of delivery (model of intravenous [IV] tubing, umbilical catheter, and/or endotracheal tube may be used).

PERINATAL PERFORMANCE GUIDE

ACTIONS	REMARKS

Epinephrine (Adrenalin) Use: Cardiac Stimulant; Vasoconstrictor

Equipment and Medication

- 1-mL syringe, marked in tenths
- 3- or 5-mL syringe
- Epinephrine in 1:10,000 concentration

Preparation

- Draw up 1 mL of 1:10,000 epinephrine.
- Draw up 3 mL of 1:10,000 epinephrine in the 3- or 5-mL syringe.
- Label the syringe as 1:10,000 epinephrine, route for administration, time and date.

Administration

IV Dose:	0.1 to 0.3 mL/kg of 1:10,000 (0.01-0.03 mg/kg)
Endotracheal dose:	0.5 to 1 mL/kg of 1:10,000 (0.05-0.1 mg/kg)
Route:	*Preferred:* Umbilical venous catheter (UVC) by IV push
	Acceptable: Endotracheal tube as UVC is being placed
Rate:	Rapidly; may be repeated every 3 to 5 minutes if necessary
Note:	If IV access is not quickly available, epinephrine may be given into the trachea, through an endotracheal tube, using the higher dosage.

Use only epinephrine 1:10,000 concentration.

Use a vial of epinephrine only once.

Epinephrine should be injected only into a vein or an endotracheal tube, NEVER into an artery.

To avoid medication errors,

1. Use different-sized syringes for intravenous (IV) and endotracheal doses: 1-mL syringe for IV doses and 3- or 5-mL syringe for endotracheal doses.

2. Use different-colored labels.

3. Call out what is being done, such as "drawing up 0.2 mL of epinephrine for IV administration" for a baby with estimated weight of 2 kg (dosage of 0.1 mL/kg), or for a baby of same weight and dosage, "drawing up 2 mL of epinephrine for endotracheal administration."

4. Be sure all team members know the differences in administration routes and dosages.

Endotracheal administration of epinephrine has been shown to give unreliable effects, and should be given only while IV access is being obtained. A higher dose likely will be required.

ACTIONS	REMARKS
Normal Saline	*Use: Blood Volume Expander*

Equipment and Medication
- Two 20-mL syringes
- Normal saline for IV use

Preparation
- Draw up 10 mL/kg of saline.
- Label the syringe as normal saline, administration route, time and date.

Administration

Dose: 10 mL/kg of baby's estimated weight

Route: IV

Rate: Slowly, steadily over 5 to 10 minutes

Ringer's lactate or O Rh-negative emergency release blood cross-matched against the mother's blood (if time permits) are also acceptable volume expanders.

Dose may be repeated as indicated by clinical response and blood pressure measurements.

Too rapid and excessive blood volume expansion may be associated with intracranial hemorrhage, particularly in preterm babies or those who experienced perinatal compromise.

ACTIONS	REMARKS
Naloxone HCl (Narcan)	*Use: Counteracts Narcotic Drugs Given to the Mother*

Equipment and Medication
- 1-mL syringe, marked in tenths
- Naloxone HCl 1 mg/mL

Preparation
- Draw up 0.1 mL/kg of the baby's weight.
- Label the syringe as naloxone HCl 1 mg/mL, administration route, time, and date.

Administration

Dose: 0.1 mg/kg
     (0.1 mL/kg of a 1 mg/mL concentration)

Route: IM, IV

Rate: Rapidly

NALOXONE IS NOT A RESUSCITATION DRUG.

A baby needing resuscitation should receive all necessary steps in the resuscitation sequence, and be stabilized, before administration of naloxone HCl is considered.

Because the duration of narcotic effect may be longer than the naloxone counter effect, a repeated dose(s) may be needed if respiratory depression recurs in the baby.

Intravenous administration is preferred. Intramuscular (IM) route will not have as rapid an effect as IV administration. Assisted ventilation may need to be continued for a longer period.

Naloxone should NOT be given to a newborn whose mother is
- *Suspected of being addicted to narcotics*
- *Receiving methadone*

Otherwise, signs of severe withdrawal, including neonatal seizures, may occur.

211

How to Care for Emergency Medications

1. *Medication:* Always use a new vial or bottle for each resuscitation. Medications often come in different concentrations. Use only the concentrations specified here for neonatal resuscitation.

2. *Point of IV Administration:* When giving emergency medications intravenously, always inject the drug at the point closest to the baby. If these medications are mixed with IV fluid in the bottle or in the IV tubing far from the baby, they will not reach the baby quickly enough to be effective.

3. *Speed of Delivery:* Emergency medications need to be given promptly, but some slower than others. Epinephrine is given rapidly; volume expanders are infused slowly and steadily, as rapid infusions of fluid are associated with intraventricular hemorrhage and should be avoided.

4. *Usable Time Frame:* Discard any medications not used within 1 hour. After that time, the drugs may begin to decompose and lose their effectiveness.

5. *Syringe Labels:* Never use an unlabeled syringe of medication. Use labels of different colors to distinguish between medications of similar appearance or different route of administration.

6. *Dosage Calculation:* Estimate a newly born baby's weight to calculate dosages. An actual weight may be obtained later, after the baby's condition has been stabilized. You may want to establish a chart of calculated dosages for babies of different weights so those calculations do not need to be done at the time resuscitation is being carried out.

Keep a copy of the following table with the supply of emergency medications in each delivery room nursery and postpartum unit.

Emergency Medications for Neonatal Resuscitation*				
Syringe Label (Medication in Final Concentration)	Syringe Size	Concentration	Administration	Remarks
Epinephrine 1:10,000	1 mL, marked in tenths OR 3 or 5 mL for endo-tracheal use	1:10,000	**IV Dose:** (0.01-0.03 mg/kg) 0.1-0.3 mL/kg **Endotracheal dose:** 0.5-1.0 mL/kg of 1:10,000 (0.05-0.1 mg/kg) **Rate:** As quickly as possible	1. Preferred route is umbilical venous cathe-ter; never inject into an artery. Endotracheal route may be used while umbilical venous cath-eter (UVC) is placed. 2. Always use 1:10,000 concentration 3. Give rapidly. 4. May repeat every 3-5 minutes.
Normal saline	10, 20, or 30 mL (dependent on baby's weight)	0.9% sodium chloride	**Dose:** 10 mL/kg **Route:** IV **Rate:** Slowly, steadily over 5-10 minutes	1. Dose may be repeated if history and/or clinical findings (pallor, weak pulses, poor perfusion, low blood pressure) indicate need. 2. Avoid rapid or excessive vol-ume expansion because either may be associ-ated with intracranial hemorrhage, particularly in preterm babies.

*IV, intravenously; IM, intramuscularly; SC, subcutaneously.

Emergency Medications for Neonatal Resuscitation* *(continued)*				
Syringe Label (Medication in Final Concentration)	**Syringe Size**	**Concentration**	**Administration**	**Remarks**
Naloxone HCl (Narcan) *The resuscitation sequence should be carried out, and the baby stabilized, BEFORE naloxone HCl administration is considered.*	1 mL, marked in tenths	1 mg/mL	**Dose:** (0.1 mL/ kg of 1 mg/mL) **Route:** IV or IM **Rate:** IV rapidly	1. Narcotic effect may outlast naloxone counter-effect, so dose may be repeated to prevent/ treat recurrent apnea. 2. Do not use if maternal narcotic addic- tion or metha- done use is suspected.

*IV, intravenously; IM, intramuscularly; SC, subcutaneously.

SKILL UNIT

Apgar Score

Please read this unit carefully to learn how to perform all aspects of determining a baby's Apgar score. The value of the Apgar score is diminished if any of the components are assigned incorrectly.

You do not need to memorize the Apgar scoring chart, and may have a copy with you when you demonstrate the skill. To master the skill, you must assign an Apgar score correctly for at least 2 babies (either in mock situations or at actual deliveries) by doing the following:

1. Score each sign correctly.
2. Describe why you gave a 0, 1, or 2 score for each sign.
3. Calculate the composite score.

PERINATAL PERFORMANCE GUIDE

ACTIONS   REMARKS

What Is an Apgar Score?

An Apgar score is a number based on a newborn's appearance, activity, and certain vital signs. A baby is given scores of 0, 1, or 2 for each of 5 signs. The sum of these 5 scores is the total Apgar score. The best score is 10; the worst is 0. The score should be assigned by an individual not involved with delivering or resuscitating the baby being scored. The signs and scores are shown below.

The score is named for Virginia Apgar, MD, the anesthesiologist who devised the score. The letters of her surname can be used to remember the components of the score: A = appearance (color), P = pulse (heart rate), G = grimace (reflex irritability), A = activity (muscle tone), and R = respirations (respiratory effort).

Sign		Score		
		0	1	2
A	**Appearance** (color)	Blue, gray, or pale	Body pink, extremities blue	Completely pink
P	**Pulse** (heart rate)	Absent	Below 100 beats per minute	Above 100 beats per minute
G	**Grimace** (reflex irritability)	No response	Grimace	Cough, sneeze, or cry
A	**Activity** (muscle tone)	Flaccid, limp	Some flexion of extremities	Well-flexed, active movement
R	**Respirations** (respiratory effort)	Absent	Slow, irregular	Good, crying

A copy of the Apgar scoring chart, in large print, should be posted prominently in each delivery room.

How Is an Apgar Score Used?

An Apgar score is useful to document a newborn's condition and response to resuscitative measures, if needed, at specific points in time after birth.

If a baby needs resuscitation, appropriate actions should be started *immediately* after birth. Do *not delay* resuscitative efforts to assign an Apgar score. The Apgar score should not be used to dictate resuscitation actions, but can be used to summarize a baby's response to resuscitation.

ACTIONS	REMARKS

When Do You Assign an Apgar Score?

If the heart rate is low, respiratory effort is inadequate, and/or baby is cyanotic, begin resuscitation IMMEDIATELY.

1. At 1 minute of age.

2. Again at 5 minutes of age.

3. If the 5-minute score is less than 7, additional scores are obtained every 5 minutes for a total of 20 minutes.

Do NOT delay resuscitation to determine an Apgar score.

Look at a clock as soon as a baby is completely delivered. Assign an Apgar score 1 minute after head and body are born.

This score reflects the baby's condition after initial stabilization or resuscitation measures.

How Do You Score Appearance (Color)?

4. *Look* at the baby.

   a. If the baby is *pink all over,* give a *score of 2.*

   b. If the baby's *hands and feet are blue,* but the *body and mucous membranes are pink,* give a *score of 1.*

   c. If the *entire body* and mucous membranes are *blue, gray, or severely pale,* give a *score of 0.*

Blue hands and feet alone may mean the baby is cold. Check for routes of heat loss and measure the baby's temperature.

How Do You Score Pulse (Heart Rate)?

5. *Listen* to the chest with a stethoscope and tap your finger each time the baby's heart beats. This allows another observer to see how fast the heart is beating.

   and/or

6. *Feel* the umbilical cord pulsation or the femoral pulse and count the heart rate out loud.

7. Determine the baby's heart rate.

   a. If the heart rate is *above 100 beats per minute (bpm),* give a *score of 2.*

   b. If the heart rate is *below 100 bpm,* give a *score of 1.*

   c. If the heart rate is *absent,* give a *score of 0.*

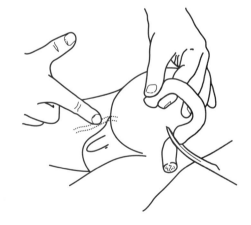

ACTIONS   REMARKS

How Do You Score Grimace (Reflex Irritability)?

8. *Stimulate* by inserting a catheter into the nose.

   a. If the baby *coughs or sneezes* when a catheter is placed *in the nose,* give a *score of 2.*

   b. If the baby only *grimaces* or "makes a face" when a *catheter* is placed *in the nose,* give a *score of 1.*

   c. If the baby has *no response* to this stimulus, give a *score of 0.*

Insert catheter into the NOSE ONLY.

Care must be taken not to stimulate the back of the throat excessively because this may lead to bradycardia or even cardiac arrest.

How Do You Score Activity (Muscle Tone)?

9. *Look* at the baby and *feel* the extremities.

   a. If the extremities are *well-flexed,* give a *score of 2.*

   b. If the extremities are only *slightly flexed* and the baby feels *somewhat limp,* give a *score of 1* (not illustrated).

   c. If the extremities are completely *extended and limp,* give a *score of 0.*

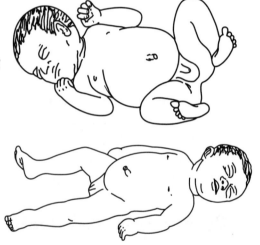

How Do You Score Respirations (Respiratory Effort)?

10. *Look* at the baby.

    a. If the baby has good respirations or is *crying,* give a *score of 2.*

    b. If the baby is taking *weak or slow, irregular breaths,* give a *score of 1.*

    c. If the baby is making *no respiratory effort* at all, give a *score of 0.*

ACTIONS **REMARKS**

Recording the Apgar Score

11. Use a form similar to the one below to record
    - The individual components of the score
    - Whatever resuscitation measures are being performed at each time point
    - A narrative describing the activities of the resuscitation, when each action occurred, which personnel were present and the role of each person

The Apgar score is often referred to later as an indication of how compromised the baby was during the few minutes following birth. Each of the components will be affected by resuscitation activities taking place at the time the score is assigned. For example, a pink color will have different implications if a baby is not being resuscitated versus a baby who is receiving chest compressions and positive-pressure ventilation with 100% oxygen.

APGAR SCORE Gestational Age _____ weeks

SIGN	0	1	2	1 minute	5 minutes	10 minutes	15 minutes	20 minutes
Color	Blue or Pale	Acrocyanotic	Completely Pink					
Heart Rate	Absent	<100 minute	>100 minute					
Reflex Irritability	No Response	Grimace	Cry or Active Withdrawal					
Muscle Tone	Limp	Some Flexion	Active Motion					
Respiration	Absent	Weak Cry; Hypoventilation	Good, crying					
TOTAL								

Comments:	Resuscitation					
	Minutes	1	5	10	15	20
	Oxygen					
	PPV/NCPAP					
	ETT					
	Chest Compressions					
	Epinephrine					

Reproduced with permission from The Apgar Score. ACOG Committee Opinion No. 333. American College of Obstetricians and Gynecologists. *Obstet Gynecol.* 2006;107(5):1209-1212.

Unit 6: Gestational Age and Size and Associated Risk Factors

221

Objectives

In this unit you will learn to

A. Define gestational aging and sizing of newborns.

B. Perform a systematic physical and neuromuscular examination of a newborn.

C. Use this physical and neuromuscular examination to estimate a baby's gestational age.

D. Determine if a baby is small, appropriate, or large for gestational age.

E. Recognize risk factors associated with each size and gestational age category of newborns.

F. Respond to risk factors with appropriate monitoring measures and screening tests.

G. Identify special measures that should be taken for late preterm and extremely preterm babies.

Unit 6 Pretest

Before reading the unit, please answer the following questions. Select the *one* best answer to each question (unless otherwise instructed). Record your answers on the test and check them against the answers at the end of the book.

1. **True   False**   All babies weighing less than 2,500 g (5 lb, 8 oz) are preterm.

2. Preterm babies are those babies whose gestational age is less than
   - **A.** 36 weeks
   - ✓ **B.** 37 weeks
   - **C.** 40 weeks
   - **D.** 42 weeks

3. For which of the following problems is a large-for-gestational-age baby, born at term, at *highest* risk?
   - **A.** Hypothermia (low body temperature)
   - **B.** Hypocalcemia (low blood calcium)
   - **C.** Hyperbilirubinemia
   - **D.** Hypoglycemia (low blood glucose)

Use the chart below to answer questions 4, 5, and 6.

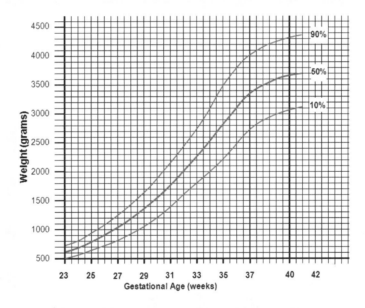

4a. A baby weighs 1,500 g (3 lb, 5 oz) at an estimated gestational age of 30 weeks, by physical and neuromuscular examination. What is the age category of this baby?
   - **A.** Preterm
   - **B.** Term
   - **C.** Post-term

4b. What is the size category of this baby?
   - **A.** Small for gestational age
   - **B.** Appropriate for gestational age
   - **C.** Large for gestational age

223

4c. Which of the following would you do for this baby?
 A. Begin early nipple feedings.
 B. Give sodium bicarbonate.
 C. Check the baby's temperature frequently.
 D. Obtain a baseline chest x-ray.

5a. A baby weighs 1,900 g (4 lb, 3 oz) and, by neuromuscular and physical examination, is at 40 weeks' gestational age. What is the age category of this baby?
 A. Preterm
 B. Term
 C. Post-term

5b. What is the size category of this baby?
 A. Small for gestational age
 B. Appropriate for gestational age
 C. Large for gestational age

5c. For which of the following problems is this baby at *highest* risk?
 A. Polycythemia (excess number of red blood cells)
 B. Apnea
 C. Hypernatremia
 D. Respiratory distress syndrome

6a. A baby weighs 1,200 g (2 lb, 10 oz) at birth and has a gestational age of 35 weeks, based on neuromuscular and physical examination. What is the size and gestational age category of this baby?
 A. Preterm, small for gestational age
 B. Term, appropriate for gestational age
 C. Term, small for gestational age
 D. Post-term, appropriate for gestational age

6b. For which of the following problems is this baby at *highest* risk?
 A. Hypercalcemia (high blood calcium)
 B. Birth injury
 C. Hypoglycemia (low blood glucose)
 D. Hyponatremia (low blood sodium)

1. What Is Gestational Age and Size?

Gestational age is a way of judging the maturity and relative size (compared to other newborns of the same maturity) of a newborn soon after birth. It can help you anticipate the problems a baby may develop. Knowing risk factors and using appropriate screening tests and care practices are the keys to prevention, or early detection and prompt treatment of, these problems.

Gestational age is the number of weeks that have passed between the

- First day of the mother's last menstrual period
- Date the baby is born

2. How Is Gestational Aging and Sizing Done?

A specialized 10-minute physical and neuromuscular examination gives an estimate of the baby's gestational age. This examination usually is quite reliable (particularly when confirmed by serial ultrasound), while a mother's dates are sometimes uncertain. The skill unit presents details of this examination.

Several signs, such as the baby's resting posture and the amount of breast tissue, are examined and noted on a chart. After completing the chart, you will have accurately determined (within 2 weeks) the gestational age of the baby being examined.

Term babies score between the beginning of the 37th week and completion of the 42nd week on the gestational-age examination. Preterm babies have immature physical signs, muscle tone,

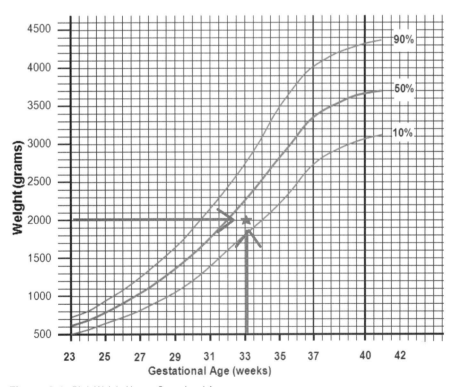

Figure 6.1. Birth Weight Versus Gestational Age.

225

and reflexes, and score below 37 weeks' gestational age on the examination. Post-term babies score above 42 completed weeks' gestational age on the examination.

Sizing of babies is done by weighing a baby soon after birth and then using a special graph to relate birth weight to gestational age.

3. How Do You Determine if a Baby Is Appropriate for Gestational Age, Small for Gestational Age, or Large for Gestational Age?

When you complete the examination, you know the baby's

- Gestational age in weeks
- Weight

Using these 2 factors (gestational age and weight), you determine if a baby is appropriate for gestational age (AGA), small for gestational age (SGA), or large for gestational age (LGA). Although other aspects of growth, such as length and head circumference, are also important factors to consider in a comprehensive assessment of fetal and neonatal health, this unit will focuses only on weight.

Plot the baby's gestational age and birth weight on the graph (Figure 6.1).* Babies with birth weights falling above the 90th percentile for their gestational ages are LGA. Likewise, babies with birth weights falling below the 10th percentile are SGA. Those babies with weights falling between 10% and 90% for their gestational ages are considered AGA (Figure 6.1).

Example:	You examine Baby Short and find he has a gestational age of 33 weeks. He weighs 2,000 g (4 lb, 6½ oz).
Problem:	Determine if Baby Short is AGA, SGA, or LGA.
Solution:	1. Find Baby Short's weight on the left side of the graph: 2,000 g.
	2. Find Baby Short's gestational age on the bottom of the graph: 33 weeks.
	3. Imagine a line running across the graph at 2,000 g.
	4. Imagine a line running up the graph at 33 weeks.
	5. Mark where the 2 lines meet. This is shown by the star (★) on the graph.
	6. The star lies between the 10th and 90th percentile lines, meaning Baby Short is AGA.
Answer:	Baby Short is preterm and AGA.

4. Which Babies Should Have Gestational Age and Size Assessment?

All babies should have their risks assessed. Gestational age and size determination is one component of risk assessment. Babies at particular risk because of their gestational age or size include

- Preterm or post-term
- Birth weight less than 2,500 g (5 lb, 8 oz)
- Birth weight greater than 4,000 g (8 lb, 13 oz)

---

*All growth curves in this unit are adapted with permission from Olsen IE, Groveman SA, Lawson ML, Clark RHH, Zemel BS. New intrauterine growth curves based on United States data. *Pediatrics*. 2010;125;e214-e224.

5. Why Do You Assess Gestational Age and Size in Newborns?

Determining gestational age and size will help you *anticipate* potential problems and *plan* for a baby's care.

- Babies who are preterm (<37 weeks), term (37 to 42 weeks), or post-term (>42 weeks) have certain characteristic problems.
- Babies who are LGA or SGA also have certain characteristic problems.
- Babies may be preterm or post-term *and* large or small for gestational age. These babies are at risk of developing the problems characteristic of their gestational age and the problems characteristic of their size.

All babies who are small are not necessarily preterm. They may be preterm OR they may be term or post-term and SGA.

All babies who are big are not necessarily term. They may be preterm and LGA.

The common problems associated with babies of different gestational ages and sizes are described in the remainder of this unit. The details for managing these problems are covered in subsequent units. For example, in this unit, you will learn which babies are at risk of developing hypoglycemia (low blood glucose), but the prevention, detection, and treatment of hypoglycemia are given in Unit 8, Hypoglycemia, in this book, and babies who are born preterm are likely to have immature lungs, but the identification and management of respiratory distress are covered in Book III: Neonatal Care, Unit 1, Oxygen, and Unit 2, Respiratory Distress.

6. When Should the Gestational Aging and Sizing Examination Be Performed?

The *Guidelines for Perinatal Care* states that each newborn's status and risks should be assessed no later than 2 hours after birth.* Sick or at-risk babies should have a gestational age and size examination as soon as possible after birth to prevent problems and plan care. History (maternal, labor, and delivery), physical examination, gestational age and size determination, and clinical tests (such as glucose screening test) are used to assess a baby's status and identify risks. For stable babies, gestational age and size determination is usually included as part of a baby's first examination shortly after birth.

The maturational assessment of gestational age (new Ballard score) shown in the skill unit may be used for all babies, whether they are sick, at risk, or well. The scoring system may be inaccurate, however, in babies who are lethargic as a result of illness or drugs. Gestational age may be estimated in such babies by eliminating the neuromuscular examination and doubling the physical maturity score, as will be described in the skill unit. When the baby's tone has improved, a complete examination may be done.

---

*American Academy of Pediatrics, American College of Obstetricians and Gynecologists. Care of the neonate. In: Lockwood CJ, Lemons JA. *Guidelines for Perinatal Care*. 6th ed. Elk Grove Village, IL: American Academy of Pediatrics; 2007:217.

Self-test

Now answer these questions to test yourself on the information in the last section. Use the chart to find the answers to the questions.

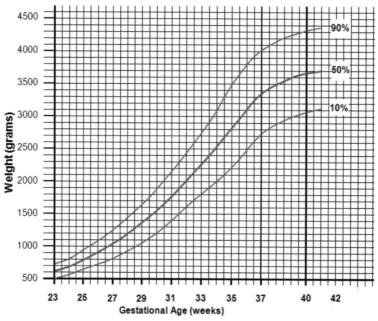

A1. You examine Baby Virginia and find she has a gestational age of 33 weeks. She weighs 3,000 g (6 lb, 10 oz). Is Baby Virginia preterm, term, or post-term? _____

Is she small for gestational age, appropriate for gestational age, or large for gestational age?

_____

A2. Baby Cook's examination shows she has a gestational age of 43 weeks. She weighs 2,500 g (4 lb, 6½oz). Is Baby Cook preterm, term, or post-term? _____

Is she small for gestational age, appropriate for gestational age, or large for gestational age?

_____

A3. Baby Ray's gestational age is 39 weeks. He weighs 2,800 g (6 lb, 3 oz).

Is Baby Ray preterm, term, or post-term? _____

Is he small for gestational age, appropriate for gestational age, or large for gestational age?

_____

A4. After a baby is born, the best way to determine the gestational age is by

_____.

A5. You can determine whether the baby is large, small, or of appropriate size by knowing the baby's gestational age and _____.

A6. It is important to know a baby's size and gestational age so that you can

_____

A7. **True**   **False**   Sick babies may have their gestational age estimated by eliminating the neuro-muscular examination and doubling the physical maturity score.

A8. **True**   **False**   All newborns should have their status and risks assessed between 6 and 12 hours after birth.

Check your answers with the list that follows the Recommended Routines. Correct any incorrect answers and review the appropriate section in the unit.

7. What Should You Think About When a Baby Is Term?

The shaded part of Figure 6.2 is the gestational age range that is technically defined as "Term," that is, 37 weeks, 0 days, through a completed 42 weeks (42 weeks, 7 days). However, the American College of Obstetricians and Gynecologists generally considers any gestation that proceeds beyond 41 weeks to be an indication for delivery and also recommends not performing an elective delivery (induction or cesarean section) before 39 weeks, unless there is a medical reason for doing so.

8. What Should You Think About When a Baby Is Preterm?

The shaded part of Figure 6.3 represents preterm babies regardless of size. Preterm babies have certain characteristic problems requiring attention. They are as follows:

A. Respiratory Distress

Difficulty breathing may be due to respiratory distress syndrome (RDS). This problem comes from immature lungs and may lead to low blood oxygen.
- Evaluate respiratory status.
- Consider surfactant therapy and ventilatory support.
- Monitor arterial blood gases and use continuous pulse oximetry for babies receiving oxygen therapy.
- Provide adequate nutrition and consider intravenous fluids.
- Screen for retinopathy of prematurity according to guidelines given later in this unit (Section 15J and in Book IV: Specialized Newborn Care, Unit 6, Continuing Care for At-Risk Babies).

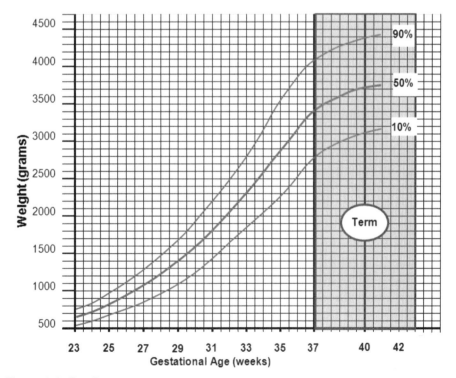

Figure 6.2. Term Zone.

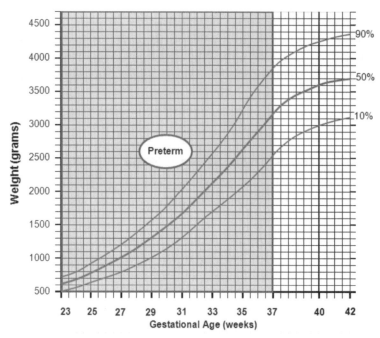

Figure 6.3. Preterm Zone.

B. Hypoglycemia (low blood glucose)

Preterm babies have low glucose stores and may become hypoglycemic. If this is not corrected, the baby may develop neurologic injury.
- Obtain blood glucose screening tests.
- Provide enteral or intravenous fluids and nutrition.

C. Hypothermia (low body temperature)

A preterm baby can become cold very easily. Just the right environmental temperature will be needed so the baby does not need to use extra energy to keep warm.
- Use neutral thermal environment. (See Unit 7, Thermal Environment, in this book.)
- Take temperature frequently.
- Minimize conductive, convective, evaporative, and radiant heat loss.

D. Feeding Difficulties

A preterm baby may be able to suck but not be able to coordinate sucking with breathing and swallowing. If the baby cannot coordinate these actions, milk may go into the lungs instead of the stomach. Babies who are less than 32 to 34 weeks' gestational age usually cannot coordinate sucking, swallowing, and breathing.
- Feed by orogastric or nasogastric tube and intravenous (IV) fluids.

E. Hypotension (low blood pressure)

A preterm baby may have low blood pressure from having received insufficient blood from the placenta, loss of blood at the time of delivery, an infection, or too much acid in the blood.
- Take blood pressure measurements.
- Consider volume expansion or pressor medications.

230

F. Anemia (low red blood cell count)

Preterm babies may have a lower red blood cell count than other babies. Because red blood cells carry oxygen, sick preterm babies may need a blood transfusion.
- Check hematocrit and/or hemoglobin.

G. Hyperbilirubinemia (high blood bilirubin level)

Preterm babies frequently become jaundiced because their livers are immature and do not get rid of bilirubin as well as more mature livers in older babies. Hyperbilirubinemia can lead to brain damage.
- Observe for jaundice.
- Check bilirubin levels.

H. Apnea (abnormally long breathing pauses)

Preterm babies may develop apnea. At times, these spells may cause the baby to have bradycardia (heart rate less than 80 beats per minute), become blue, need oxygen, or require assisted ventilation.
- Continuously monitor heart rate and respiratory pattern with electronic equipment.

I. Sepsis (blood infection)

One of the common causes for preterm labor and delivery is maternal infection. This infection may be passed to the fetus. Although a baby may not appear sick immediately at birth, preterm newborns should be considered at high risk of developing sepsis.
- Observe for signs of sepsis.
- Consider obtaining cultures and starting antibiotics.

J. Maternal Substance Use

Maternal cocaine use has been associated with preterm labor and delivery. Investigate maternal substance use, particularly if there are no other clearly identifiable risk factors for preterm delivery.
- Obtain thorough history regarding substance use.
- Consider social service referral.

9. What Should You Think About When a Baby Is Post-term?

Note: Technically, the official designation of "post-term" is defined as any gestation beyond 42 completed weeks (ie, 42 weeks + 7 days). However, the American College of Obstetricians and Gynecologists generally considers any gestation that proceeds beyond 41 weeks to be an indication for delivery.

Typical problems of babies born post-term include the following:

A. Perinatal Compromise

Post-term babies often do not tolerate labor well and may require resuscitation at birth. They may have had a period of hypoxia or decreased blood flow during labor or delivery.
- Evaluate for possible complications following resuscitation.

B. Respiratory Distress

Babies who are post-term are more likely to be born through meconium-stained amniotic fluid. They may have aspirated meconium and developed pneumonia. These babies also may develop a pneumothorax (ruptured lung) soon after delivery, especially if assisted ventilation is needed. Post-term babies are also at higher risk of developing persistent pulmonary hypertension of the newborn (PPHN), especially if they experienced an episode of low blood oxygen and/or acidosis.

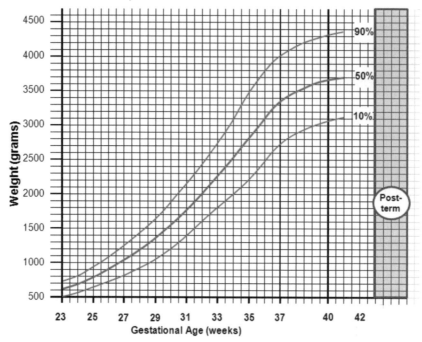

Figure 6.4. Post-term Zone.

- Evaluate respiratory status.
- Maintain normal blood oxygen levels and pH; do not remove a baby who requires oxygen therapy from the oxygen for even a few seconds for *any reason*.

C. Hypoglycemia (low blood glucose)

Placental function often begins to deteriorate in post-term pregnancies, resulting in inadequate nutrients going to the fetus. The fetus's own glucose stores may then be used for growth and energy. Therefore, a post-term baby may be born with low glucose stores and be more likely to develop hypoglycemia. Hypoglycemia can cause brain damage.

- Obtain blood glucose screening tests.
- Provide fluids and nutrition.

D. Fetal abnormalities

Fetal abnormalities, especially of the central nervous system, are among the causes of delayed onset of labor.

10. What Should You Think About if a Baby Is Small for Gestational Age?

Babies who are SGA are at risk of developing certain typical problems requiring action, including the following:

A. Hypoglycemia (low blood glucose)

Babies who are small for gestational age may have low glucose stores. This may lead to hypoglycemia and then to neurologic damage.

- Obtain blood glucose screening tests.
- Provide fluids and nutrition.

Weight (grams)
4500
4000
3500
3000
2500
2000
1500
1000
500
90%
50%
10%
SGA
23
25
27
29
31
33
35
37
40
42
Gestational Age (weeks)

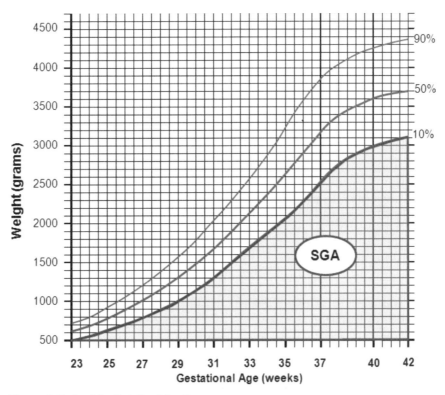

Figure 6.5. Small-for-Gestational-Age Zone.

B. Respiratory Distress

Babies who are SGA often tolerate labor poorly and may require resuscitation at birth. They may develop a pneumothorax (ruptured lung) or inhale fluid or meconium into their lungs.

- Evaluate for possible complications following resuscitation.
- Evaluate respiratory status.

C. Congenital Malformations and/or Congenital Infections

Babies who are SGA may have been born to women who had an infection during pregnancy. There are more congenital defects noted in babies who are SGA than in other babies.

- Evaluate for malformations.
- Evaluate for congenital infection.

D. Polycythemia (high red blood cell count)

Babies who are SGA frequently have thick blood from an increased number of red blood cells and, therefore, have high hematocrit and hemoglobin levels. Polycythemia may lead to severe problems by clogging vessels in the brain, lungs, and intestines.

- Check hematocrit and/or hemoglobin.

E. Maternal Substance Use

Babies who are SGA may have been born to women who use alcohol, cigarettes, heroin, amphetamines, cocaine, and/or other street drugs.

- Investigate maternal history for substance use.
- Consider social service referral.

11. What Should You Think About if a Baby Is Large for Gestational Age?

Babies who are LGA have certain typical problems requiring attention, including the following:

A. Birth Injury

Babies who are LGA may be of sufficient size to lead to a difficult labor and delivery; birth injury can result.
- Evaluate for birth injuries.
- Evaluate for possible complications following resuscitation.

B. Hypoglycemia (low blood glucose)

Babies who are LGA are often born to women with diabetes mellitus or abnormal glucose tolerance during pregnancy. These babies are not diabetic themselves and may have high insulin levels in response to their mothers' high glucose levels. After they are born, and no longer have their mothers' blood glucose supply, their high insulin levels may cause their blood glucose to fall. Even if a woman is not a known diabetic, every baby who is LGA should be checked carefully for low blood glucose. Hypoglycemia can lead to brain damage.
- Obtain blood glucose screening tests.
- Provide fluids and nutrition.

C. Respiratory Distress Syndrome

Babies born to women with diabetes mellitus have a higher incidence of RDS, even at gestational ages when most babies would not develop RDS.
- Evaluate respiratory status.

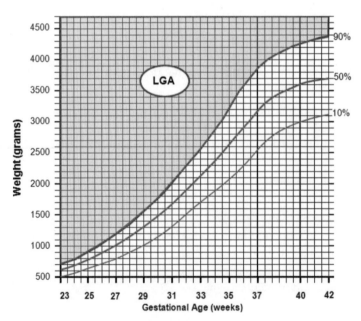

Figure 6.6. Large-for-Gestational-Age Zone.

12. What Should You Think About if a Baby Is Preterm and Small for Gestational Age?

Some babies may be preterm and smaller than expected for their gestational age. These babies are likely to have problems of prematurity and of being SGA. Anticipate and monitor for these characteristic problems, including

- Breathing difficulties (RDS, pneumothorax, or aspiration pneumonia)
- Hypothermia
- Hypoglycemia
- Feeding difficulty
- Hypotension
- Hyperbilirubinemia
- Apnea
- Anemia or polycythemia
- Congenital infection and/or malformation
- Sepsis
- Possible exposure to maternal substance use

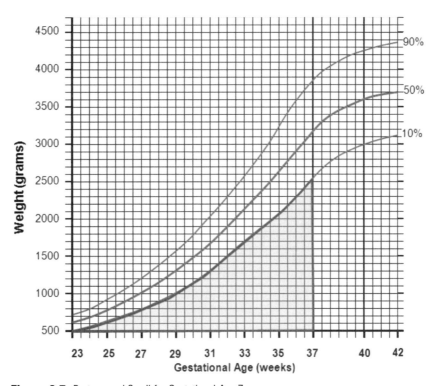

Figure 6.7. Preterm and Small-for-Gestational-Age Zone.

13. What Should You Think About if a Baby Is Preterm and Large for Gestational Age?

Some babies may be big babies, but also may be preterm (Figure 6.8).

These babies are likely to have problems of prematurity and of being LGA. Anticipate and monitor for these characteristic problems, including

- Respiratory distress syndrome
- Hypothermia
- Hypoglycemia
- Feeding difficulty
- Hypotension
- Hyperbilirubinemia
- Apnea
- Anemia
- Sepsis

Study Table 6.1 and Table 6.2. Table 6.1 lists the common problems of babies who are preterm, post-term, SGA, and LGA. Table 6.2 lists the actions that you should take *routinely* to screen and monitor babies for these typical problems.

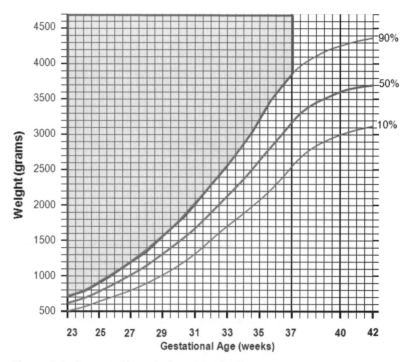

Figure 6.8. Preterm and Large-for-Gestational-Age Zone.

Table 6.1. Risk Factors for Babies of Different Sizes and Gestational Ages*

	SGA	AGA	LGA
Preterm	Combination of preterm and SGA ⟶ problems ↓	1. Respiratory distress syndrome (RDS) 2. Hypoglycemia 3. Hypothermia 4. Feeding difficulties 5. Hypotension 6. Anemia 7. Hyperbilirubinemia 8. Apnea 9. Sepsis 10. Maternal substance use	Combination of ⟵preterm and LGA problems ↓

Term	1. Hypoglycemia
	2. Perinatal compromise
	3. Respiratory distress
	  a. Pneumothoraces
	  b. Aspiration pneumonia
	4. Congenital malformations and/or congenital infections
	5. Polycythemia
	6. Maternal substance use
			1. Hypoglycemia
			2. Birth injury
			3. Perinatal compromise
			4. Respiratory distress syndrome (RDS)

Post-term	↑ Combination of post-term and ⟶ SGA problems	1. Perinatal compromise
		2. Respiratory distress
		  a. Pneumothoraces
		  b. Aspiration pneumonia
		  c. Persistent pulmonary hypertension of the newborn (PPHN)
		3. Hypoglycemia
			↑ Combination of ⟵ post-term and LGA problems

*SGA, small for gestational age; AGA, appropriate for gestational age; LGA, large for gestational age; RDS, respiratory distress syndrome.

Table 6.2. Actions to Evaluate Babies of Different Sizes and Gestational Ages*		
	SGA	AGA	LGA
Preterm	Combination of actions for → preterm and SGA ↓	1. Evaluate respiratory status. 2. Obtain blood glucose screening tests. 3. Determine neutral thermal environment; take temperature frequently. 4. Evaluate ability to feed orally. 5. Take blood pressure measurements. 6. Check hematocrit. 7. Observe for jaundice. 8. Continuously monitor heart rate and/or respiratory pattern (especially <1,800 g and/or <35 weeks). 9. Evaluate for signs of sepsis. 10. Investigate maternal history for substance use.	Combination of ← actions for preterm and LGA ↓
Term	1. Evaluate for possible complications following resuscitation. 2. Evaluate respiratory status. 3. Obtain blood glucose screening tests. 4. Evaluate for malformations/congenital infections. 5. Check hematocrit. 6. Evaluate maternal history for substance use.		1. Obtain blood glucose screening tests. 2. Evaluate for birth injuries. 3. Evaluate for possible complications following resuscitation. 4. Evaluate respiratory status.
Post-term	↑ Combination of actions for → post-term and SGA	1. Evaluate for possible complications following resuscitation. 2. Evaluate respiratory status. 3. Obtain blood glucose screening tests. 4. Evaluate ability to feed orally. 5. If supplemental oxygen needed, monitor oxygenation and pH.	↑ Combination of ← actions for post-term and LGA

*SGA, small for gestational age; AGA, appropriate for gestational age; LGA, large for gestational age; RDS, respiratory distress syndrome.

Self-test

Now answer these questions to test yourself on the information in the last section.

B1. Which of the following problems are more likely to occur in preterm babies who are appropriate for gestational age?

Yes	No	
____	____	Congenital malformations
____	____	Apnea
____	____	Meconium aspiration
____	____	Anemia

Use the chart below to answer the questions that follow it.

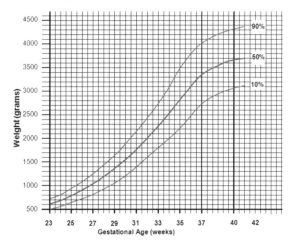

B2a. A newborn weighs 3,430 g (7 lb, 9 oz) and is estimated to be at 32 weeks' gestation. Describe the baby as appropriate for gestational age, large for gestational age, or small for gestational age, and term, preterm, or post-term.

_____

B2b. Which of the following problems are more likely to occur in this baby?

Yes	No	
____	____	Sepsis
____	____	Respiratory distress syndrome
____	____	Hypertension
____	____	Hypoglycemia

B3a. A baby weighs 1,390 g (3 lb, 1 oz) and, by neuromuscular/physical examination, was estimated to be at 36 weeks' gestational age. Describe the baby as appropriate for gestational age, large for gestational age, or small for gestational age, and term, preterm, or post-term.

_____

B3b. Which of the following is important to do for *all* babies of this category?
   A. Restrict fluid intake.
   B. Obtain blood glucose screening tests.
   C. Place in supplemental oxygen.

Check your answers with the list that follows the Recommended Routines. Correct any incorrect answers and review the appropriate section in the unit.

As well as the 6 categories described to this point (preterm, term, post-term, SGA, AGA, and LGA), 2 additional categories require special attention. These are both subcategories of "Preterm."

- Late Preterm (34 0/7 weeks to 36 6/7 weeks)
- Extremely Preterm (less than 28 weeks' gestation)

14. What Should You Think About When a Baby Is Late Preterm?

Babies born after 33 completed weeks of gestation, but before term, may initially appear healthy, but are at risk of developing many of the problems associated with prematurity (Figure 6.9). In particular, they should be evaluated and treated as necessary for the following problems:

- Respiratory distress (RDS, transient tachypnea, or pneumonia)
- Hypothermia from low fat stores
- Hypoglycemia from low liver glycogen
- Poor feeding from immature suck patterns
- Exaggerated jaundice from an immature liver

15. What Should You Think About if a Baby Is Extremely Preterm?

Babies born extremely preterm (<28 weeks' gestation), often weighing less than 1,000 g (2 lb, 3 oz), have the characteristic problems of any preterm baby, as well as special problems related to being extremely preterm. The particular points listed in the following text are *in addition* to care considerations listed earlier for all preterm newborns.

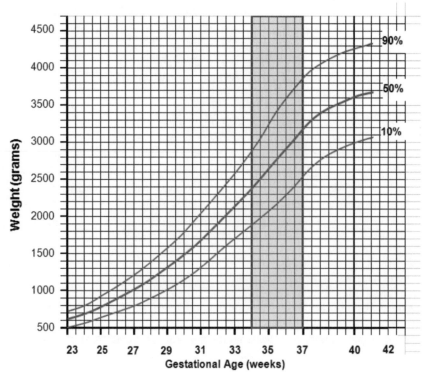

Figure 6.9. Late Preterm Zone.

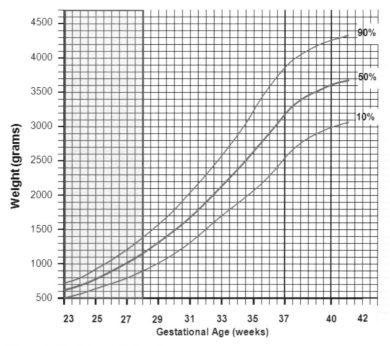

Figure 6.10. Extremely Preterm Zone.

While almost all tiny babies will require management in a regional intensive care nursery, they could be born in *any* hospital. The care these tiny babies receive during the first few hours after birth is vitally important to their long-term outcome.

A. Respiratory Distress

A very small baby who has respiratory distress at birth is likely to have RDS. Extremely preterm babies may, however, have more problems than usual in clearing lung secretions. These small babies tire easily and quickly. Even mild RDS can cause them to develop low blood oxygen (Pao_2 and Spo_2) and high carbon dioxide ($Paco_2$). Many of these very small babies will require assisted ventilation.

- Evaluate respiratory status.
- Monitor arterial blood gases; use continuous pulse oximetry.
- Provide CPAP or intubate for assisted ventilation when necessary.
- Consider administering surfactant therapy.

B. Hypoglycemia (low blood glucose)/Hyperglycemia (high blood glucose)

Very preterm babies have low glucose stores and may become hypoglycemic; any stress increases the likelihood of this occurring. If hypoglycemia is not corrected, brain damage can occur.

When given intravenous (IV) fluids, however, very tiny babies may develop *high* blood glucose. High blood glucose can cause an increase in urine glucose and may result in excessive fluid losses in the urine.

In general, IV fluid therapy of D5W with amino acids should be used initially for extremely preterm babies. After several days of age, an extremely preterm baby may be able to tolerate glucose higher than D5W without spilling glucose into the urine.

Because tiny babies can easily become hypoglycemic or hyperglycemic, glucose monitoring is especially important.
- Monitor blood glucose.
- Monitor urine glucose.
- Use D5W IV fluid initially (with amino acids if available); adjust according to blood and urine glucose monitoring.

C. Hypothermia (low body temperature)

Extremely preterm babies can become cold easily and quickly. Even slight cold stress can cause a tiny baby to become sick or worsen already-existing problems such as low blood oxygen or hypoglycemia.

Great care must be taken to minimize heat loss from the moment a baby is born. Because these babies usually require intensive intervention and monitoring, they are best cared for initially under radiant warmers with servo control.
- Use plastic wrap and chemically activated warming mattress in the delivery room.
- Use radiant warmer with servo control.
- Take temperature frequently.
- Minimize conductive, convective, evaporative, and radiant heat loss.
- Avoid nonessential procedures.

 Preventing hypothermia is critically important in the management of tiny babies.

D. Hydration (fluid intake)

Tiny babies, even if they are not sick, should not be fed immediately by mouth or tube. They should have IV fluids started.

Because tiny babies have thin skin and a large surface area-to-weight ratio, they lose a great deal of fluid through their skin. Fluid requirements are greater than for larger babies. Tiny babies require extra fluids to prevent dehydration. For babies who are under radiant warmers, placing plastic wrap across the sides of the warmer bed, over the baby (or using a clear plastic "body tent"), helps decrease water losses and maintain temperature.
- Feed by tube when clinically stable, and introduce oral feeds when developmentally appropriate.
- Weigh the baby so accurate fluid requirements can be calculated (weigh *carefully*— avoid over-handling the baby and/or causing cold stress).
- Start IV fluids; if a tiny baby will stay in your hospital for longer than several hours, consult regional center staff because fluid and nutrition management are complex.
- Place a clear plastic covering over the baby. (Be sure this does not pose a hazard to the baby's airway.)

E. Hypotension (low blood pressure)

An extremely preterm baby's blood pressure may seem dangerously low when, in fact, it is normal for the baby's size. If there is no history of blood loss, the baby does not have a metabolic acidosis or appear poorly perfused (paleness or a mottled color of the skin), and the volume of urine output is acceptable (1 to 2 mL/kg/hr), the arterial blood pressure is likely adequate.

As a general guideline for extremely preterm babies (24 to 28 weeks' gestation), a baby's acceptable *mean* arterial pressure will be about the same as the baby's gestational age. For example, a mean blood pressure of 26 mm Hg may be appropriate for a baby of 26 weeks' gestation.
- Monitor blood pressure frequently.
- Correct hypotension very carefully and slowly.

F. Anemia (low red blood cell count)
Extremely preterm babies may have a lower red blood cell count than other babies. Because their blood volume is so small (<3 oz or 90 mL/kg), even small amounts of blood drawn for laboratory tests may make the baby anemic and, possibly, hypotensive.
- Check hematocrit and/or hemoglobin.
- Withdraw smallest volumes of blood needed to perform laboratory tests; record and tally amount withdrawn.
- Consider a transfusion of packed red blood cells if large amounts of blood are withdrawn or if the baby becomes hypotensive.

G. Hyperbilirubinemia (high blood bilirubin level)
Very preterm babies usually become jaundiced because their livers are immature and do not get rid of bilirubin as well as the livers of older babies. Preterm babies bruise easily, and bruising also can contribute to increased bilirubin. Increased amounts of bilirubin may cause brain damage. Very preterm babies are at risk of developing brain damage at lower bilirubin levels than older babies.
- Consider checking bilirubin levels before jaundice is seen, especially if bruising is present.
- Check bilirubin levels frequently.
- Initiate phototherapy at lower levels of bilirubin than recommended for moderately preterm newborns.

H. Apnea (breathing pauses longer than 20 seconds or associated with bradycardia and/or oxygen desaturations)
Extremely preterm babies have a nearly 100% chance of developing apnea. At times, these spells can cause the baby to have bradycardia (heart rate less than 80 beats per minute), become blue, and require oxygen. Occasionally, a tiny baby will have life-threatening apnea that requires vigorous stimulation, ventilation with a bag and mask, or intubation. Babies with severe spells must have the underlying cause(s) investigated and treated. If no cause is found or if treatment is initiated but a baby still has severe spells, the baby usually will require assisted ventilation or medication administration.
- Monitor heart rate continuously with electronic equipment.
- Investigate cause(s) of apnea.
- Consider respiratory stimulants, such as caffeine.
- Assist baby's ventilation if apnea is severe.

I. Intracranial Hemorrhage (bleeding in the brain)
An extremely preterm baby is more likely than other babies to develop bleeding in the brain or in the ventricles (fluid-filled chambers within the brain). This bleeding can cause brain damage. Possible causes of intracranial bleeding include sudden changes in blood pressure, rapid infusion of blood replacement or volume expanders, inadequate blood

supply from placenta, rapid infusion of high concentrations of glucose or other hypertonic solutions, high serum sodium, and pneumothorax (lung rupture).

- Monitor hematocrit and/or hemoglobin.
- Handle the baby gently.
- Avoid sudden changes in fluid management, ventilatory management, and other care practices.

J. Retinopathy of Prematurity (ROP) (eye disease of prematurity)
Tiny babies are at great risk of developing some degree of ROP, an eye condition that can progress to total blindness, or go away completely. Some factors associated with the development of ROP are extreme prematurity, prolonged oxygen treatment, high blood oxygen levels, and the severity of certain complications of prematurity (such as sepsis and apnea).

- Monitor arterial blood gases and use continuous pulse oximetry.
- Adjust inspired oxygen concentration (FIO_2) to avoid excessively high blood oxygen (PaO_2 or SpO_2).
- Arrange for an eye examination with an ophthalmologist experienced with ROP who can perform a dilated funduscopic examination for babies. (See Book IV: Specialized Newborn Care, Unit 8, Continuing Care.)

K. Chronic Lung Disease (CLD, formerly known as bronchopulmonary dysplasia)
Extremely preterm babies frequently require ventilator support and supplemental oxygen for prolonged periods. These babies are likely to develop CLD, and sometimes need a protracted course of supplemental oxygen and medications for their lung disease.

- Consider early administration of surfactant.
- Use ventilator support that is as gentle as possible.
- Use lowest concentration of supplemental oxygen that maintains adequate blood oxygenation.

 All care providers should keep in mind that it is important to handle preterm babies gently, especially extremely preterm babies, and to avoid unnecessary handling of these tiny babies.

The appropriate techniques for developmental care of extremely preterm babies is an evolving practice. Long-term care of such tiny babies usually is provided in regional medical centers and, therefore, is not addressed in this program.

Self-test

Now answer these questions to test yourself on the information in the last section.

C1. For which of the following problems is an *extremely* preterm baby at *highest* risk?
  A. Meconium aspiration
  B. Intracranial hemorrhage
  C. Hyperthermia
  D. Hypercalcemia

C2. In which of the following babies is retinopathy of prematurity *most* likely to develop?
  A. Preterm baby
  B. Small-for-gestational-age baby
  C. Large-for-gestational-age baby
  D. Extremely preterm baby

C3. **True** **False** The only glucose problem seen in very tiny preterm babies is hypoglycemia.

C4. **True** **False** A blood transfusion may be needed if a total of 5 mL or more of blood is withdrawn from a tiny baby for laboratory tests.

C5. The risk of intracranial hemorrhage can be reduced in tiny babies if _____ infusion of blood, volume expanders, and concentrated intravenous solutions are *avoided*.

Check your answers with the list that follows the Recommended Routines. Correct any incorrect answers and review the appropriate section in the unit.

Gestational Age and Size and Associated Risk Factors

Recommended Routines

All the routines listed below are based on the principles of perinatal care presented in the unit you have just finished. They are recommended as part of routine perinatal care.

Read each routine carefully and decide whether it is standard operating procedure in your hospital. Check the appropriate blank next to each routine.

Procedure Standard in My Hospital	Needs Discussion by Our Staff	
_____	_____	1. Establish a policy of performing a gestational aging and sizing examination on all newborns within 2 hours of birth.
_____	_____	2. Establish a policy of classifying each baby as small for gestational age, appropriate for gestational age, or large for gestational age, and preterm, term, or post-term, and recording the findings in each baby's medical record.
_____	_____	3. Develop standing orders to implement appropriate actions for each gestational age and size category.
_____	_____	4. Develop special procedures for identifying and caring for babies born late preterm or extremely preterm.
_____	_____	5. Establish a policy of evaluating the status and assessing risk (including history, gestational age and size, and clinical tests [as appropriate]) of each newborn within 2 hours after birth.
_____	_____	6. Establish a policy to discourage elective cesarean section prior to 39 weeks' gestation, without specific medical indication.

247

Self-test Answers

These are the answers to the self-test questions. Please check them with the answers you gave and review the information in the unit wherever necessary.

A1. Baby Virginia is preterm and large for gestational age.

A2. Baby Cook is post-term and small for gestational age.

A3. Baby Ray is term and appropriate for gestational age.

A4. Physical and neuromuscular examination

A5. Weight

A6. *Anticipate* problems common to the baby's size and gestational age and *plan* appropriate care measures.

A7. True

A8. False.　Assessment of each baby's status and risks should be made no later than 2 hours after birth.

B1.
Yes	No	
___	X	Congenital malformations
X	___	Apnea
___	X	Meconium aspiration
X	___	Anemia

B2a. Preterm, large for gestational age

B2b.
Yes	No	
X	___	Sepsis
X	___	Respiratory distress syndrome
___	X	Hypertension
X	___	Hypoglycemia

B3a. Preterm, small for gestational age

B3b. B.　Obtain blood glucose screening tests.

C1. B.　Intracranial hemorrhage

C2. D.　Extremely preterm baby

C3. False.　Hyperglycemia (high blood glucose) may occur. This can cause glucose to spill into the urine and lead to excessive fluid losses.

C4. True

C5. Rapid

Unit 6 Posttest

If you are applying for continuing education credits, a posttest for this unit is available online. Completion of unit posttests and the book evaluation form are required to achieve continuing education credit. For more details, go to www.cmevillage.com.

SKILL UNIT

Estimating Gestational Age by Examination of a Newborn

This skill unit will teach you how to determine a baby's gestational age using physical and neuromuscular signs. You will learn how to use the Ballard scoring system. The Ballard scoring system shown in this skill unit may be used for all babies, but may be temporarily inaccurate in babies who are lethargic as a result of illness or drugs. Gestational age may be estimated in such babies by eliminating the neuromuscular examination and doubling the physical maturity score. When the baby's tone has improved, a complete examination may be done.

You may be asked to watch a videotape showing the scoring system and/or attend a skill demonstration.

Jeanne L. Ballard, MD, the developer of the score, has produced a video titled, *New Ballard Score: A Maturational Assessment of Gestational Age Using the New Ballard Score.* The "new" score includes extremely preterm babies. The video is available at www.ballardscore.com.

Hard copies of the video and related materials are available through:

> Trihealth
> Corporate Educational Services
> 619 Oak St
> Cincinnati, OH 45206
> Phone: 513/569-6323
>   513/569-5470
> Fax: 513/569-5479

To master the skill, you will need to estimate correctly the gestational age and determine the size of at least 2 babies in your nursery. The accuracy of your physical and neuromuscular examinations, as well as your calculations of the babies' sizes, should be checked by comparison with results obtained independently by your coordinator(s) or others skilled in performing the examination and determining preterm, term, or post-term, and small-for-gestational-age, appropriate-for-gestational-age, or large-for-gestational-age status.

Use the charts on the following pages to record your findings while examining babies in your nursery. You should bring them to the bedside for reference during a skill session.

The charts also may be copied, or multiple copies may be purchased from the American Academy of Pediatrics (www.aap.org/bookstore).

MATURATIONAL ASSESSMENT OF GESTATIONAL AGE (New Ballard Score)

NAME_____   SEX _____

HOSPITAL NO. _____   BIRTH WEIGHT _____

RACE_____   LENGTH _____

DATE/TIME OF BIRTH _____   HEAD CIRC._____

DATE/TIME OF EXAM _____   EXAMINER _____

AGE WHEN EXAMINED _____

APGAR SCORE: 1 MINUTE _____5 MINUTES_____10 MINUTES_____

NEUROMUSCULAR MATURITY

NEUROMUSCULAR MATURITY SIGN	SCORE							RECORD SCORE HERE
	-1	0	1	2	3	4	5	
POSTURE								
SQUARE WINDOW (Wrist)	>90°	90°	60°	45°	30°	0°		
ARM RECOIL		180°	140–180°	110–140°	90–110°	<90°		
POPLITEAL ANGLE	180°	160°	140°	120°	100°	90°	<90°	
SCARF SIGN								
HEEL TO EAR								

TOTAL NEUROMUSCULAR MATURITY SCORE

PHYSICAL MATURITY

PHYSICAL MATURITY SIGN	SCORE							RECORD SCORE HERE
	-1	0	1	2	3	4	5	
SKIN	sticky friable transparent	gelatinous red translucent	smooth pink visible veins	superficial peeling &/or rash, few veins	cracking pale areas rare veins	parchment deep cracking no vessels	leathery cracked wrinkled	
LANUGO	none	sparse	abundant	thinning	bald areas	mostly bald		
PLANTAR SURFACE	heel-toe 40–50 mm: -1 < 40 mm: -2	>50 mm no crease	faint red marks	anterior transverse crease only	creases ant. 2/3	creases over entire sole		
BREAST	imperceptible	barely perceptible	flat areola no bud	stippled areola 1–2 mm bud	raised areola 3–4 mm bud	full areola 5–10 mm bud		
EYE / EAR	lids fused loosely: -1 tightly: -2	lids open pinna flat stays folded	sl. curved pinna; soft; slow recoil	well-curved pinna; soft but ready recoil	formed & firm instant recoil	thick cartilage ear stiff		
GENITALS (Male)	scrotum flat, smooth	scrotum empty faint rugae	testes in upper canal rare rugae	testes descending few rugae	testes down good rugae	testes pendulous deep rugae		
GENITALS (Female)	clitoris prominent & labia flat	prominent clitoris & small labia minora	prominent clitoris & enlarging minora	majora & minora equally prominent	majora large minora small	majora cover clitoris & minora		

TOTAL PHYSICAL MATURITY SCORE

SCORE
Neuromuscular _____
Physical _____
Total _____

MATURITY RATING

SCORE	WEEKS
-10	20
-5	22
0	24
5	26
10	28
15	30
20	32
25	34
30	36
35	38
40	40
45	42
50	44

GESTATIONAL AGE (weeks)

By dates _____
By ultrasound _____
By exam _____

Adapted from Ballard JL, Khoury JC, Wedig K, Wang L, Eilers-Walsman BL, Lipp R. New Ballard Score, expanded to include extremely premature infants. *J Pediatr.* 1991; 119:417-423, with permission from Elsevier.

4500
4000
3500
3000
2500
2000
1500
1000
500
Weight (grams)
LGA
AGA
SGA
90%
50%
10%
23
25
27
29
31
33
35
37
40
42
Gestational Age (weeks)
Preterm
Term
Post-term

4500
4000
3500
3000
2500
2000
1500
1000
500
Weight (grams)
90%
50%
10%
23
25
27
29
31
33
35
37
40
42
Gestational Age (weeks)

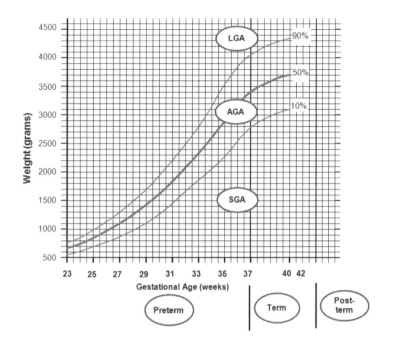

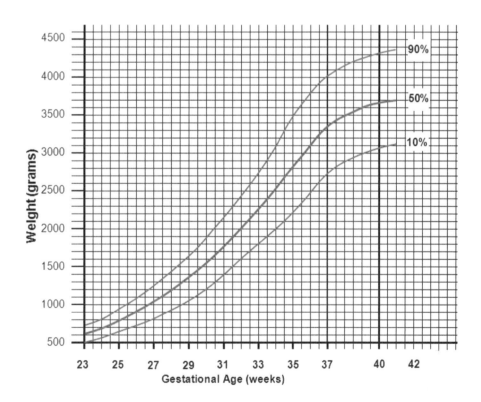

Unit 7: Thermal Environment

Objectives

In this unit you will learn

A. The causes and consequences of hypothermia (low body temperature) and hyperthermia (high body temperature)

B. How to minimize heat loss in newborns

C. How to control thermal environment to keep metabolic expenditure by a newborn to a minimum (neutral thermal environment)

D. How to operate radiant warmers and incubators

Unit 7 Pretest

Before reading the unit, please answer the following questions. Select the *one best* answer to each question (unless otherwise instructed). Record your answers on the test and check them against the answers at the end of the book.

1. An axillary temperature of 35.8°C (96.6°F) in a preterm newborn represents
   A. Hypothermia (low body temperature)
   B. Normal body temperature
   C. Hyperthermia (high body temperature)

2. Which of the following babies does *not* need to have his or her temperature checked more often than normal routine?
   A. A term baby with hypoglycemia
   B. A baby born at 32 weeks' gestation who is appropriate weight for gestational age
   C. A baby born at 40 weeks' gestation who is small for gestational age
   D. A baby born at 41 weeks' gestation who is appropriate weight for gestational age

3. Which of the following methods is *most* appropriate to regulate the temperature of a term baby who is small for gestational age, with hypoglycemia?
   A. Clothed, in a crib with blankets
   B. In an incubator, with the air temperature set at 36.0°C (96.8°F)
   C. Under a radiant warmer, with the servo control sensor set to keep the skin temperature of the baby's trunk at 36.5°C (97.8°F)
   D. In an incubator, with the air temperature set at 37.0°C (98.6°F)

4. Which of the following is *most* appropriate when a baby is receiving care under a radiant warmer?
   A. Set the radiant warmer to the baby's neutral thermal environment temperature and tape the servo control probe to the exposed side of his trunk.
   B. Set the servo control sensor to 36.5°C (97.8°F) and tape the probe to the exposed side of his trunk.
   C. Set the servo control sensor to 36.5°C (97.8°F) and tape the probe to the side of his trunk that is resting on the mattress.
   D. Set the servo control sensor to 35.5°C (97.0°F) and tape the probe to the side of his trunk that is resting on the mattress.

5. Which of the following methods of taking a baby's temperature is *not* recommended for frequent vital signs?
   A. Rectal
   B. Axillary
   C. Abdominal skin
   D. Any of the above methods is appropriate for frequent vital signs

6. True False A baby whose temperature is 35.2°C (95.4°F) should have a blood glucose screening test checked.

7. True False When a baby is in the appropriate neutral thermal environment temperature range in an incubator, the baby's rectal or axillary temperature will always be normal (37.0°C or 98.6°F).

8. True False An elevated temperature is most commonly caused by an infection in a baby.

9. True **False**   Incubator portholes that are left open can result in conductive heat loss.

10. True **False**   A newborn who has a skin temperature of 35.0°C (95.0°F) will have a higher metabolic rate than a baby who has a skin temperature of 36.5°C (97.8°F).

11. True **False**   Delayed drying of a baby after delivery promotes evaporative heat loss.

12. True **False**   A baby with a slightly low body temperature requires fewer calories and less oxygen than a baby with a normal temperature.

13. True **False**   During the first week after birth, the neutral thermal environmental range is the same for all babies of the same birth weight, regardless of gestational age.

1. What Is Temperature Control?

Temperature control means regulating a baby's body temperature with external equipment. If the thermal environment is properly controlled, a baby will not have to use extra oxygen and calories to produce heat. An otherwise healthy baby can become sick if cold stressed.

2. How Does a Baby Produce Heat?

Babies produce heat in a different way from adults. Babies have a special substance called brown fat. They use oxygen and calories to break down this brown fat to produce heat. Preterm and small-for-gestational-age babies have less brown fat than term babies and appropriate-for-gestational-age babies.

 Babies who are cold do not shiver to warm themselves.

Checking body temperature is the only way to know if a baby is cold.

3. How Does a Baby Lose Heat?

Babies can lose body heat *very* quickly. Body heat may be lost in any combination of 4 ways.

A. Conduction

Conductive heat loss occurs when a baby is in contact with cold objects. Examples of *preventing* conductive heat loss are
- Pre-warm receiving bed in the delivery room.
- Cover cold scale surface when weighing a baby.
- Change wet diapers and bed linens.

B. Convection

Convective heat loss occurs when cold air circulates around a baby. Examples of *preventing* convective heat loss are
- Keep delivery room warm.
- Put a hat on the baby soon after delivery.
- Keep the baby out of the draft of air conditioners.
- Keep incubator portholes closed when not working with the baby; work through portholes for procedures rather than opening the side of the incubator.
- Warm and humidify the oxygen/air mixture for babies receiving oxygen therapy.

C. Evaporation

Evaporative heat loss occurs when a liquid evaporates from a warm surface. When a baby is wet, evaporative heat loss increases significantly. Examples of *preventing* evaporative heat loss are
- Dry a baby quickly after delivery.
- Delay bathing a baby until body temperature is normal and stable for several hours.
- Change wet linen promptly.
- Warm and humidify the oxygen/air mixture for babies receiving oxygen therapy.

D. Radiation

Radiant heat loss occurs when a baby is near, but not in direct contact with, a cold object. The baby radiates heat to the nearest solid object. Adults experience radiant heat loss in a warm room on a cold day when they go near a closed window and feel a chill. They do not touch the window, but some of their body heat is transmitted or radiated to the cold windowpane. In much the same way, babies in incubators lose heat to the incubator wall, which has been cooled by the room temperature. Following are examples of *preventing* radiant heat loss:

• Keep nursery warm, even if a baby is in an incubator.
• Keep a baby away from cold windows and walls, especially if the baby is in an open crib or a single-walled incubator.*
• Use double-walled incubators whenever possible.*

In addition to the actions listed above, some babies may benefit from special measures to prevent heat loss. For example, chemically activated warming mattresses (commercially available) or a transport incubator may be useful while transporting sick or small babies from a delivery room to the nursery.

 Hypothermia (low body temperature) is hazardous for a baby.† Becoming chilled after delivery should not be an expected occurrence.

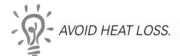 *AVOID HEAT LOSS.*

Self-test

Now answer these questions to test yourself on the information in the last section.

A1. How do babies produce heat to keep themselves warm?

_____

A2. **True**   **False**   Babies can keep themselves warm by shivering, as can adults.

A3. **True**   **False**   Babies use oxygen and calories to produce body heat.

A4. Give an example of conductive heat loss.

_____

A5. Give an example of convective heat loss.

_____

A6. Give an example of evaporative heat loss.

_____

A7. Give an example of radiant heat loss.

_____

Check your answers with the list that follows the Recommended Routines. Correct any incorrect answers and review the appropriate section in the unit.

---

*Radiant heat loss is more common with single-walled incubators. Double-walled incubators are designed to reduce radiant heat loss significantly because a layer of warm air between the walls keeps the inner wall at the neutral thermal environment temperature, while the outer wall may be much colder.

†One exception may be a baby born at term who experiences an asphyxial event may benefit from therapeutic hypothermia instituted within 6 hours of the event. (See Unit 5, Resuscitating the Newborn, in this book.)

4. How Are Temperatures Taken?

There are 3 acceptable ways to measure a baby's temperature.

A. Rectal

This is usually the first temperature taken after delivery. It gives a good estimate of deep body or core temperature, and checks patency of the anus.

Rectal measurement of a baby's temperature is seldom indicated after the initial measurement. Use of rectal thermometers may cause perforation of the colon or may result in cardiorespiratory instability due to vagal nerve stimulation.

 Measuring temperature rectally is not recommended for frequent or routine vital signs.

B. Axillary

This is the best way to take a baby's temperature for frequent vital signs. In most circumstances, an axillary temperature can be considered the same as the rectal temperature, as long as the baby's arm is kept next to his or her side while the temperature is being taken.

C. Skin

This is a convenient way to measure the temperature of a baby requiring a skin probe, such as when an incubator or radiant warmer is used in servo control mode. Skin temperatures are lower than axillary or rectal temperatures. Therefore, a baby's temperature also should be checked intermittently with an axillary measurement or, in some cases, a rectal measurement.

Note: Temperature measurements taken with an ear probe are a quick way to check a baby's temperature. Tympanic measurements, however, have *not* been shown to be reliable in neonates and, therefore, are *not* recommended.

5. How Should a Baby's Temperature Be Interpreted?

A. Normal

All babies (large, small, preterm, post-term, term) have the same normal temperature.
- Axillary or rectal: 37.0°C (98.6°F)
- Skin: 36.5°C (97.8°F)

 Although a single "normal" temperature is given above, it is clear that all babies will not have this exact temperature at all times. However, this normal value should be your goal when regulating any newborn's temperature.

B. Hyperthermia

An elevated or higher-than-normal temperature

Reasons for high body temperatures in newborns include the following:

1. Directly Overheating a Baby
   - Under a radiant warmer with the warmer set incorrectly
   - Under certain types of phototherapy lights

2. Overheating a Baby's Environment
   - In an incubator with the temperature set incorrectly
   - In a bassinet and over-bundled in a warm room

3. Blood Infection (Sepsis): In contrast to adults or older children, newborns usually do *not* have a fever when an infection is present. Some infected babies, however, will have elevated temperatures.

An overheated baby uses excessive oxygen and calories as the body's metabolism is increased. Because of a reduced ability to sweat, overheated babies may appear normal. Touching a baby's skin is not a reliable way to determine if a baby's body temperature is elevated. The only way to know if a newborn is overheated is to take the baby's temperature.

C. Hypothermia

A lower-than-normal temperature

Reasons for low body temperatures in newborns include the following:

1. Blood Infection (Sepsis): Hypothermia is more commonly a sign of sepsis than hyperthermia in a newborn.

2. Heat Loss to the Environment (by conduction, convection, evaporation, and/or radiation)

A cold baby cannot shiver and may appear normal. Low body temperature cannot be identified reliably by feeling a baby's skin. The only way to know if a newborn is hypothermic is to take the baby's temperature.

 Monitor each baby's temperature. If an abnormal temperature is found, investigate the cause.

Self-test

Now answer these questions to test yourself on the information in the last section.

B1. What are 3 acceptable ways to measure a baby's temperature?

_____

_____

B2. Which method of taking a baby's temperature is not recommended for routine vital signs?

_____

B3. Which 2 methods of taking a baby's temperature will show approximately the same body temperature?

_____ and _____

B4. What is the abdominal skin temperature of a normal, healthy baby?

_____

B5. Which of the following is the *most* common reason for an elevated temperature in a newborn?
  A. An infection
  B. Incubator air temperature set too high
  C. Being born preterm

B6. What are 2 common reasons a baby will have a lower-than-normal temperature?
  A. A blood infection (sepsis)
  B. Excess caloric intake
  C. Heat loss to the environment

Check your answers with the list that follows the Recommended Routines. Correct any incorrect answers and review the appropriate section in the unit.

6. What Happens When a Baby Is Chilled or Cold Stressed?

When babies are chilled, their metabolic rate increases. Three consequences of an increased metabolic rate are

- Hypoglycemia (low blood glucose)
- Acidosis (low blood pH)
- Hypoxia (inadequate oxygen for brain and body tissue)

A baby does not need to be severely cold stressed to develop hypoglycemia, acidosis, and/or hypoxia. Some babies will demonstrate these findings if their temperatures drop only 1 or 2 degrees. Tiny babies are especially vulnerable to cold stress.

A. Hypoglycemia

When a baby is chilled, his or her metabolic rate will increase to produce heat. This increased metabolic rate consumes glycogen stores and blood glucose faster than normal. A chilled baby may, therefore, develop hypoglycemia. A screening test value below 45 mg/dL requires evaluation and some form of treatment. (See Unit 8, Hypoglycemia, in this book.)

B. Acidosis

When a baby is chilled, brown fat is converted to heat and fatty acids. These fatty acids, and lactic acid from incomplete glucose breakdown, are released into the bloodstream, resulting in lower blood pH. A chilled baby may, therefore, become acidotic. Acidosis, in turn, can cause vasoconstriction of pulmonary blood vessels, resulting in low blood oxygen levels.

C. Hypoxia

When a baby is chilled, extra oxygen is needed to produce heat. For example, when a baby's temperature drops to 35.0°C (95.0°F), twice as much oxygen is needed than at 37.0°C (98.6°F).

Chilled babies with normal lungs will increase their respiratory rates to get extra oxygen and may show signs of respiratory distress (grunting, nasal flaring, retractions, and/or tachypnea). Allowing a baby to become hypothermic, or not warming a baby who has become chilled, can make an otherwise healthy baby sick.

Chilled babies with diseased lungs may become so ill that they are not able to get enough oxygen to maintain brain and body functions. Hypothermia in a baby with respiratory disease can significantly worsen the baby's condition.

 Hypothermia can cause a healthy baby to become ill and a sick baby to deteriorate dramatically.

7. What Happens When a Baby Is Overheated?

Babies who become overheated will increase their respiratory rates, heart rates, and metabolic rates. This added stress might compromise an already sick or at-risk baby.

8. Which Babies Have Difficulty Controlling Their Own Temperatures?

Some babies are at greater risk of being cold stressed, while others are at increased risk of being overheated. All of these babies should have their temperatures taken frequently.

A. Babies More Likely to Be Cold Stressed

  1. Preterm Babies

     Preterm babies have not had time to build up white fat for insulation or brown fat for heat production. Compared with term babies, preterm babies also have a greater surface area in relation to body weight from which to lose heat.

     They are *very* susceptible to temperature insults from the relatively cool air of delivery rooms, bathing, drafts, and inadequately warmed incubators. The smaller the baby, the greater the risk of cold stress.

     Extremely low birth weight (ELBW) newborns need special consideration in the delivery room. Protocols for delivery room resuscitation of ELBW newborns include

     - Setting the delivery room temperature to 26°C (80°F).
     - Use of plastic wrap or polyethylene bags (Figure 7.1). For extremely low birth weight babies (less than 29 weeks' gestation), immediately after birth, you should place them in a plastic bag, below the shoulders, without drying. (See American Academy of Pediatrics. *Textbook of Neonatal Resuscitation.* Kattwinkel J, ed. 6th ed. Elk Grove Village, IL. American Academy of Pediatrics: 2011.)
     - Use of chemically activated exothermic mattresses. Warmth also can be provided by commercially available, chemically activated warming mattresses, made for this purpose.* Follow manufacturers' instructions.

     Linens and clothing should be pre-warmed, and chemical mattresses should be activated before placing these items next to the baby.

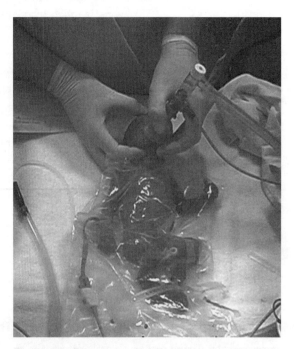

Figure 7.1. Extremely Low Birth Weight Newborn With Plastic Wrap to Maintain Temperature.
Reprinted with permission from Professor Colin Morley, University of Melbourne.

---

*Caution: Chemically activated warming mattresses should be stored at room temperature, or they may overheat or under-heat when activated.

Temperature should be closely monitored if using both plastic/polyethylene wraps and exothermic mattresses, because of the risk of hyperthermia.

2. Small-for-Gestational-Age (SGA) Babies

Because they are malnourished, SGA babies do not have as much brown fat for heat production or white fat for insulation. Also, they have a relatively large surface area, for their body weight, from which to lose body heat. However, their metabolic rate may be higher than in preterm babies of comparable size. Small-for-gestational-age babies are more likely to become either hypothermic or hyperthermic.

3. Sick Babies*

Sick babies use extra oxygen and calories just to maintain normal body functions. Their organ systems and metabolism may not be able to tolerate the additional stress of being chilled.

 While some babies are particularly vulnerable to cold stress, any newborn—even term, healthy babies—can quickly become chilled.

It is important to protect the thermal environment of all babies.

B. Babies More Likely to Be Overheated
   1. Babies in incubators
   2. Babies under radiant warmers
   3. Babies under phototherapy lights

Self-test

Now answer these questions to test yourself on the information in the last section.

C1. What are 3 problems that may develop if a baby is chilled?

_____

_____

_____

C2. Which babies should have their temperatures taken more often?

_____

_____

_____

C3. **True** **False** A baby in respiratory distress can become critically ill from being chilled.

C4. **True** **False** Chilled babies have increased metabolic rates.

C5. **True** **False** Overheated babies have increased metabolic rates.

Check your answers with the list that follows the Recommended Routines. Correct any incorrect answers and review the appropriate section in the unit.

---

*Cooling of term gestation babies following an asphyxial event has been shown to be beneficial under certain conditions. Cooling of such babies should be instituted within 6 hours of the event and coordinated by institutions with multidisciplinary expertise. (See Unit 5, Resuscitating the Newborn, in this book, and Book III: Neonatal Care, Unit 10, Preparation for Neonatal Transport.)

9. How Does Temperature Control Help to Minimize Oxygen and Caloric Requirements?

The best way to minimize oxygen and caloric requirements is to put a baby in an incubator or under a radiant warmer and supply enough heat so that heat losses and heat production are balanced at the lowest possible levels. This environment is called the neutral thermal environment (NTE). In an incubator, there is a narrow range of air temperature that provides an NTE. Under a radiant warmer, NTE is accomplished by maintaining a normal skin temperature with servo control.

 Neutral thermal environment (NTE) is an environment in which a baby uses the least amount of energy to maintain a normal body temperature. Different amounts of external heat are required to establish NTE for babies of different sizes and ages.

10. How Do You Determine a Baby's Neutral Thermal Environment?

A. Incubator

A baby in the appropriate NTE incubator air temperature range should maintain a skin temperature close to 36.5°C (97.8°F) and a rectal or axillary temperature close to 37.0°C (98.6°F). The details of adjusting an incubator to NTE are described in Skill Unit: Incubators and Neutral Thermal Environment, at the end of this unit. Briefly, the procedure for determining a baby's NTE is as follows:

1. Birth to 6 Days Old
   - Estimate the baby's gestational age. (See Unit 6, Gestational Age and Size and Associated Risk Factors, in this book.)
   - Look at Figure 7.2 and find the appropriate temperature band on the graph for the baby's gestational age and postnatal age (days since birth).

2. Baby 7 Days or Older
   - Determine the baby's weight in kilograms.
   - Look at Figure 7.3 and find the appropriate temperature band on the graph for the baby's current weight and postnatal age.

Example: Baby Jefferson is born at 33 weeks' gestational age and is appropriate size. What temperature should his incubator air temperature be on day 3 to provide NTE?

- Turn to Figures 7.2 and 7.3. Figure 7.2 shows that the NTE temperature for a 33-week gestation baby at 3 days of age is 35.0°C (95.0°F). Set the incubator temperature to 35.0°C and monitor the baby's temperature.

At 14 days of age Baby Jefferson weighs 1.5 kg. What should the incubator air temperature be on day 14?

- Figure 7.3 shows that the NTE temperature for a 1.5-kg baby at 14 days postnatal age is 33.5°C (92.4°F). Set the incubator temperature to 33.5°C and continue to monitor the baby's temperature.

Note: The NTE temperatures in the graphs are given as guidelines and should be considered close estimates of a baby's NTE. The NTE for an individual baby may vary a few tenths of a degree from the graph temperatures.

B. Radiant Warmer

A baby's NTE is provided by a radiant warmer when normal skin temperature is maintained using servocontrol. When skin temperature is maintained close to 36.5°C (97.8°F) (slightly lower in very big babies and slightly higher in very small babies), core or rectal temperature will be close to 37.0°C (98.6°F), and oxygen requirements will be minimal. The details of using a radiant warmer are described in Skill Unit: Radiant Warmers. Briefly, the procedure is as follows:

1. *Keep the baby unclothed, or with only a small diaper.* This is to allow the baby's skin to absorb the radiant heat. A thin, transparent plastic sheet placed over the baby may help to decrease convective and evaporative heat losses in small preterm babies. (Take care not to obstruct the baby's airway.)

2. *Cover the tip of the probe so it is* not *directly exposed to the radiant heat.* Usually, a commercially available reflective cover is used for this. The adhesive side holds the probe tip in place and the exposed side reflects the radiant heat so the probe measures only the baby's body temperature. Be sure the tip is completely in contact with the baby's skin.

3. *Tape the probe to the side of the baby away from the mattress.* If the baby is lying on his or her back, tape the servo control probe to the baby's abdomen. Tape the probe to the baby's lower back if the baby is lying on his or her stomach.

   The probe should not be placed between the baby and the mattress. That location will result in falsely high skin temperature readings and cause the baby to be *under*-heated. The servo control mechanism will stop providing heat in response to the false temperature, until the temperature registered drops below the preset temperature. The baby's actual temperature may be significantly lower.

4. *Be sure the probe is taped to a fleshy area of the baby's trunk.* Avoid the extremities and bony prominences, such as the spine, sternum, and scapula. The probe will register falsely low temperatures when taped in these areas.

5. *Set the servo control mechanism to 36.5°C, "automatic" control.* This will cause the radiant warmer to turn on or off as the baby's skin temperature falls below or rises above 36.5°C (97.8°F).

C. Supplemental Oxygen

Inspired oxygen/air temperatures below a baby's NTE can cool a baby. Babies who require oxygen therapy should have the oxygen/air mixture humidified and heated to the baby's NTE temperature. This is true whether a baby is in an incubator or under a radiant warmer.

Heat from an incubator or radiant warmer will *not* adequately warm an oxygen/air mixture. A separate heated humidifier is required. The temperature setting for the heated humidifier is determined from the NTE charts, the same way that incubator temperatures are determined.

Excessively high temperatures (particularly higher than 37.0°C [98.6°F]) for oxygen/air mixture also should be avoided because they can overheat a baby.

Self-test

Now answer these questions to test yourself on the information in the last section. Use the charts and flow diagram in the next section, as necessary.

D1. Providing neutral thermal environment with an incubator includes
   A. Setting the incubator air temperature to 37.0°C (98.6°F).
   B. Setting the incubator air temperature according to the baby's weight.
   C. Setting the incubator air temperature according to the baby's age and weight.

D2. The purpose of the neutral thermal environment is to
   A. Prevent overheating a baby.
   B. Individualize a baby's care.
   C. Minimize the oxygen and calories a baby needs.
   D. Increase a baby's metabolic rate.

D3. What is the neutral thermal environment incubator air temperature for a baby born at 32 weeks' gestation on the first day after birth?
   _____°C

D4. What is the neutral thermal environment incubator air temperature for a 10-day-old baby who weighs 1,300 g?
   _____°C

D5. A 1,500-g (3 lb, 5 oz) newborn under a servo-controlled radiant warmer has a skin temperature of 36.4°C (97.6°F) and a rectal temperature of 37.0°C (98.6°F). Is this baby in a neutral thermal environment?
   Yes _____ No _____

Check your answers with the list that follows the Recommended Routines. Correct any incorrect answers and review the appropriate section in the unit.

11. Will Providing a Neutral Thermal Environment Always Work?

A. Incubator

The NTE incubator air temperature (Figures 7.2 and 7.3) will keep a baby's temperature normal only if the baby
   • Is naked in an incubator
   • Does not have an infection (is not septic)
   • Is appropriate size for gestational age
   • Is *not* extremely small (<1,000 g or 2 lb, 3 oz)

AND sources of heat loss are controlled

   • Wet diapers are removed promptly.
   • Oxygen (if used) is humidified and warmed to the baby's NTE temperature.
   • Incubator portholes are closed after each entry into the incubator.
   • Outside walls of the incubator are not unusually cold (eg, in a cold nursery, in front of an air conditioner, or by an outside window during the winter).

If a baby is hypothermic in the appropriate environmental temperature, consider that there are abnormal routes of heat loss or the baby has an infection.

B. Radiant Warmers (See Figure 7.4)

Under a radiant warmer, a baby's skin temperature will be maintained in the normal range, even if there are extra heat losses. You should routinely check for possible sources of heat loss (cold, non-humidified oxygen, wet diapers or linens, etc) for newborns under radiant warmers, even when a baby's temperature is normal. In addition, you should monitor closely for other signs of infection (see Book III: Neonatal Care, Unit 8, Infections) because the temperature changes seen with infection also will be masked.

 When using a radiant warmer, remember to check for sources of heat loss and have a high index of suspicion for infection.

If the servo control probe is taped incorrectly (tip is not entirely in contact with the baby's skin) or positioned incorrectly (taped to a bony prominence or to the mattress side of the baby), the skin temperature may register "normal," but the baby's actual axillary or rectal temperature may be high or low.

 Do not rely on the skin temperature registered on a radiant warmer as the measure of a baby's temperature. Periodically use a standard thermometer to check the axillary temperature.

12. Will Managing a Baby's Temperature With Servo Control in an Incubator Provide a Neutral Thermal Environment?

Not necessarily. Many incubators are equipped with an optional servo control mechanism. This mechanism can be used, with a probe taped to the baby's trunk, in much the same way that radiant warmers are used to maintain a baby's skin temperature at a set temperature. All of the possible problems with radiant warmers are also possible when servo control is used with an incubator.

While a baby's temperature will be normal, the baby may be using extra calories and oxygen to produce heat, with the incubator environmental temperature supplying only a small portion of the total heat the baby needs to stay warm. In addition, temperature changes associated with infection or abnormal heat loss may be masked.

To minimize these problems, it is important to use the correct technique for incubator servo control, which is similar to the technique used for radiant warmers. While the details of managing a baby's temperature with servo control in an incubator are not discussed in this unit, the main points are as follows:

1. Keep the baby unclothed, or with only a small diaper.
2. Position the probe on the side of the baby away from the mattress. If the baby is lying on his or her back, tape the servo control probe to the baby's abdomen. Tape the probe to the baby's lower back if the baby is lying on his or her stomach.

   The probe should not be placed between the baby and the mattress. That location will result in falsely high skin temperature readings and cause the baby to be *under*-heated. The servo control mechanism will respond to the falsely high temperature and stop providing heat until the false temperature drops below the preset temperature. The baby's actual temperature may be significantly lower.

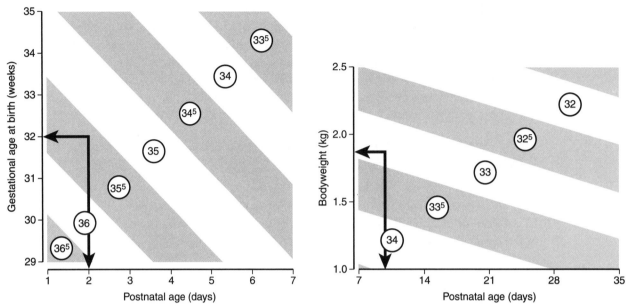

Figure 7.2. Neutral Thermal Environment (°C) During the First Week. **Figure 7.3.** Neutral Thermal Environment (°C) From Day 7 to Day 35.

Reprinted from Sauer PJJ, Dane HJ, Visser HKA. *Arch Dis Child*. 1984;59:18-22 with permission from BMJ Publishing Group Ltd.

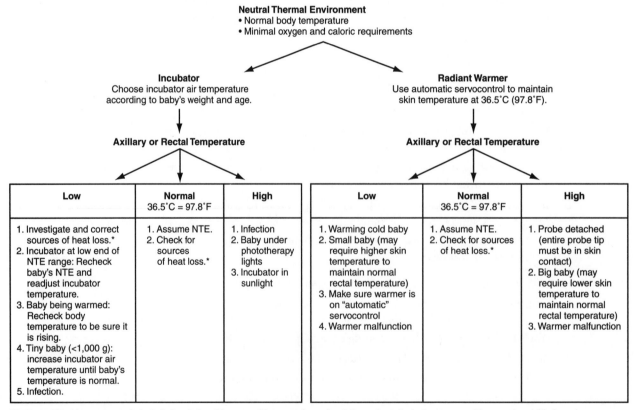

*Routes of heat loss commonly include incubator side opened for procedures (work through portholes), oxygen cold or non-humidified, cool nursery, wet linen, incubator near cold window, etc.

Figure 7.4. Control of Thermal Environment for Newborns.

3. Tape the tip of the probe so it is completely in contact with the baby's skin. Be sure the entire tip is in contact with the baby's skin so the temperature registered accurately indicates the baby's skin temperature. Tape or commercially available foam pads (with adhesive back) may be used to secure the probe tip.

4. Be sure the probe is taped to a fleshy area of the baby's trunk. Avoid the extremities and bony prominences, such as the spine, sternum, and scapula. The probe will register falsely low temperatures when taped in these areas.

5. Set the servo control mechanism to 36.5°C, skin temperature. This will cause the incubator heater to turn on or off as the baby's skin temperature falls below or rises above 36.5°C (97.8°F). When a servo control probe is taped to a baby, be sure the mechanism is set to register skin temperature, *not* incubator air temperature.

13. If a Sick or Small Baby Has a Normal Body Temperature, Do You Still Have to Provide a Neutral Thermal Environment?

Yes. A baby will use minimal energy to maintain a normal temperature *only* in the NTE that is appropriate to the baby's age and weight.

A baby may have a normal rectal/axillary temperature even when not in the appropriate NTE. In this case, the baby must use considerable energy (calories and oxygen) to maintain a normal body temperature.

Self-test

Now answer these questions to test yourself on the information in the last section.

E1. A baby is in the appropriate incubator neutral thermal environment air temperature but has an axillary temperature of 35.0°C (96.0°F). What are 2 possible reasons why the baby is cold?

_____

_____

E2. **True** **False** As long as a baby is in an incubator set at the appropriate neutral thermal environment air temperature, the baby's body temperature will remain normal (37.0°C [98.6°F]).

E3. **True** **False** If a 1,800-g (4 lb) baby with respiratory distress has a normal body temperature (37.0°C [98.6°F]), he does not need to be put in a neutral thermal environment.

E4. A baby is in an incubator, with the air temperature set for the appropriate neutral thermal environment. What are 3 conditions that must be met before the baby's temperature can be expected to remain normal?

_____

_____

E5. What does placing a baby in a neutral thermal environment do for the baby?
  A. Ensures that the baby will not get sick
  B. Ensures that the baby's body temperature will remain normal
  C. Ensures that the baby is using minimum energy (oxygen and calories) to maintain a normal body temperature

Check your answers with the list that follows the Recommended Routines. Correct any incorrect answers and review the appropriate section in the unit.

14. How Should a Baby's Temperature Be Regulated?

A. Clothed in a Bassinet With Nursery Temperature at 74°F to 76°F
   - Full-term, well babies
   - Preterm babies weighing approximately 1,600 to 1,700 g (3 lb, 8 oz to 3 lb, 12 oz), who are not sick
   - Small-for gestational-age, term babies who are not sick

B. Incubator Adjusted to Appropriate NTE Air Temperature
   - Preterm, appropriate-for-gestational-age babies weighing less than 1,600 to 1,700 g (3 lb, 8 oz to 4 lb)
   - Sick babies who do *not* require multiple procedures

C. Radiant Warmer With Automatic Servo Control
   - Sick babies who require many procedures
   - Babies whose axillary/rectal temperatures cannot be maintained at 37.0°C (98.6°F) in an incubator adjusted to NTE air temperature (abnormal routes of heat loss have been ruled out); these may include sick SGA babies, very small babies, or septic babies

D. Skin-to-Skin With Baby's Mother or Father

   1. Healthy, Term Newborns

      Skin-to-skin contact between mother and baby soon after delivery will help keep a healthy, term newborn warm, provided the baby is dried thoroughly and the exposed side of the baby is covered. In this situation, most women can serve as safe and effective heat sources for their babies.

   2. Small or Sick Babies, in Stable Condition

      Skin-to-skin contact between mothers or fathers and their babies also has been used for sick and preterm babies, after a baby's condition has been stabilized. For selected babies, this seems to be a safe way to provide close contact between parent and baby, while maintaining the baby's temperature. The technique carries hazards (hypothermia, disruption of therapy, etc), however, and cannot be assumed to be safe for all small or sick babies.

      Consider the risks and benefits, parental desire and preparation, and the stability of the baby's condition before undertaking skin-to-skin contact for sick or small babies. Provide ongoing monitoring of the baby's temperature and condition.

15. What Do You Do When a Baby Has a Low Body Temperature?

First, *warm the baby*. How this is done will depend on how cold the baby is.

A. Slightly Chilled Baby

   A baby with a moderately low body temperature (such as 35.0°C to 36.0°C or 95.0°F to 96.8°F) usually can be warmed adequately in an incubator adjusted to the appropriate NTE temperature. If the baby's body temperature does not rise over 1 to 2 hours, increase the incubator temperature *slightly*, until the baby becomes warm. Warming the incubator air too quickly may induce apnea, especially in preterm newborns. Once the baby's temperature is normal, reestablish the NTE incubator air temperature. If a baby becomes chilled in the appropriate NTE, increase the incubator temperature, even if this means going above the NTE range. After you have begun to warm the baby, search for routes of abnormal heat loss and evaluate the baby for signs of infection (see Book III: Neonatal Care, Unit 8, Infections), and monitor the baby for signs of cold stress (eg, hypoglycemia, acidosis, hypoxia).

B. Severely Cold-Stressed Baby

1. In an Incubator
   • Place the baby in an incubator with the air temperature set 1°C to 1.5°C (2°F to 3°F) higher than the baby's body temperature.
   • As the baby's temperature increases, increase the environmental (air) temperature to keep it 1°C to 1.5°C (2°F to 3°F) above the baby's temperature.
   • When the baby's temperature reaches 37.0°C (98.6°F), set the incubator air temperature to the appropriate NTE temperature.

2. Under a Radiant Warmer
   • Attach the probe to the baby's skin and set the servo control to 36.5°C (97.8°F). The baby's skin temperature will rise quickly to 36.5°C, while rectal (core) temperature will rise more slowly to 37.0°C.
   • Monitor rectal temperature frequently until it is normal, and then intermittent axillary temperatures may be taken.

Self-test

Now answer these questions to test yourself on the information in the last section.

F1. A baby is born at home during the winter. Her temperature at admission to the nursery is 33°C (91.4°F). How would you warm this baby using an incubator?

_____

_____

F2. When a baby is under a radiant warmer, what temperature should be set for the servo control mechanism?

_____ °C or _____ °F

F3. What method for controlling the thermal environment is recommended for each of the following babies?
   A. Normal, full-term, well baby: _____
   B. Stable, 1,500-g, preterm baby: _____
   C. Sick, full-term baby *not* requiring many procedures: _____
   D. Sick, preterm baby requiring many procedures: _____
   E. Stable, small-for-gestational-age, term baby: _____
   F. Sick, small-for-gestational-age, term baby: _____

F4. A baby is admitted to your nursery. You take her temperature and discover it is 35.0°C (95.0°F). How would you warm this baby?

_____

_____

F5. **True   False**   Rapid warming of incubator air temperature may lead to apnea attacks, especially in preterm newborns.

Check your answers with the list that follows the Recommended Routines. Correct any incorrect answers and review the appropriate section in the unit.

Thermal Environment

Recommended Routines

All the routines listed below are based on the principles of perinatal care presented in the unit you have just finished. They are recommended as part of routine perinatal care.

Read each routine carefully and decide whether it is standard operating procedure in your hospital. Check the appropriate blank next to each routine.

Procedure Standard in My Hospital   **Needs Discussion by Our Staff**

_____   _____   1. Establish a routine of measuring body temperature frequently in all sick and at-risk babies.

_____   _____   2. Establish a policy of withholding baths from all sick babies.

_____   _____   3. Establish a policy of withholding baths from any baby until the baby's temperature has been measured and has remained normal for several hours.

_____   _____   4. Establish a policy that will ensure the continuous availability of a radiant warmer or pre-warmed incubator for any unexpected admission to the nursery.

_____   _____   5. Post the neutral thermal environment graphs and establish a policy of adjusting the environmental temperature of any occupied incubator to the appropriate neutral thermal environment temperature.

_____   _____   6. Use equipment to monitor and adjust the temperature of supplemental oxygen.

Self-test Answers

These are the answers to the self-test questions. Please check them with the answers you gave and review the information in the unit wherever necessary.

A1. They use oxygen and calories to break down brown fat.

A2. False.   Babies cannot shiver to help warm themselves.

A3. True

A4. Any condition where a baby is in direct contact with a cold object (such as a cold scale, delivery room bed, etc)

A5. Any condition where cold air moves over a baby (such as cold oxygen flow, draft from an open window or air conditioner, incubator portholes left open, etc)

A6. Any condition where a liquid is allowed to evaporate from a baby's skin (such as remaining wet after delivery, giving a bath, etc)

A7. Any condition where a baby is close to a cold, solid object (such as a cold wall or closed window, cold wall of a single-walled incubator, etc)

B1. Rectal, axillary, skin

B2. Rectal

B3. Rectal and axillary

B4. 36.5°C (97.8°F)

B5. B. Incubator air temperature set too high. (Note: Infection can cause a fever in a newborn, but it is uncommon.)

B6. A. A blood infection (sepsis)
    C. Heat loss to the environment

C1. Hypoglycemia, acidosis, hypoxia

C2. Babies more likely to be cold stressed, including preterm, small-for-gestational-age, sick babies
    Babies more likely to be overheated, including babies in incubators, under radiant warmers or under phototherapy lights

C3. True

C4. True

C5. True

D1. C. Setting the incubator air temperature according to the baby's age and weight

D2. C. Minimize the oxygen and calories a baby needs.

D3. 35.5°C (96.0°F)

D4. 34.0°C (93.2°F)

D5. Yes

E1. The baby is septic and/or there are abnormal routes of heat loss.

E2. False.   The body temperature may go higher or lower than 37.0°C (98.6°F) while in an appropriate neutral thermal environment temperature range. If they occur, such changes should be investigated to determine the cause for the abnormal temperature.

E3. False.   The purpose of neutral thermal environment is to minimize oxygen and caloric consumption, as well as to keep a baby's temperature normal.

E4. Any 3 of the following:
    • Baby is naked in an incubator.
    • Baby does not have an infection (is not septic).
    • Baby is appropriate size for gestational age.
    • Baby is *not* extremely small (<1,000 g or 2 lb, 3 oz).

Sources of heat loss are controlled
- Wet diapers are removed promptly.
- Oxygen (if used) is humidified and warmed to appropriate neutral thermal environment temperature.
- Incubator portholes are closed after each entry into the incubator.
- Incubator walls are not unusually cold.

E5. C. Ensures the baby is using minimum energy (oxygen and calories) to maintain a normal body temperature

F1. Put baby in an incubator set at 34°C to 35.5°C. Increase incubator air temperature in increments of 1°C to 1.5°C until baby's rectal/axillary temperature reaches 37.0°C (98.6°F). Set incubator air temperature to neutral thermal environment temperature after body temperature reaches 37.0°C, or put baby under a radiant warmer with skin temperature set for 36.5°C (97.8°F). Monitor rectal temperature until normal, then use axillary measurements.

F2. 36.5°C or 97.8°F

F3. A. Normal, full-term, well baby: clothed in crib with blanket, nursery temperature set at 74°F to 76°F
      B. Stable, 1,500-g, preterm baby: Incubator set at the baby's neutral thermal environment temperature
      C. Sick, full-term baby not requiring many procedures: Incubator set at the baby's neutral thermal environment temperature
      D. Sick, preterm baby requiring many procedures: Radiant warmer, servo control set for 36.5°C skin temperature
      E. Stable, small-for-gestational-age, term baby: Clothed in crib with blanket, nursery temperature set at 74°F to 76°F
      F. Sick, small-for-gestational-age, term baby: Incubator with environmental temperature adjusted to keep the baby's body temperature at 37.0°C, or under a radiant warmer with servo control set for 36.5°C skin temperature

F4. Place the baby in an incubator with the air temperature set for her neutral thermal environment temperature, or under a radiant warmer with the skin temperature set at 36.5°C (97.8°F). Be sure to evaluate baby for possible consequences of hypothermia (hypoglycemia, acidosis, hypoxia).

F5. True

Unit 7 Posttest

If you are applying for continuing education credits, a posttest for this unit is available online. Completion of unit posttests and the book evaluation form are required to achieve continuing education credit. For more details, visit www.cmevillage.com.

SKILL UNIT

Radiant Warmers

This skill unit will teach you how to operate a radiant warmer and regulate a baby's temperature using servo control.

Study this skill unit. Then attend a skill practice and demonstration session.

To master the skill, you will need to demonstrate correctly each of the following steps:

1. Select mode of operation.
2. Attach servo control probe to baby.
3. Determine temperature setting.
4. Set high and low temperature alarms.
5. Keep baby unclothed.
6. Position transparent plastic cover, if used.
7. Minimize heat loss.

PERINATAL PERFORMANCE GUIDE

Operating Radiant Warmers

ACTIONS	REMARKS

Deciding to Use a Radiant Warmer

1. Do you anticipate the admission of a sick or at-risk baby?

    Yes: Prepare to use the radiant warmer for this baby.

    No: Make sure the radiant warmer is clean and in operating condition.

It is generally easier to observe babies and carry out special procedures (eg, umbilical catheterization) when they are under radiant warmers than when they are in incubators.

Preparing to Use a Radiant Warmer

2. Collect the proper equipment.

• Radiant warmer
• Servo control probe
• Cover for the tip of the servo control probe

3. Plug in the radiant warmer.

4. Connect the servo control probe to the radiant warmer.

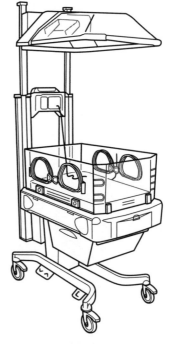

Adapted from *Lippincott's Nursing Procedures and Skills,* with permission from Lippincott Williams & Wilkins. 2012.

5. Place the radiant warmer on *automatic* mode.

•

Automatic mode means the warmer turns on and off in response to the baby's skin temperature, as it is registered by the servo control probe, to maintain the baby's skin temperature at the preset temperature (servo control).

Manual mode means that the radiant warmer will continue heating unless you turn it off. A baby can be quickly overheated.

280

ACTIONS	REMARKS

Using a Radiant Warmer

6. The baby should be unclothed to absorb the radiant heat. Leaving clothes on the baby will decrease the efficiency of heat input from the warmer.

If the baby is extremely preterm, a sheet of thin plastic placed over a baby below the neck, will help to decrease convective and evaporative losses, without interfering with the radiant heat needed to keep the baby warm.

If thin plastic wrap is used, be sure to keep it away from the baby's airway.

7. Decide where to place the temperature probe.
   • On the baby's abdomen (if baby is lying on back)
   • On the baby's lower back (if baby is lying on stomach)

Avoid placing the probe over bony prominences (sternum, ribs, scapula, etc) or on the baby's arms or legs. These locations will not give an accurate skin temperature, but will instead register a relatively low temperature, causing the radiant warmer to put out excess heat, which may, in turn, overheat the baby.

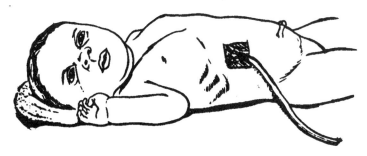

8. Securely tape the temperature probe to the baby.

Care must be taken to keep the servo control probe tip in constant contact with the baby's skin.

9. Cover the tip of the probe so that it is not directly exposed to the radiant heat.

To protect a baby's skin, a piece of clear adhesive dressing may be used to hold the probe tip in place on the baby's skin. A piece of opaque cloth tape or a commercially available reflective cover is then taped to the clear adhesive, over the probe tip.

10. Set the appropriate servo control skin temperature (36.5°C or 97.8°F).

281

ACTIONS	REMARKS

Using a Radiant Warmer (continued)

Check rectal temperature to make sure it is close to 37.0°C (98.6°F). If low, continue to check the baby's rectal temperature until it is normal. Then use axillary temperatures for routine monitoring.

It is important to check a baby's axillary temperature, in addition to the skin temperature registered by the servo control probe. A loose or incorrectly placed probe, or an incorrectly set warmer, can cause a baby to be severely overheated or under-heated, even though the probe registers the desired skin temperature.

Adjust the servo control preset temperature higher or lower as needed to keep the axillary/rectal temperature at 37.0°C (98.6°F).

It is important to recognize a change in temperature quickly because the baby can be chilled or overheated within a short period. Know the operation and meaning of the alarms on the warmer you are using.

If your radiant warmer has "high" and "low" temperature alarms, set these at 0.5°C (1.0°F) above and below the preset temperature. (Many warmers have internal alarms that cannot be set manually.)

11. Keep the sides of the radiant warmer bed in the upright position. Minimize drafts in the room.

This is to minimize the baby losing heat by convection and evaporation. (See step number 6.)

12. Radiant warmers can increase the baby's insensible water loss by as much as 100%. If a baby is to stay under a radiant warmer for more than several hours, it is important to increase the baby's fluid intake.

A clear plastic covering is particularly useful for decreasing insensible water losses in babies with birth weights less than 1,500 g (3 lb, 5 oz).

What Can Go Wrong?

1. Radiant warmer is placed on manual rather than automatic mode of operation.

The heating mechanism will not turn off automatically. The baby will become overheated.

2. The servo control probe may malfunction and the baby may be chilled or overheated when all other settings are correct.

This is rare. However, if you suspect this to be the problem, try another temperature probe. Continue frequent monitoring of the baby's temperature with a standard thermometer.

3. The baby's desired temperature is set inaccurately.

The baby will be chilled or overheated.

4. The temperature probe becomes dislodged.

ACTIONS	REMARKS
What Can Go Wrong? (continued)	
5. The probe is taped over a bony prominence or on an extremity.	The temperature registered may be lower than the baby's actual skin temperature, causing the warmer to put out more heat than necessary and resulting in the baby being overheated. Be sure the probe is taped to a fleshy part of the baby's trunk.
6. The baby is lying on the probe. The baby will become overheated. Check the baby's temperature with a second thermometer. Re-tape the probe.	While the probe should be covered to prevent *direct* exposure to the radiant heat, it should be taped to the exposed side of the baby. If the probe is between the baby and the mattress, the temperature recorded is likely to be inaccurate.

SKILL UNIT

Incubators and Neutral Thermal Environment

This skill unit will teach you how to determine a baby's neutral thermal environment (NTE) and how to operate an incubator to provide a baby's NTE.

Study this skill. Then attend a skill practice and demonstration session.

To master this skill, you will need to demonstrate each of the following steps correctly:

1. Determine baby's NTE.
2. Preheat incubator to NTE.
3. Prepare water reservoir (if present and appropriate for specific incubator).
4. Transfer baby from radiant warmer to incubator.
5. Settle baby in incubator.
6. Check baby's temperature.
7. Record NTE in baby's bedside chart.

PERINATAL PERFORMANCE GUIDE

Operating Incubators and Setting Neutral Thermal Environment

ACTIONS	REMARKS

Deciding to Use an Incubator

1. Is there a sick or at-risk baby who will stay in your nursery rather than be transferred to a regional intensive care nursery within the next few hours?

   Yes: Move this baby from a radiant warmer to an incubator as soon as any special procedures have been completed.

   No: Make sure at least one incubator is clean and in operating condition.

Keep babies who will be transferred under a radiant warmer until special procedures, such as umbilical catheterization, are complete or the baby is ready to be transported.

It is recommended to keep a clean incubator plugged in and warm, ready to receive a baby, at all times.

Preparing to Use an Incubator

2. Prepare the bed of the incubator with clean linen.

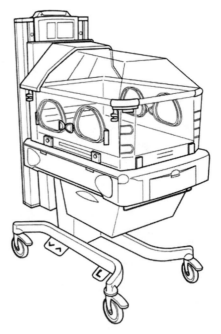

From *Lippincott's Nursing Procedures and Skills,* with permission from Lippincott Williams & Wilkins. 2012.

3. Check water reservoir (if present).
   - Be sure reservoir is clean.
   - Fill only with *distilled* water.
   - Cleanse the reservoir in between patients (following manufacturer's recommendation).

Beware: Water in a reservoir can become contaminated. Follow manufacturer's recommendation regarding cleaning.

ACTIONS **REMARKS**

Setting the Neutral Thermal Environment

4. Use the neutral thermal environment (NTE) figures 7.2 and 7.3 in this unit, and repeated in Figures 1 and 2 here. Find the appropriate temperature band for the baby in your care.
   - To determine NTE for babies 0 to 6 days of age, estimate the baby's gestational age.

Example

Baby Thomas is 2 days old and has an estimated gestational age of 32 weeks. Find the baby's gestational age on the vertical scale (see horizontal arrow).

Now find the baby's postnatal age (days since birth) on the horizontal scale (see vertical arrow).

Find the area of the graph where straight lines drawn from these 2 points meet (see arrows).

For Baby Thomas, this intersection falls in the temperature band labeled 35.5. Baby Thomas's NTE is 35.5°C.

- To determine NTE for babies 7 or more days of age, determine the baby's weight in kilograms.

Example

Baby Thomas is now 10 days old and weighs 1,850 g (1.85 kg). Find the baby's age on the horizontal scale (see vertical arrow).

Now find the baby's current weight on the vertical scale (see horizontal arrow).

Find the area of the graph where straight lines drawn from these 2 points meet (see arrows).

Baby Thomas's NTE is now 33.0°C.

Gestational age at birth (weeks)
35
34
33
32
31
30
29
33^5
34
34^5
35
35^5
36
36^5
1
2
3
4
5
6
7
Postnatal age (days)

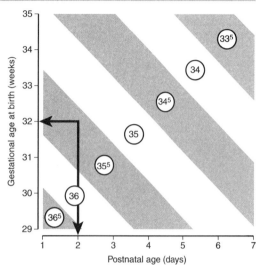

Figure 1. Neutral Thermal Environment (°C) During the First Postnatal Week (0 to 6 Days of Age).

Bodyweight (kg)
2.5
2.0
1.5
1.0
32
32^5
33
33^5
34
7
14
21
28
35
Postnatal age (days)

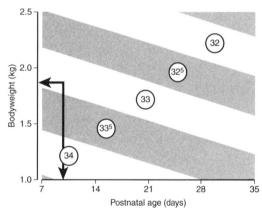

Figure 2. Neutral Thermal Environment (°C) From 7 to 35 Days of Age.

Reproduced from Sauer PJJ, Dane HJ, Visser HKA. *Arch Dis Child.* 1984;59:18-22 with permission from BMJ Publishing Ltd.

ACTIONS	REMARKS

Caring for a Baby in an Incubator

5. Preheat the incubator to the NTE temperature, which you have determined from the graphs.

   - Check the temperature inside the incubator.
   - Adjust the incubator temperature higher or lower as required to reach the NTE.
   - Wait 15 or 20 minutes.
   - Recheck the air temperature inside the incubator.
   - Readjust the incubator setting if necessary, wait again, and recheck the incubator temperature.

For many incubators, the desired temperature can be set digitally. It is still important, however, to check the actual air temperature inside the incubator and readjust the temperature setting, as necessary, to achieve the desired incubator air temperature.

6. *Plan* how you will transfer the baby and any attached monitoring equipment, intravenous tubing, etc, to the incubator.

This is a *critical step* and must be done to ensure a smooth transfer with minimum stress to the baby.

If the baby is requiring oxygen via an oxyhood, have someone hold the tubing over the baby's nose during the entire transfer. If the baby is requiring PPV, continue the assisted ventilation, for the baby during the entire transfer using the appropriate concentration of oxygen. Be prepared to resume the pre-transfer oxygen therapy *immediately,* as soon as the baby has been placed in the incubator.

Removing an oxygen-dependent baby from oxygen for even a very brief period can make the baby's condition deteriorate severely.

7. When the incubator has reached the correct temperature, place the baby inside.

   - Open the incubator door.
   - Place the baby inside.
   - Close the incubator door as quickly as possible.
   - Work through the portholes to settle the baby.
   - Close the portholes.

Sick and at-risk babies exposed to room temperature can be chilled very quickly. After you have settled the baby, recheck his or her temperature.

8. Check and record the incubator temperature and the baby's temperature every 30 minutes until both are stable.

9. Recheck the graphs every day and adjust the incubator setting appropriately as the baby grows.

Record the NTE temperature in the baby's bedside chart each day.

ACTIONS   **REMARKS**

Caring for a Baby in an Incubator (continued)

10. Continue to keep a baby in the appropriate NTE until the baby

    - Is no longer sick
    - Weighs more than 1,600 to 1,700 g (about 3 lb, 8 oz to 3 lb, 12 oz),
    - Can maintain a normal body temperature in a bassinet with shirt, diaper, and blankets
    - Continues to gain weight steadily

What Can Go Wrong?

1. Neutral thermal environment is set incorrectly.

   Recheck the graph for the temperature for the baby's current age and weight.

2. Some incubators are designed so that the warm air flows up the sides of the incubator. This may mean the air reaching an incubator wall thermometer is warmer than the air in the center of the incubator next to the baby.

   If this is the design of incubators in your nursery, suspend a temperature probe directly over the baby. Adjust the baby's NTE according to the temperature recorded there.

3. The baby is cold or hot in the appropriate NTE.

   - Check for routes of heat loss or gain.
     - Room temperature too cold, thus causing the baby to have excessive radiant heat loss to cold incubator walls (less likely to occur with double-walled incubators)
     - Incubator close to cold windows (heat loss) or in direct sunlight (heat gain)
     - Wet mattress or linens
     - Incubator portholes left open
     - Oxygen (if needed) not warmed to appropriate NTE (too hot or too cold)
   - Suspect sepsis.
   - Very small (<1,000 g or 2 lb, 3 oz) preterm babies *may* require special techniques to maintain their body temperatures. Care of these tiny babies is not discussed here.
   - Small-for-gestational-age babies may become slightly overheated or underheated in an incubator adjusted according to the graphs. Raise or lower the incubator temperature as needed to keep an SGA baby's body temperature normal.

289

ACTIONS	REMARKS

What Can Go Wrong? (continued)

4. The incubator is set to "skin" rather than "air" temperature control.

When providing NTE as outlined in this skill unit, you are controlling the temperature of the *air* inside the incubator.

If you wish to servo control a baby's temperature, you need to

- Set the incubator to "skin" (not "air").
- Set the temperature of the servo control probe to 36.5°C (98.6°F).
- Tape the probe to the baby, as you would if using a radiant warmer.

Unit 8: Hypoglycemia

Objectives

In this unit you will learn to

A. Understand the hazards of hypoglycemia.

B. Identify babies at risk for hypoglycemia.

C. Institute monitoring and preventive measures for babies at risk for hypoglycemia.

D. Recognize the signs of hypoglycemia.

E. Obtain accurate blood glucose screening test results.

F. Treat hypoglycemia and monitor babies receiving treatment.

Unit 8 Pretest

Before reading the unit, please answer the following questions. Select the *one best* answer to each question (unless otherwise instructed). Record your answers on the test and check them against the answers at the end of the book.

1. **True   False**   Untreated hypoglycemia in a newborn can cause neurologic injury.

2. **True   False**   Intravenous therapy for hypoglycemia should be stopped as soon as the blood glucose screening test results become normal.

3. **True   False**   A baby who is hypoglycemic may have a seizure.

4. **True   False**   Large-for-gestational-age babies are at risk for the development of hypoglycemia.

5. **True   False**   Babies of diabetic women also have diabetes mellitus and, therefore, are at risk for hypoglycemia.

6. **True   False**   A newborn's blood glucose screening test result of 32 mg/dL requires evaluation.

7. Which of the following term babies is at *highest* risk for hypoglycemia?
    A. Baby whose mother last ate 14 hours prior to delivery
    B. Baby with intrauterine growth restriction
    C. Breastfed baby
    D. Baby who was delivered by planned cesarean section

8. The legs of a term, appropriate-for-gestational-age baby shake uncontrollably for a minute or 2. What should you do?
    A. Begin intravenous therapy with 25% glucose.
    B. Wrap the baby in an extra blanket.
    C. Obtain a blood glucose screening test.
    D. Watch the baby to see if the shaking happens again.

9. A baby weighing 3,780 g (8 lb, 5 oz) is born at 38 weeks' gestation to a woman with diabetes mellitus. What is the most appropriate time for this baby's *first* feeding?
    A. Within 1 hour of age
    B. 4 to 6 hours of age
    C. 8 to 10 hours of age
    D. On demand

10. A baby is being treated for hypoglycemia. The baby's intravenous (IV) infiltrates at 3:00 am. What should you do?
    A. Pull out the IV and have a new one started immediately.
    B. Leave in the IV and slow the rate.
    C. Pull out the IV and have a new one started when rounds are made at 8:00 am.
    D. Pull out the IV and feed the baby 15% glucose by mouth.

11. A baby has a blood glucose screening test result of 10 mg/dL and is jittery. What should you do next?
    A. Begin feedings of formula or breast milk immediately.
    B. Give 2 mL/kg of 25% glucose intravenously, and then run a 10% glucose infusion at 5 mL/kg per hour.
    C. Draw a blood sample for laboratory analysis of blood glucose. If the test confirms a low blood glucose level, begin treatment as soon as the test result is known.
    D. Give 2 mL/kg of 10% glucose intravenously, and then run a 10% glucose infusion at 5 mL/kg per hour.

1. What Is Hypoglycemia?

Hypoglycemia means low blood sugar (glucose). The blood glucose level is maintained by the body converting glycogen stores to glucose. When glycogen reserves are used up, the blood glucose level drops.

 Untreated persistent hypoglycemia in babies can result in death or permanent neurological damage, particularly in babies who have experienced hypoxic-ischemic injury and/or are hyperinsulinemic (eg, infants of inadequately controlled diabetic mothers).

2. Which Babies Are More Likely to Develop Hypoglycemia?

A. Infants of Diabetic Mothers (IDM)

Women with diabetes mellitus often have elevated blood glucose levels. This excess glucose is passed to the fetus through the placenta.

The fetus is not diabetic and, therefore, appropriately increases insulin production to counteract the high blood glucose levels. At delivery, the baby is suddenly separated from the woman's glucose supply. The baby still has very high insulin levels. This causes hypoglycemia to develop in the baby.

Very tight control of maternal diabetes throughout pregnancy may minimize, or eliminate, these effects on the fetus and newborn.

B. Large-for-Gestational-Age (LGA) Babies

Some women develop gestational diabetes mellitus (GDM)—a condition unique to pregnancy. This may not be detected. Babies born to women with abnormal glucose tolerance, whether they have diabetes mellitus or GDM, are often LGA. Therefore, all LGA babies should be considered at risk for developing hypoglycemia.

C. Small-for-Gestational-Age (SGA) Babies

These babies have been malnourished in utero and, therefore, have not built up glycogen stores. Their meager glycogen stores are quickly used up after birth. SGA babies also have a relatively greater metabolic rate and, therefore, use more glucose than appropriate-for-gestational-age babies of the same size.

D. Preterm Babies, including Late Preterm Babies

These babies have had less time to build up glycogen stores. They are also likely to be more stressed at birth than term newborns. Their small glycogen reserves may be quickly exhausted after birth.

E. Post-term Babies

Placental function may begin to deteriorate in post-term gestation. This limits the supply of nutrients from the pregnant woman to the fetus. The fetus may then begin to use fetal glycogen stores to meet metabolic demands. Therefore, when the baby is born, there is a reduced glycogen reserve, which may be used up quickly.

F. Sick or Stressed Babies

Babies may be stressed because the woman has problems during pregnancy (eg, pregnancy-specific hypertension). Babies also may be stressed if problems develop during labor and/or delivery (eg, abruptio placentae). Babies are stressed after birth if they are sick or have been chilled.

Sick or stressed babies have a higher metabolic rate and need extra energy to keep their body functions as close to normal as possible. Babies use glucose and glycogen stores to produce this extra energy. This may deplete the glycogen stores more quickly than normal, and hypoglycemia may develop.

G. Fasted Babies

Babies who must be kept npo or who cannot take adequate amounts orally may become hypoglycemic as their glycogen stores are depleted. Supplementation with glucose-containing intravenous (IV) fluids is essential for all sick babies and for many at-risk babies.

H. Babies With Polycythemia

Babies whose hematocrit exceeds 65% to 70% are at risk for hypoglycemia, although the mechanism is unclear.

I. Babies with congenital anomalies

Some babies with midline craniofacial defects may have abnormal hormonal control of blood glucose (low growth hormone and/or cortisol). Therefore, babies with a cleft palate, a small penis, or ambiguous genitalia should have glucose screening performed.

Self-test

Now answer these questions to test yourself on the information in the last section.

A1. True   False   Babies with hypoglycemia often have low glycogen reserves.

A2. What can happen to a baby who develops hypoglycemia and is not treated properly?

_____

A3. Name 9 categories of babies who are at risk for hypoglycemia.

1. _____
2. _____
3. _____
4. _____
5. _____
6. _____
7. _____
8. _____
9. _____

A4. Babies of diabetic women often have adequate glycogen stores, but are at risk for hypoglycemia because of the high _____ levels they develop in response to their mothers' high blood glucose levels.

Check your answers with the list that follows the Recommended Routines. Correct any incorrect answers and review the appropriate section in the unit.

Note: The following recommendations differ slightly from those published in Pediatrics *(American Academy of Pediatrics, Committee on Fetus and Newborn. Clinical Report—Postnatal glucose homeostasis in late preterm and term infants. Pediatrics. 2011;127:575-579).*

3. How Is Hypoglycemia Detected?

A. Babies With Signs of Hypoglycemia

The most common signs of hypoglycemia include the following, either individually or in combination:

- *Jitteriness:* The baby is hyperreactive to sudden stimuli.
- *Tremors:* An arm or leg shakes uncontrollably.
- *Seizures:* A part of the body shakes rhythmically or becomes rigid.
- *Lethargy:* The baby responds sluggishly or not at all to normal stimuli.
- *Apnea:* Breathing stops suddenly; the baby may turn blue.
- *Cyanosis:* The baby may turn blue.
- *Tachypnea:* The baby may have rapid respirations.
- *High-pitched cry.*
- *Poor feeding*: The baby is reluctant to breastfeed or bottle-feed.
- *Eye rolling*: May be associated with lethargy or seizure activity.
- *No signs:* Blood glucose levels can be very low without giving any clinical indication.

 Some babies with hypoglycemia will not show any signs.

If a baby displays any signs of hypoglycemia, a blood glucose screening test should be obtained *immediately.* Varieties of small, handheld, blood glucose screening instruments are available for this purpose.

B. Babies With Risk Factors for Hypoglycemia

Asymptomatic babies at risk for hypoglycemia who do not have an IV should be fed within 1 hour of age and should have a glucose screening test 30 minutes after the feeding.

Other newborns at risk for hypoglycemia (eg, premature babies weighing under approximately 1,800 g), or sick babies, should have an IV started with a 10% glucose infusion at a rate of 5 mL/kg per hour and a blood glucose screening test obtained within 1 hour after birth.

Even if the first test result is normal, at-risk babies should have tests repeated until there is adequate glucose intake (feedings and/or IV fluids) and blood glucose levels measured before feedings are consistently above 45 mg/dL.

4. How Is Hypoglycemia Prevented in Asymptomatic, At-Risk Babies?

Treatment for at-risk babies is aimed at *prevention* of hypoglycemia. In some cases, hypoglycemia will still develop. It is, therefore, important to *continue to monitor blood glucose screening tests.*

Sick babies, babies who are unable to tolerate nipple or tube feedings or who are npo, and at-risk babies with a birth weight under approximately 1,800 g should have an IV started with D10W within the first hour following birth. (Note: Extremely preterm babies may be given higher IV fluid volumes with D5W. See Book III: Neonatal Care, Unit 5, Intravenous Therapy.)

For other at-risk babies,

- Start early, frequent feedings. Give the first feeding *within* 1 hour after birth.
- Put breastfed babies to the breast frequently, and follow blood glucose screening tests closely.
- Use formula (not glucose water) if a baby is able to tolerate nipple or tube feedings.
- Continue to check blood glucose screening tests for at-risk babies before each feeding for the first 24 hours of age.

5. How Is Hypoglycemia Treated in Babies?

There is some controversy about the specific blood glucose value that should be used to define hypoglycemia. Many experts agree, however, that blood glucose in newborns should be maintained above 45 mg/dL and that a screening test value below 45 mg/dL requires evaluation and some form of treatment. (See Figure 8.1.)

A low screening test result should be confirmed with an actual blood glucose level. Glucometers may give inaccurate readings when the baby's blood glucose is low or low normal.

Appropriate treatment depends on the degree of hypoglycemia. Early, frequent feedings are used to prevent hypoglycemia in at-risk babies, and frequent feedings are also used to treat slightly low blood glucose in any baby. If glucose levels fall, or if a baby develops signs of hypoglycemia, IV infusion of glucose is required.

 Low blood glucose must be brought up quickly. The longer a baby is left with hypoglycemia, the greater the chance of brain damage.

- *Treatment Recommendations* are given in Figure 8.1.
- *Highly Concentrated Glucose:* When bringing blood glucose levels up quickly, **do *not* use highly concentrated glucose** solutions (such as 25% or 50% glucose). Rapid infusions of such concentrated glucose may cause brain damage in small babies. Infusions of excess glucose also may cause an increase in insulin release with recurrence of the hypoglycemia.
- *Infusion of Glucose Higher Than 12.5%:* If continuous infusion of glucose in a concentration higher than 12.5% is needed, infusion through a peripheral IV should be avoided. Infiltration of IV fluids containing concentrated glucose can cause severe tissue damage.

  Infusions of concentrated glucose should be through a central line, such as an umbilical venous catheter (UVC). If a UVC is used, the tip should be placed above the diaphragm to avoid infusion of concentrated glucose solutions into the circulation of the liver. (See Book III: Neonatal Care, Unit 3, Umbilical Catheters.) The baby with an umbilical venous catheter (UVC) in place may begin or continue feeding. When an umbilical artery catheter (UAC) is in place, it is generally recommended that a baby be kept npo.
- *Stopping IV Glucose:* As feedings are tolerated, the infusion should be tapered gradually as blood glucose screening tests are checked frequently. The glucose infusion may be required for 24 to 48 hours or longer.

 Low blood glucose must be <u>treated quickly</u>, but IV glucose therapy should be <u>terminated gradually</u>, or hypoglycemia may recur.

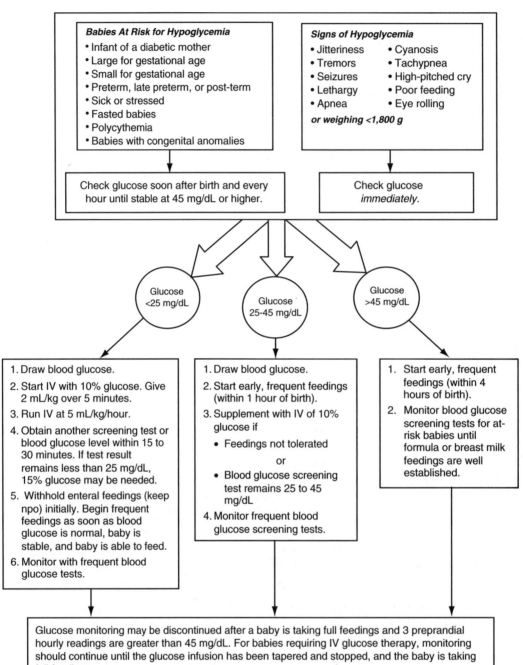

Low blood glucose must be brought up quickly.

Intravenous glucose infusion should be tapered gradually.

Figure 8.1. Prevention, Detection, and Treatment of Neonatal Hypoglycemia.

6. Do Some Babies Need Additional Blood Glucose Monitoring?

Certain babies may need blood glucose monitoring for several days after birth. Babies treated for hypoglycemia may have an undetected recurrence if monitoring is stopped too soon. At-risk babies with low glucose stores may do well initially but develop late-onset hypoglycemia at several days of age, particularly if they become sick or stressed or eat poorly.

A. Monitoring Babies At Risk for Hypoglycemia
  * Continue to obtain blood glucose screening tests until full feedings are well established. This is especially important for breastfed babies because the actual volume of milk a baby takes is unknown.
  * Obtain the blood glucose screening tests before the baby eats, because blood glucose is likely to be lowest just prior to a feeding.
  * Consider supplemental feedings for at-risk babies who are being breastfed, if they cannot maintain their blood glucose levels, drawn before feedings, in the normal range.

B. Monitoring Babies Treated for Hypoglycemia*
  * After beginning IV glucose therapy, frequently check the placement and flow of a baby's IV. If the IV becomes infiltrated, another one should be started without delay.
  * Even if a baby is receiving treatment for hypoglycemia, screening test values or blood glucose levels must be checked within 15 to 30 minutes of starting therapy and frequently thereafter. This is done to be sure the baby is receiving enough glucose.
  * If a baby has a blood glucose level (or blood glucose screening test) less than 25 mg/dL or has signs of hypoglycemia, oral feeding should be delayed until blood glucose has been increased by IV therapy and reached the normal level of >45 mg/dL. A hypoglycemic baby may not be able to coordinate swallowing and breathing and, therefore, may aspirate feedings.
  * Obtain blood glucose screening tests frequently while the glucose infusion is being tapered and until full feedings become established.

---

*Babies requiring more than 12% glucose intravenously to achieve a blood glucose level >45 mg/dL should have glucose delivery calculated as mg/kg/min to determine the amount being received and to ensure receipt of a constant infusion of glucose. This calculation is described in Book III: Neonatal Care, Unit 5, Intravenous Therapy.

Self-test

Now answer these questions to test yourself on the information in the last section.

B1. What are 5 of the most common signs of hypoglycemia?

A. _____

B. _____

C. _____

D. _____

E. _____

B2. A baby has a blood glucose screening test value of 40 mg/dL. What would you do?
   A. Prepare for a blood glucose determination.
   B. Begin early feedings and repeat the blood glucose screening test in 1 hour.
   C. No action indicated.

B3. A baby with hypoglycemia should have the low blood glucose level brought up
   A. Quickly
   B. Slowly

B4. A baby has a blood glucose level of 10 mg/dL. What is the *first* treatment that should be given to treat the hypoglycemia?
   A. Intravenous therapy with normal saline
   B. Early feedings
   C. Intravenous therapy with 10% glucose

B5. **True**   **False**   A blood glucose screening test result of 0 to 25 mg/dL should be confirmed with a blood glucose level.

B6. Which of the following solutions is correct to use for treatment of hypoglycemia?
   A. 10% glucose
   B. 25% glucose
   C. 50% glucose

B7. **True**   **False**   It is important to obtain blood glucose screening tests even while a baby is receiving intravenous glucose in the treatment of hypoglycemia.

B8. **True**   **False**   A baby with low blood glucose will always have at least one sign of hypoglycemia.

B9. A 4,000-g (8 lb, 13 oz) baby is jittery and has a blood glucose screening test result of 20 mg/dL. You draw a blood glucose level, then immediately begin treatment with an intravenous infusion of 10% dextrose.
   How much would you give initially? _____
   What rate would you set for the infusion? _____

Check your answers with the list that follows the Recommended Routines. Correct any incorrect answers and review the appropriate section in the unit.

Hypoglycemia

Recommended Routines

All the routines listed below are based on the principles of perinatal care presented in the unit you have just finished. They are recommended as part of routine perinatal care.

Read each routine carefully and decide whether it is standard operating procedure in your hospital. Check the appropriate blank next to each routine.

Procedure Standard in My Hospital	Needs Discussion by Our Staff	
_____	_____	1. Establish standing orders that will ensure blood glucose screening for all babies at risk for hypoglycemia.
_____	_____	2. Establish a policy of • Starting early feedings for well babies • Starting feedings within 1 hour of age for babies at risk for hypoglycemia • Establishing intravenous glucose within 1 hour of age for the very low birth weight or sick baby
_____	_____	3. Establish a policy of regular calibration and quality control measures for the bedside glucose screening instrument(s) used in your hospital. This procedure should follow manufacturer's instructions and be in accordance with your hospital's policy regarding point-of-care tests.

Self-test Answers

These are the answers to the self-test questions. Please check them with the answers you gave and review the information in the unit wherever necessary.

A1. True

A2. Death or permanent neurological damage,

A3. A. Infants of diabetic mothers
   B. Large-for-gestational-age babies
   C. Small-for-gestational-age babies
   D. Preterm babies
   E. Post-term babies
   F. Sick or stressed babies
   G. Fasted babies
   H. Babies with polycythemia
   I. Babies with certain congenital anomalies

A4. Insulin

B1. Any 5 of the following
   • Jitteriness
   • Tremors
   • Seizures
   • Lethargy
   • Apnea
   • Cyanosis
   • Tachypnoa
   • High-pitched cry
   • Poor feeding
   • Eye rolling

B2. A and B

B3. A. Quickly.

B4. C. Intravenous therapy with 10% glucose

B5. True.   However, treatment for the hypoglycemia should begin immediately, before the result of the blood glucose level is known.

B6. A. 10% glucose

B7. True

B8. False.   Some babies with hypoglycemia may not have any signs. Lack of signs does not mean the baby's hypoglycemia is less significant.

B9. *Initial dose* is 2 mL/kg given slowly: 2 mL $\times$ 4.0 kg = 8 mL

   Continuous infusion is 5 mL/kg/hr: 5 mL $\times$ 4.0 kg = 20 mL/hr

   You would give 8 mL of 10% glucose intravenously over 5 to 10 minutes. This should be followed by a continuous infusion of 10% glucose at a rate of 20 mL per hour.

Unit 8 Posttest

If you are applying for continuing education credits, a posttest for this unit is available online. Completion of unit posttests and the book evaluation form are required to achieve continuing education credit. For more details, go to www.cmevillage.com.

SKILL UNIT

Blood Glucose Screening Tests

This skill unit will teach you how to perform a blood glucose screening test. Several brands of glucose electronic screening instruments (glucometers) are commercially available. If your hospital uses more than one brand of glucometer in the perinatal care areas, you will need to learn how to use each brand.

Study this skill unit, and then attend a skill practice and demonstration session.

To master the skill, you will need to demonstrate each of the following steps correctly:

1. Calibrate the glucometers used in your hospital according to manufacturer's instructions.
2. Milk blood toward baby's heel and/or wrap foot in warm compress (may be optional if using an automated incision device).
3. Prepare heel.
4. Prick heel.
5. Touch drop of blood to reagent strip or microchamber.
6. Record test results.

PERINATAL PERFORMANCE GUIDE

Blood Glucose Screening Tests

Several different manufacturers produce a variety of electronic instruments designed for bedside screening of blood for blood glucose level. This skill unit will describe the general technique for obtaining a blood sample and delivering it to a glucometer, but details of the procedure are different for different brands of machines. Be sure to follow manufacturer's instructions for the testing materials and device(s) used in your hospital.

ACTIONS	REMARKS

Deciding to Use a Blood Glucose Screening Test

1. Ask yourself, "Is there any reason to suspect that the baby's blood glucose level may be low?"

   - Does the mother have diabetes mellitus?
   - Is the baby small or large for gestational age?
   - Is the baby preterm or post-term?
   - Is the baby sick or been stressed?
   - Does the baby have polycythemia (hematocrit >65%)?
   - Does the baby have any signs of hypoglycemia (lethargic, irritable, tremors, seizures, jittery, unexplained apnea spell)?
   - Is the baby not being fed enterally or not taking adequate feedings?
   - Does the baby have any congenital anomalies?

   Yes: Do a screening test.

   No: There is no indication a blood glucose screening test is needed.

Obtaining a Blood Glucose Screening Test

2. Collect the proper equipment.
   - Reagent test or microchamber strip
   - Skin antiseptic swab preferred by your hospital
   - Sterile 2 x 2 gauze
   - Adhesive bandage (optional)
   - Heel warmer (preferred)
   - Incision device for blood sampling*

Test strips gradually deteriorate after a container is opened. Always use the original container to store strips, label the bottle with the date first opened, and close the cap tightly immediately after obtaining a strip.

Select the size that matches the size of the baby.

---

*Examples are Tenderfoot, by International Technidyne Corporation (www.itcmed.com), and NeatNick, by Hawaii Medical (www.hawaiimedical.com).

ACTIONS **REMARKS**

Obtaining a Blood Glucose Screening Test (continued)

3. Prepare the glucometer according to the manufacturer's instructions and your hospital's policy regarding tests done at the bedside.

   Glucometers may require a drop of blood to be absorbed into the microchamber of a disposable test strip. The microchamber is inserted into the reader, which gives a blood glucose value in a specified number of seconds. Some glucometers require the disposable test strip to be inserted before the drop of blood is applied.

The readers, or glucometers, must be checked against a quality control standard. Usually this check is performed when

- A new bottle of test strips is opened.
- The lid was left off a bottle of test strips.
- The monitor was dropped.
- Test results do not seem to match clinical condition.
- Glucometer batteries were changed.
- A specified period of time (usually 24 hours) has elapsed since the last check was done.

Know the specific quality control procedure for the glucometer you are using.

4. Take the baby's leg in your hand. Gently milk the blood toward the heel, then gently squeeze the foot. Release your squeeze and milk again. Repeat this until the sole of the foot is bright pink.

   Note: This step is generally not needed when an automated incision device is used or when a heel warmer is applied for 5 minutes prior to procedure.

This is to ensure freshly circulated capillary blood in the baby's foot, and that blood will flow readily when the heel is pricked. If time allows, it is preferable to achieve the same effect by wrapping a warm compress or heel warmer around the baby's foot for 5 to 10 minutes.

5. Identify the spot to prick to obtain the blood sample.

   Better blood flow is obtained when the inside of the heel is pricked. The outside of the heel also may be used, but do *not* prick the

   - Sole of the foot
   - Center or the back of the heel

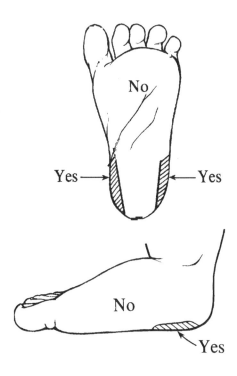

ACTIONS   **REMARKS**

Obtaining a Blood Glucose Screening Test (continued)

6. Clean the baby's heel with the skin antiseptic swab. Allow the heel to dry.

7. Stick the heel with a quick, determined thrust of the microlancet or use an automated incision device.

    Note: There is evidence that spring-loaded automatic microlancets need fewer repeat punctures and are associated with fewer newborn distress responses than manual lancets.

    (A manual lancet is illustrated.)

8. Apply gentle pressure with thumbs and fingers to the baby's leg and foot. Release to allow for capillary refill. Avoid excessive milking of the baby's leg, because it can cause hemolysis and an increase in pain.

If using a microlancet (shown in the illustration below), cautious, tiny jabs may cause trauma to the skin but not produce any blood.

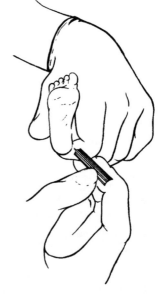

9. Wipe away first drop of blood with sterile gauze.

10. Touch the opening of the microchamber or the reagent strip to the drop of blood.

    Capillary action will fill the microchamber with blood. Be sure the chamber is completely filled.

    Be certain you know how the testing materials and glucometer(s) used in your hospital work.

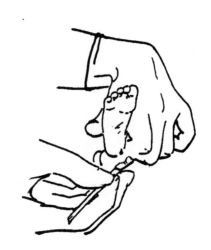

ACTIONS	REMARKS

Obtaining a Blood Glucose Screening Test (continued)

11. Put the reagent strip or microchamber into the glucometer. Some glucometers require the reagent strip to be loaded into the device before blood is applied.

The machine will take a specified time (usually a precise number of seconds) to register a reading.

12. Record the glucose screening test result and time in the baby's chart.

If you get a low blood glucose screening test result, you should confirm this by sending a blood sample to the laboratory for chemical analysis of blood glucose. However, do not wait for the laboratory result before starting therapy.

13. Soothe the baby. A variety of comfort measures can be used alone or in combination to manage heelstick pain. These include
    - Facilitated tucking (extremities flexed and held close to baby's trunk)
    - Positioning and nesting
    - Gentle, rhythmic stroking, patting, or rocking
    - Swaddling and/or holding the baby in an upright position
    - Pacifier use for nonnutritive sucking
    - Pacifier with 24% sucrose solution

Reducing pain and helping a baby to self-regulate following a painful procedure can reduce short-term physiologic and biochemical stress responses.

ACTIONS	REMARKS

What Can Go Wrong?

1. The baby's heel is not dry, thus resulting in diluted blood.

Reading will be low.

2. The test strip has deteriorated.

Reading will be false. Be sure to put the lid tightly on the bottle after obtaining a strip. Label the bottle with the date it is first opened. Discard containers according to manufacturer's recommendations and/or expiration date on the container, whichever comes sooner.

ACTIONS	REMARKS

What Can Go Wrong? (continued)

3. You prick the center or back of the baby's heel.

This may have serious, long-term consequences. Repeated pricks over the weight-bearing center of the heel can cause scar tissue formation and result in delayed walking and/or abnormal gait. Pricks over the back of the heel can damage the Achilles tendon.

However, numerous repeated blood samples may be safely obtained when the heel is pricked within the shaded areas shown in the illustrations that accompany step 5 of the previous section.

4. The baby's foot or leg is bruised after the procedure.

Excessive squeezing was used to obtain the drop of blood. Bruising should *not* occur. Good blood flow can be obtained by warming the baby's foot with a heel warmer, and by correctly using an automated incision device.

5. Quality control checks are not performed regularly.

Be sure to follow the manufacturer's directions for the quality control procedure and recommended frequency of checks for the specific glucometer used in your hospital.

You also should know your hospital's policy regarding point-of-care laboratory tests.

6. You use a manual lancet or an incorrect size of automatic incision device and go too far into the baby's flesh.

The depth of penetration of a manual lancet is variable. Automatic devices enter the skin at a controlled, standard depth, but must be the correct device for the size of the baby in your care. Devices for term babies enter the skin farther than devices designed for smaller babies. Devices are generally available in term and preterm neonatal sizes, and sometimes in a third size for extremely preterm babies.

PCEP

Perinatal Continuing Education Program

Pretest Answer Key
Book I: Maternal and Fetal Evaluation and Immediate Newborn Care

Unit 1: Is the Mother Sick? Is the Fetus Sick?

PRETEST

1. Yes   No
   - X ___ By the woman's primary care physician, in consultation with a specialist
   - ___ X By the woman's primary care physician, until she enters labor
   - X ___ Jointly by the woman's primary care physician and a specialist, with prenatal visits by the woman to both
   - X ___ Transfer of the woman's care entirely to a specialist at regional medical center

2. Yes   No
   - X ___ Ask the woman about recent intake of prescription and nonprescription drugs.
   - X ___ Check fetal heart rate.
   - X ___ Assess frequency, duration, and quality of contractions.
   - X ___ Review the course of previous labors and deliveries.
   - X ___ Assess fetal position and estimate fetal weight.

3. D
4. False
5. False
6. False
7. False
8. False
9. True
10. True
11. Yes No
    - X ___ Decreased fetal movement for 1 day, at 34 weeks' gestation
    - X ___ Occasional periods of bradycardia (heart rate <110 beats per minute)
    - X ___ Premature rupture of membranes
    - X ___ A woman with gestational hypertension
12. Yes   No
    - X ___ Gonorrhea
    - X ___ Stable renal disease
    - X ___ Abnormal glucose tolerance
    - X ___ Maternal age of 13 years

Unit 2: Fetal Age, Growth, and Maturity

1. B
2. A
3. D
4. True
5. True
6. True
7. False
8. False
9. A
10. A
11. False
12. False
13. True
14. True

Unit 3: Fetal Well-being

1. D
2. A
3. B
4. C
5. D
6. C
7. True
8. False
9. True
10. True

11. True
12. True
13. False
14. True
15. False
16. B
17. C
18. A
19. D

Unit 4: Is the Baby Sick?

NO PRETEST

Unit 5: Resuscitating the Newborn

1. C
2. C
3. B
4. A
5. D
6. A
7. B
8. B
9. C
10. D
11. A

12. A
13. D
14. B
15. True
16. False
17. True
18. False
19. True
20. True
21. False
22. True

Unit 6: Gestational Age and Size and Associated Risk Factors

1. False
2. B
3. D
4a. A
4b. B
4c. C

5a. B
5b. A
5c. A
6a. A
6b. C

Unit 7: Thermal Environment

1. A
2. D
3. C
4. B
5. A
6. True
7. False

8. False
9. False
10. True
11. True
12. False
13. False

312

Unit 8: Hypoglycemia

1. True
2. False
3. True
4. True
5. False
6. True

7. B
8. C
9. A
10. A
11. D

Glossary

ABO incompatibility: A condition that may lead to neonatal hemolytic disease. The pregnant woman has group O red cells and has antibodies to group A red cells and group B red cells. These antibodies are transferred to the fetus and cause destruction of fetal red blood cells. While this process is similar to Rh incompatibility, the hemolytic disease resulting from ABO incompatibility is less severe than the disease caused by Rh incompatibility. Unlike Rh incompatibility, ABO incompatibility cannot be prevented by giving the mother Rh immune globulin.

Abruptio placentae: Premature separation of a normally placed placenta. Placenta separation can occur at any time during pregnancy, but is most likely to occur during late pregnancy and before the onset of labor. Several risk factors are associated with abruptio placentae, but usually the cause is unknown. Depending on the degree of separation, bleeding may be slight or severe. If severe, both the woman and fetus may go into shock. Bleeding, even severe bleeding, can be completely hidden behind the placenta. In the most severe cases, the uterus is tense, board-like, and tender. The woman's blood pressure may fall, and symptoms of shock and/or disseminated intravascular coagulation may develop. Fetal distress is common, and fetal death may occur. Abruptio placentae requires an emergency response.

Abruption: Used synonymously with abruptio placentae.

Acidosis: Abnormally *low* pH of the blood. The range of blood pH in a healthy neonate is between 7.25 and 7.35. A blood pH of 7.20 or lower is considered severe acidosis. Acidosis may result from metabolic disturbances in which the serum bicarbonate is low, or from inadequate respiratory efforts in which serum carbon dioxide is high. Often metabolic and respiratory factors simultaneously influence the blood pH. Acidotic babies are usually lethargic and may have mottled or grayish-colored skin. If extremely acidotic, babies typically take deep, regular gasping breaths. If a baby is gasping, the pH is probably 7.0 or less. Acidosis should be corrected promptly, most commonly with assisted ventilation when due to inadequate respiratory effort, or occasionally by administration of sodium bicarbonate if due to metabolic factors.

Acoustic stimulation: A test in which fetal response to a sound when produced by a device placed against the maternal abdomen and triggered to give a loud, 1-second buzz is used as an estimate of fetal well-being. This test may be used during a non-stress test and during labor.

Acquired immunodeficiency syndrome (AIDS): The symptomatic stage of the illness caused by the human immunodeficiency virus (HIV).

Adrenaline: Official British Pharmacopoeia name for epinephrine. The trademark name for epinephrine preparations is Adrenalin.

Age, adjusted: *See* Age, corrected.

Age, chronological: The number of days, weeks, months, or years that have elapsed since birth.

Age, conceptional: The time elapsed between the day of conception and the day of delivery. (Note: The term conceptual age is incorrect and should not be used.) Conceptional age may be used when conception occurred as a result of assisted reproductive technology, but should *not* be used to indicate the age of a fetus or newborn. *See* Age, gestational.

Age, corrected: Chronological age in weeks or months reduced by the number of weeks born before 40 weeks of gestation. It is used only for children up to 3 years of age who were born preterm. It is the preferred term to use after neonatal hospitalization, and should be used instead of "adjusted age." *Example:* A 24-month-old child born at 28 weeks' gestation has a corrected age of 21 months.

Age, gestational: The number of weeks that have passed from the first day of the woman's last menstrual period to the time at which you estimate the age of a fetus or the birth of a baby. If pregnancy was achieved using assisted reproductive technology and, therefore, the date of fertilization or implantation is defined, gestational age may be calculated by adding 2 weeks to the conceptional age.

Age, postmenstrual: The weeks of gestational age, plus chronological age. It is the preferred term to describe the age of preterm infants during neonatal hospitalization. (Note: Postconceptional age should *not* be used.) *Example:* A baby born at 33 weeks, 1 day with a chronological age of 5 weeks, 4 days has a postmenstrual age of 38 weeks, 5 days.

Albumin: The major protein in blood.

Alkalosis: Abnormally *high* pH of the blood. The range of blood pH in a healthy neonate is between 7.25 and 7.35. Alkalosis may result from a high serum bicarbonate or, more commonly, when the carbon dioxide concentration in a baby's blood is lowered by hyperventilation (assisting the baby's breathing at an excessively fast rate). Babies who are alkalotic may not respond to stimulation intended to increase their breathing efforts until their blood carbon dioxide level rises toward the normal range.

Alpha-fetoprotein: A normal fetal serum protein. When a fetus has an open neural tube defect, such as anencephaly or meningomyelocele, increased amounts of this protein pass into the pregnant woman's blood and the amniotic fluid, thus providing the basis for an antenatal screening test. Low or high maternal serum alpha-fetoprotein levels may also indicate certain other fetal chromosomal defects or congenital malformations.

ALT: Alanine aminotransferase (alanine transaminase). The serum level of this enzyme is used as a measure of liver function. When liver cells are destroyed by disease or trauma, transaminases are released into the bloodstream. The higher the ALT, the greater the number of destroyed or damaged liver cells.

Alveoli: The numerous, small, sac-like structures in the lungs where the exchange of oxygen and carbon dioxide between the lungs and the blood takes place.

Amniocentesis: A procedure used to obtain amniotic fluid for tests to determine genetic makeup, health, or maturity of the fetus. Using ultrasound guidance, a needle is inserted through a pregnant woman's abdominal wall and into the uterus where a sample of amniotic fluid is withdrawn, usually at 16 to 20 weeks' gestation. If done earlier (11-13 weeks), there is often insufficient amniotic fluid and the complication rate is higher.

Amnioinfusion: Infusion of fluid into the amniotic cavity. Amnioinfusion may be done by either of the following procedures: (1) after membranes have ruptured, by passing a catheter through the cervix and into the uterus and infusing normal saline warmed to body temperature or (2) by infusing warmed saline through an amniocentesis needle placed through the maternal abdominal wall and into the uterus. Amnioinfusion may be used to reduce cord compression (as indicated by variable fetal heart rate decelerations) during labor when oligohydramnios is present.

Amnion: The inner membrane surrounding the fetus. The amnion lines the chorion but is separate from it. Together these membranes contain the fetus and the amniotic fluid.

Amnionitis: Infection of the amniotic fluid and amnion. If amnionitis is present, the woman will usually have a fever and, when the membranes rupture, the amniotic fluid may be foul-smelling and/or cloudy. Chorioamnionitis almost always develops if amnionitis is present.

Amniotic fluid: Fluid that surrounds the fetus and makes up the "water" in the "bag of waters." It provides a liquid environment in which the fetus can grow freely and serves as insulation, protecting the fetus from temperature changes. It also protects the fetus from a blow to the uterus by distributing equally in all directions any force applied to the uterus. Amniotic fluid is composed mainly of fetal urine, but also contains cells from the fetus's skin and chemical compounds from the fetus's respiratory passages.

Amniotic fluid analysis: Evaluation of various compounds in the amniotic fluid that relate to fetal lung maturity and fetal health. Fetal skin cells that normally float in the amniotic fluid may also be obtained with amniocentesis and grown in a culture to allow determination of fetal chromosomal status.

Amniotic fluid embolism: Amniotic fluid that escapes into the maternal circulation, usually late in labor or immediately postpartum. Rather than causing a mechanical blockage in the circulation as emboli of other origin might do, amniotic fluid embolism is thought to cause an anaphylactic-type response in susceptible women. This response is dramatic and severe, with sudden onset of hypoxia and hypotension. Seizures and/or cardiac arrest may occur. If a woman survives the initial phase, disseminated intravascular coagulation often follows. Although rare, it is one of the more common causes of maternal death in industrialized countries.

Amniotic fluid index (AFI): A way of estimating the relative volume of amniotic fluid from ultrasound measurement of a fluid pocket in each uterine quadrant. The 4 measurements are summed and compared to a chart of normal values for each week of gestation.

Analgesia: The relative relief of pain without loss of consciousness. Administration of specific medication(s) is the most common way to provide analgesia.

Anemia: Abnormally low number of red blood cells. The red blood cells may be lost due to bleeding, destroyed due to disease process, or produced in insufficient numbers. Anemia is determined by measuring the hemoglobin or hematocrit.

Anencephaly: A lethal congenital defect of neural tube development where there is partial or complete absence of the skull and brain.

Anesthesia: The total relief of pain, with or without loss of consciousness. Usually requires more invasive techniques than that required for analgesia. General inhalation anesthesia produces loss of consciousness while major conduction anesthesia, such as spinal or epidural injection of long-lasting local anesthetics, produces total loss of pain in a specific area of the body without loss of consciousness.

Anomaly, congenital: Malformation resulting from abnormal development during embryonic or fetal growth. For example, a cleft lip is a congenital anomaly, as is gastroschisis, anencephaly, and countless others. Used synonymously with congenital malformation.

Antenatal testing: Techniques used to evaluate fetal growth and well-being prior to the onset of labor. Examples include non-stress test, biophysical profile, and ultrasonography.

Antenatal: Period during pregnancy before birth. Synonymous with prenatal.

Antepartum: Period of pregnancy before delivery. Most often used for period of pregnancy preceding the onset of labor. (Intrapartum is used to refer to the time during labor.) Used in reference to the woman.

Antibody: A type of blood protein that is produced by the body's lymph tissue in response to an antigen (a protein that is foreign to the bloodstream). Each specific antibody is formed as a defense mechanism against a specific antigen.

Antibody screening test: A test of maternal serum against a large variety of blood group antigens as a screening test for possible blood group incompatibility between a pregnant woman and her fetus. If the antibody screening test is positive, the individual blood group incompatibility should be identified. *See also* Coombs test.

Antibody titers: A test used to indicate the relative concentration of a particular antibody present in a person's blood. *Example:* A high rubella titer indicates a person has been exposed to rubella (German measles) and has formed a significant amount of antibody against the rubella virus and, therefore, will most likely be able to ward off another attack of the virus without becoming ill.

Anticonvulsants: Drugs given to prevent the occurrence of seizures (convulsions). The most common anticonvulsants used in infants are phenobarbital and Dilantin (phenytoin). Anticonvulsant therapy, with certain medications, for a pregnant woman with a seizure disorder may affect the health of the fetus.

Antiphospholipid antibody syndrome (APS): Development of antibodies to naturally occurring phospholipids in the blood, causing abnormal phospholipid function. Antiphospholipid antibodies may be present in healthy women but are more commonly associated with a generalized disease (eg, lupus erythematosus). They have a strong association with recurrent abortion, fetal growth restriction, preeclampsia, and other factors adversely affecting fetal and/or maternal health.

Aorta: The main artery leaving the heart and feeding the systemic circulation. It passes through the chest and abdomen, where it branches into smaller arteries. In a newborn, an umbilical arterial catheter passes through one of the arteries in the umbilical cord and into the abdominal section of the aorta.

Apgar score: A score given to newborns and based on heart rate, respiratory effort, muscle tone, reflex irritability, and color. The score is given 1 minute after the baby's head and feet are delivered (not from the time the cord is cut) and again when the baby is 5 minutes old. If the 5-minute score is less than 7, additional scores are given every 5 minutes for a total of 20 minutes. The 1-minute Apgar score indicates a baby's immediate condition; the 5-minute score reflects the baby's condition and the effectiveness of re-suscitative efforts. A low 5-minute score is a worrisome sign. It is not, however, a certain indicator of damage. Likewise, a high score is not a guarantee of a healthy baby. The score is named for Dr Virginia Apgar, who developed it. The 5 letters of her name may also be used to signify the 5 components of the score: A = appearance (color), P = pulse (heart rate), G = grimace (reflex irritability), A = activity (muscle tone), and R = respirations.

Apnea: Stoppage of breathing for 15 seconds or longer; or stoppage of breathing for less than 15 seconds if also accompanied by bradycardia or cyanosis.

Appropriate for gestational age (AGA): Refers to a baby whose weight is above the 10th percentile and below the 90th percentile for babies of that gestational age.

Arrhythmia: Abnormal rhythm of the heartbeat. *Fetal* arrhythmias are rare. One of the more common ones is congenital heart block, which occurs almost exclusively with maternal systemic lupus erythema-tosus, although it is uncommon even in that situation. With a *maternal* arrhythmia, the more persistent the arrhythmia and the farther the rate is from normal (either faster or slower), the more likely it is that there will be a deleterious effect on maternal cardiac output and, thus, on blood flow to the uterus.

Artery: Any blood vessel that carries blood away from the heart.

Asphyxia: A condition resulting from inadequate oxygenation and/or blood flow and characterized by low blood oxygen, high blood carbon dioxide, metabolic acidosis, and organ injury.

Aspiration: (1) Breathing in or inhaling of a fluid (such as formula, meconium, or amniotic fluid) into the lungs. Aspiration usually interferes with lung function and oxygenation. If inhaled, meconium is irritat-ing as well as obstructing, resulting in meconium aspiration syndrome, which often causes serious and sometimes fatal lung disease. (2) The removal of fluids or gases from a cavity, such as the stomach, by suction. *Example:* A nasogastric tube is inserted and an empty syringe is attached to the tube and used to suck out or aspirate air and gastric juices from the stomach.

Assisted ventilation: Use of mechanical devices to help a person breathe. Bag and mask with bag-breathing, endotracheal tube with bag-breathing, or a respirator machine may each be used to assist ventilation.

AST: Aspartate aminotransferase (aspartate transaminase). The serum level of this enzyme is used as a measure of liver function. As with alanine aminotransferase, liver damage causes transaminases to be re-leased into the bloodstream.

Atelectasis: Condition in which lung alveoli have collapsed and remain shut.

Atony: Loss of muscle tone or strength. Uterine atony is a leading cause of postpartum hemorrhage.

Axillary: Refers to the axilla, or armpit.

Bacteriuria: The presence of bacteria in the urine. May also be spelled bacteruria.

Bag-breathing: Artificially breathing for a person by inflating the lungs with a resuscitation bag and mask or resuscitation bag and endotracheal tube.

Ballooning of lower uterine segment: A sign of impending labor, either term or preterm. The process leading to labor produces thinning of the lower uterine segment of myometrium, so that the lower seg-ment "balloons out" into the anterior fornix of the vagina. The "ballooned" segment may be seen during speculum examination or palpated during digital examination.

BCG: Bacille Calmette-Guérin. Vaccine made from the Calmette-Guérin strain of *Mycobacterium bovis* for immunization against tuberculosis.

Beta human chorionic gonadotropin (ß-hCG): A hormone produced by the trophoblastic cells of the chorionic villi. It is the first biochemical marker of pregnancy and is produced in increasing amounts until maximal levels are reached at 8 to 10 weeks. When present in the blood or urine of a woman, she is pregnant. High titers are found with multifetal gestation and erythroblastosis fetalis, extremely high titers may be seen with hydatidiform mole and choriocarcinoma, while declining or low levels are found with spontaneous abortion and ectopic pregnancy.

Betamimetic: A drug that stimulates beta receptors of smooth muscle, such as the myometrium (uterine muscle), causing decreased contractions. Used to suppress the onset of premature labor. A betamimetic drug is also called a beta-agonist. An example is terbutaline.

Bilirubin: A substance produced from the breakdown of red blood cells. High blood bilirubin level causes the yellow coloring of the skin (and sclera) that is termed jaundice.

Biophysical profile (BPP): A combination of measures used to evaluate fetal well-being. Each of the 5 components ([1] non-stress test, [2] ultrasound evaluation of amniotic fluid volume, [3] fetal body movements, [4] muscle tone, and [5] respirations) are scored. Each measure is given 2 points if present, zero if absent (there is no score of 1). The scores are added together for the final BPP score.

Biparietal diameter (BPD): Diameter of the skull, measured as the distance between the parietal bones, which lie just above each ear. Ultrasonography is used to determine the BPD of the fetal skull. Serial BPD measurements are used to assess fetal growth and to estimate fetal gestational age.

Bishop score: A system that scores cervical dilation, effacement, consistency, and position, as well as station of the presenting part to assess the "readiness" of a cervix for labor. Scores correlate with the likelihood that an attempt at induction of labor will be successful.

Blood gas measurement: Determination of the pH and concentration of oxygen, carbon dioxide, and bicarbonate in the blood.

Blood group: There are numerous blood groups in humans, each defined by their antigenic responses. The major blood groups are A, B, AB, and O, which are then further defined by their Rh type, positive or negative, as well as various other minor antigens.

Note: Every person is exposed to the major blood group antigens (A and B) soon after birth, because the antigens are found in the air, food, and water. Each person who lacks one or both of the major blood group genes (A or B) will make antibodies against the antigen(s) they lack. Thus persons with blood group O develop anti-A and anti-B antibodies and keep them throughout life. If given a blood transfusion with group A or B blood, a person with group O blood will have a transfusion reaction, which may in some cases be fatal. Similar reactions occur when a person with group B blood is given group A blood, or vice versa. Group "AB" persons do not make antibodies against either A or B because they have both antigens on their red blood cells. Persons with group AB blood can receive blood from people with any major blood group, but AB blood should be transfused only into persons with AB blood. Persons with group O blood should receive only blood transfusions with O blood, but O blood may be used to transfuse a person with any major blood group. This is why a person with AB blood is called a "universal recipient" and a person with O blood is called a "universal donor."

Blood pressure, diastolic: The lowest point of the blood pressure between heartbeats, when the heart is relaxed.

Blood pressure, mean: The average blood pressure about halfway between the systolic and diastolic blood pressures.

Blood pressure, systolic: The highest point of the blood pressure. The blood pressure during the heartbeat, when the heart is contracted.

Blood smear: A thin layer of blood spread across a glass slide and studied under a microscope to determine the types of blood cells present.

Blood glucose screening test: Any of several commercially available, small, thin, plastic reagent strips designed to estimate blood glucose level with a single drop of blood. A color change caused by a drop of blood placed on the reagent pad provides an estimate of the blood glucose level. In addition, several handheld devices are designed to draw in a tiny amount of blood and give a digital readout of the glucose level.

Blood type: *See* Blood group.

Bloody show: Bloody mucus passed from the vagina in late pregnancy, usually associated with cervical effacement. It often heralds the onset of labor and is a normal finding. Any bleeding in pregnancy, however, should be investigated.

bpm: Abbreviation for beats per minute. Used primarily in relation to fetal heart rate.

Brachial plexus nerve injury: Paralysis of the arm that results from injury to the upper brachial plexus. Is associated with shoulder dystocia or a difficult breech delivery when traction is applied to the shoulder, stretching the nerve trunks exiting from the cervical spinal cord (brachial plexus). However, about half of these injuries occur in children in which there was no evidence of either shoulder dystocia or breech delivery. The injury, therefore, may be initiated before birth by deformation of the neck and shoulder by abnormal positioning of the fetus. Many such palsies will recover within the first few years of life.

Bracht maneuver: A method of delivering breech presentations in cases where delivery is imminent and neither a practitioner skilled in vaginal breech delivery nor cesarean section is immediately available.

Bradycardia: Slow heart rate. (1) *Fetal:* Considered to be a baseline heart rate of less than 110 beats per minute for 2 minutes or longer. Bradycardia alone may or may not indicate fetal distress. (2) *Neonatal:* Considered to be a sustained heart rate less than 100 beats per minute.

Breech presentation: The feet-first or buttocks-first presentation of a fetus. *Frank:* buttocks present, with the fetus's legs extended upward alongside the body; *footling:* one foot can be felt below the buttocks; *double footling:* both feet can be felt below the buttocks; *complete:* buttocks present, with the knees flexed.

Bronchopulmonary dysplasia (BPD): Also called chronic lung disease (CLD). A form of CLD sometimes seen in infants who have required ventilator therapy for any of a variety of lung problems, including respiratory distress syndrome, meconium aspiration syndrome, etc. BPD is thought to result from the combined effects of oxygen free-radical injury of premature lungs and trauma to the lungs produced by high airway pressures generated by ventilators.

Brow presentation: The brow (forehead) of the fetus is the presenting part. On vaginal examination, the anterior fontanel can be felt, but the posterior fontanel cannot. Management depends on whether the presentation stays brow, changes to face, or the baby's neck flexes and the presentation becomes vertex.

BUN: Blood urea nitrogen. A blood chemistry test of renal function. The higher the BUN, the more urinary excretion has been impaired.

Caput succedaneum: Edema of the fetal scalp that develops during labor. This swelling crosses the suture lines of the skull. Caput succedaneum may occur with a normal, spontaneous vaginal delivery but a lengthy labor or delivery by vacuum extraction increases the risk of occurrence.

Cardiac massage: *See* Chest compressions.

Cardiac output: The output of the left ventricle in milliliters per minute.

Central nervous system depression: Condition in which the body is less reactive than normal to stimuli, such as a pinprick. Central nervous system depression may be characterized by delayed reflexes, lethargy, or coma. It may result from a variety of causes, including certain drugs, certain metabolic disorders, or asphyxia.

Cephalhematoma: Also cephalohematoma. Hematoma under the periosteum of the skull and limited to one cranial bone (does not cross suture lines) of the newborn. It is usually seen following prolonged labor and difficult delivery, but may also occur with uncomplicated birth. Delivery with forceps or vacuum extraction increases the risk of occurrence.

Cephalopelvic disproportion (CPD): *See* Fetopelvic disproportion.

Cerclage of the cervix: The procedure of placing a suture around the cervix to prevent it from dilating prematurely. There are several different techniques for placing the suture. Cervical cerclage is used as a treatment for incompetent cervix.

Cervix: The cervix of the uterus is the lower, narrow end of the uterus, which opens into the vagina.

Cesarean delivery (or section): Surgical delivery of the fetus through an abdominal incision. The uterine incision may be classical (vertical, cutting through both the contractile and non-contractile segments) or confined to the non-contractile lower uterine segment (either vertical or transverse incision).

Chest compressions: Artificial pumping of the blood through the heart by a bellows effect created from intermittent compression of the sternum, over the heart, during resuscitation.

Chickenpox: *See* Varicella-zoster.

Chlamydia: A type of microorganism with several species. Capable of producing a variety of illnesses, including eye infection, pneumonia, and infection of the genitourinary tract.

Choanal atresia: Congenital blockage of the nasal airway. Because babies breathe mainly through their noses, a baby with choanal atresia will have severe respiratory distress at birth. The immediate treatment is insertion of an oral airway. Surgical repair when the baby is stable is required for permanent correction.

Chorioamnionitis: Inflammation of the fetal membranes, also known as intra-amniotic infection, or IAI. The fetus may also become infected.

Chorion: Fetal membrane that surrounds the amnion, but is separate from it, and lies against the decidual lining of the uterine cavity (endometrium). During embryonic development the chorion gives rise to the placenta.

Chorionic villus sampling (CVS): A highly specialized technique in which a tiny portion of the chorionic villi, which contains the same genetic material as the fetus, is obtained in a manner similar to a needle biopsy. The cells obtained may be analyzed for chromosomal defects. CVS may be done as early as 9 weeks' gestation, with the results available within 2 days, allowing earlier and more rapid detection of chromosomal disorders than is possible with amniocentesis. The incidence of complications is low but somewhat higher than the risks associated with amniocentesis.

Chromosome: The material (DNA protein) in each body cell that contains the genes, or information regarding hereditary factors. Each normal cell contains 46 chromosomes. Each chromosome contains numerous genes. A baby acquires half of the chromosomes from the mother and half from the father. A chromosomal defect results from an abnormal number of chromosomes or structural damage to the chromosomes. *Example:* Each cell in the body of a baby with Down syndrome (trisomy 21) contains 47 instead of 46 chromosomes.

Circulatory system: The system that carries blood through the body and consists of the heart and blood vessels. The systemic circulatory system carries blood to and from the head, arms, legs, trunk, and all body organs except the lungs. The pulmonary circulatory system carries blood to the lungs, where carbon dioxide is released and oxygen is collected, and returns the oxygenated blood to the systemic circulatory system.

Cirrhosis: Chronic degeneration of the hepatic cells, replacing them with fibrosis and nodular tissue and resulting in liver failure. Chronic hepatitis and alcoholism are common causes.

CLD: Chronic lung disease. *See* Bronchopulmonary dysplasia.

CMV: Cytomegalovirus. The virus that causes cytomegalic inclusion disease.

Coagulation: The process of blood clot formation.

Colon: The large intestine, which is between the small intestine and the rectum.

Colonization: Persistent, asymptomatic presence of bacteria in a particular area of the body. If symptoms develop, it becomes an infection. *Example:* Many women have vaginal and/or rectal colonization with group B streptococci (GBS) but are entirely without symptoms, although maternal GBS colonization poses a risk for life-threatening neonatal infection.

Compliance (of lung): Refers to the elastic properties of the lungs. Babies with certain lung diseases have decreased compliance (stiff lungs) and thus cannot expand their lungs well during inhalation.

Comprehensive ultrasound: Detailed ultrasound examination designed to review all parts of fetal anatomy. Done when congenital malformation(s) is suspected.

Condyloma: Warty growth of the skin in the genital area caused by human papillomavirus (HPV).

Congenital: Refers to conditions that are present at birth, regardless of cause. Congenital defects may result from a variety of causes, including genetic factors, chromosomal factors, diseases affecting the pregnant woman, drugs taken by the woman, etc. The cause, however, of most congenital defects is unknown. *Note:* Congenital and hereditary are not synonymous. Congenital means present at birth. Hereditary means the genetic transmission from parent(s) to child of a particular trait, which may be the trait for a specific inheritable disease and associated malformation(s). Some defects are congenital and hereditary, but many are simply congenital with no genetic link.

Congestive heart failure: A condition that develops when the heart cannot pump as much blood as it receives. As a result, fluid backs up into the lungs and other tissues, causing edema and respiratory distress. Congestive heart failure may result from a diseased or malformed heart, severe lung disease, or too much fluid given to the patient.

Conjugation of bilirubin: Process that occurs in the liver and combines bilirubin with another chemical so it may be removed from the blood and pass out of the body in the feces. Failure of bilirubin conjugation is one cause of jaundice.

Conjunctivitis: Inflammation of the membrane that covers the eye and lines the eyelids. Certain genital tract infections, particularly *Chlamydia* and gonorrhea, in a pregnant woman can cause severe conjunctivitis and eye damage in a newborn, unless proper neonatal treatment is given.

Continuous positive airway pressure (CPAP): A steady pressure delivered to the lungs by means of a special apparatus or mechanical ventilator. CPAP may be used for babies with respiratory distress syndrome to prevent alveoli from collapsing during expiration.

Contraction stress test (CST): Termed oxytocin challenge test (OCT) when oxytocin is used to induce contractions. A brief period of uterine contractions (either spontaneous or induced with nipple stimulation or with intravenous oxytocin administration) during which the fetal heart rate and uterine contractions are monitored with an external monitor. It is a test used in certain high-risk pregnancies to assess fetal well-being.

Coombs test: Test to determine the presence of antibodies in blood or on red cells. There are 2 forms of the test. The direct Coombs test detects antibodies attached to the red blood cells; the indirect Coombs test detects antibodies within the serum. *Example:* The direct test is used to detect antibodies present on the red cells of Rh-positive babies born to Rh-negative sensitized women. The indirect test is used on a woman's blood to detect antibodies to fetal Rh-positive cells. *See also* Antibody screening test.

Cord presentation: A situation when the umbilical cord lies against the membranes over the cervix, beneath the fetal presenting part. This poses a risk for cord injury or prolapse when the membranes rupture.

Cordocentesis: *See* Percutaneous umbilical blood sampling (PUBS).

Corticosteroids: Refers to any of the steroids of the adrenal cortex. Betamethasone and dexamethasone are artificially prepared steroids that may be given to a woman to speed up the process of lung maturation in her fetus when preterm delivery is unavoidable.

CPD: Cephalopelvic disproportion. *See* Fetopelvic disproportion (FPD).

Creatinine: A chemical in the blood excreted in urine and used as an indication of renal function.

Cryoprecipitate: A concentrated form of plasma. In a much smaller volume, it contains fibrinogen, Factor VIII, and some, but not all, of the other clotting factors found in fresh frozen plasma. Used in the treatment of severe disseminated intravascular coagulation.

CVS: Chorionic villus sampling.

Cyanosis: Bluish coloration of the skin. (1) *Central cyanosis:* Bluish coloration of the skin and mucous membranes due to inadequate arterial blood oxygen concentration. Sometimes babies with central cyanosis are described as appearing dusky. (2) *Acrocyanosis:* Cyanosis of the hands and feet only, which is generally not associated with low blood oxygen concentration.

Cytomegalic inclusion disease: An infection with cytomegalovirus. Maternal infection may go unnoticed but fetal infection, especially early in gestation, can damage every organ system. The disease commonly causes an enlarged liver and spleen, encephalitis, microcephaly, intracranial calcification, and visual or hearing defects.

Cytomegalovirus (CMV): The specific virus that causes cytomegalic inclusion disease.

Debridement: Removal of dead tissue and foreign matter from a wound.

Deceleration: *See* Fetal heart rate deceleration.

Decidua: Endometrium that has undergone the hormonal effects of pregnancy; the endometrium during pregnancy.

Deflexed head: The fetal head is not round. It is longer from front to back (occipitomental diameter is approximately 13.5 cm at term) than it is from side to side (biparietal diameter is approximately 9.5 cm at term). When the fetal head is well flexed with the chin on the chest, the top of the head, with a maximum diameter of 9.5 to 10 cm, is presented to the pelvis. In most cases, the pelvis is larger than this, allowing the head (largest part of the fetus) to pass through it. When the head is deflexed, as it is in brow and face presentations, the farther the chin is from the chest, the larger the diameter presented to the pelvis. These presentations make vaginal delivery difficult or impossible without risk of serious damage to the fetus and/or the woman.

Deformation: Structural defect of a fetus caused by mechanical force, rather than by abnormal embryonic development or from an inherited disease. External factors, such as uterine tumors or amniotic bands, may produce a deformity by compressing parts of the fetus. Prolonged oligohydramnios can also cause deformities, due to lack of the amniotic fluid cushion normally provided to a growing fetus. Sometimes these deformities, such as an angulated spine or flattened head, straighten out spontaneously over time. In other cases, cosmetic surgery will be needed for correction. Malformation and deformation are not synonymous. *Malformation* is the term used when a congenital anomaly is due to *abnormal development* of the fetus. *Deformation* is the term used when a congenital anomaly is due to *external mechanical force* applied to a growing fetus.

Dehiscence: Separation of an incision that had been surgically united. The separation may be partial, involving only the outer layer, or complete through all tissue layers. In perinatal care, this term is most commonly applied to the postoperative separation of an abdominal incision or the development of an opening in a uterine scar from a previous cesarean section.

Diabetes mellitus: A metabolic disorder in which the body's ability to use glucose is impaired due to a disturbance in normal insulin production. This leads to high blood glucose levels and to other metabolic imbalances. Diabetes mellitus during pregnancy places the woman and fetus at risk for certain serious problems and may affect the health of the newborn.

Diabetes, gestational: Also called glucose intolerance of pregnancy or gestational diabetes mellitus (GDM). Disturbance of glucose metabolism that mimics diabetes mellitus and first appears during pregnancy and, in many cases, disappears after delivery. Women with this condition are more likely than the general population, however, to develop insulin-dependent diabetes later in life. Because normal control of blood glucose during pregnancy is important for fetal well-being, and because this metabolic problem is fairly common, screening tests for abnormal glucose tolerance are recommended for every prenatal patient.

Diaphragm: The muscular membrane that separates the chest cavity from the abdominal cavity.

Diaphragmatic hernia: A defect in the diaphragm through which the abdominal organs slip and enter the chest, where they compress the lungs. If the abdominal organs enter the chest cavity early in gestation, the development of one or both of the lungs can be severely inhibited.

DIC: Disseminated intravascular coagulation.

Digital examination: Examination of the cervix and, during labor, the presenting part of the fetus, with a sterile, gloved hand (examination is done using your fingers, or digits), as opposed to a vaginal examination using a speculum to view the cervix.

Digitalis: A drug that increases the contraction force of the heart while at the same time decreases the rate at which the heart beats. Sometimes used to treat congestive heart failure.

Dilatation: The condition of being stretched beyond normal dimensions. In perinatal care this most commonly refers to the degree of opening in the cervical os. Synonymous with dilation.

Dipstick: Thin, narrow paper or plastic strip (or "stick") with chemical reagent(s) that changes color in the presence of certain specific conditions in the liquid being tested. There are different types of dipsticks to test for different substances, and some dipsticks have several reagent patches to test for several substances on the same stick. Dipsticks are used to test body fluids, such as vaginal secretions, gastric aspirate, or urine. Examples of their use in perinatal care include testing vaginal secretions for pH to help identify rupture of the membranes and urine for protein in women with hypertension.

Disseminated intravascular coagulation (DIC): An acquired disturbance of the body's blood clotting processes in which clotting factors are consumed, leaving the blood incapable of coagulating. Certain serious illnesses may trigger the onset of DIC in neonates or adults. Most commonly in neonates, DIC may accompany severe sepsis, hypoxia, acidosis, and/or hypotension. In pregnant women, DIC may accompany placental abruption, retained dead fetus syndrome, or sepsis. Blood platelets and clotting factors are activated abnormally by the release of thromboplastic substances into the circulation. As a result, numerous fibrin clots are formed in the capillaries. Red blood cells may be broken down as blood flow pushes the cells through the clogged capillaries, which may lead to hemolytic anemia. In addition, oozing from puncture sites, surgical incisions or other wounds, and easy bruising may occur as the platelets and clotting factors are consumed by the fibrin clots and are no longer available to maintain normal blood clotting. Neonates with DIC, especially preterm babies, are also at risk for pulmonary or intracranial hemorrhage. Treatment, which is complex, is directed at correcting the underlying disease process and providing emergency management to correct the clotting deficit.

Diuretics: Drugs (furosemide, thiazides, spironolactone, etc) given to prevent or decrease fluid buildup in the lungs and body by increasing urine output.

DNA testing: Also called genetic testing. Samples of tissues (blood, urine, skin, etc) are treated, using a highly technical process, to extract the DNA of chromosomes (and mitochondria). Tests can then reveal defective genes that cause specific diseases. Most disease-causing genes, however, have not yet been identified.

Dolichocephalic: Long-headed; typically refers to the elongated head of a fetus in breech position when ultrasonography is used to measure the fetal skull biparietal diameter (BPD). This head shape reduces the accuracy of BPD measurements.

Doppler instrument: A device used to detect changes of blood flow through a blood vessel. A Doppler instrument may be used to detect fetal heartbeats.

Double setup: A vaginal examination performed in an operating room, with everything in readiness for either a vaginal or cesarean delivery. Used in cases of suspected placenta previa during labor, where the examination itself may trigger such profuse hemorrhage that immediate surgery is required.

Down syndrome: Trisomy 21. A chromosomal abnormality resulting in a typical facial appearance, mental retardation, and sometimes other congenital defects, particularly cardiac defects. In the past, this condition was sometimes referred to as mongolism. Individuals with Down syndrome have 47 instead of the normal 46 chromosomes.

Ductus arteriosus: The ductus arteriosus is a blood vessel in the fetus that connects the pulmonary artery and the aorta. This allows less blood to go to the fetal lungs and more blood to go to the systemic and placental circulation. Normally this vessel closes shortly after birth, thus redirecting blood flow to the lungs. A patent ductus arteriosus means that the ductus arteriosus persistently remains open after birth. As a result, and with the changes in pressure that occur within the circulatory system once placental circulation is eliminated, blood may flow from the aorta into the pulmonary artery, resulting in too much blood directed to the lungs. This may cause congestive heart failure in the baby.

Dusky: *See* Cyanosis.

Dye test: In perinatal care, this usually refers to a test done to determine if the amniotic membranes are ruptured. There is no indication for a dye test unless there is reason to suspect that rupture of membranes has occurred, other tests are negative, *and* the diagnosis of ruptured membranes will affect clinical management. Amniocentesis is done under ultrasound guidance. If indicated, a sample of amniotic fluid is withdrawn for testing. A dye, usually indigo carmine, is then introduced through the amniocentesis needle. A sterile gauze pad (4 x 4) is placed high in the woman's vagina. If no dye appears on the pad after 20 to 30 minutes of sitting or walking, it is most likely that the membranes are intact and have not ruptured.

Dyspnea: Difficult breathing, labored breathing. This may accompany any variety of disease states or be a result of physical exertion in a healthy person.

Dystocia: Difficult labor. Types: (1) *Uterine:* Abnormal labor, particularly prolonged labor. Used to refer to weak or ineffective uterine contractions. Usually used to describe a labor that is so obstructed that a cesarean section is necessary. (2) *Shoulder:* Situation in which the shoulders of a baby in vertex presentation become trapped after delivery of the head. This is an emergency, requiring immediate intervention to avoid severe fetal hypoxia.

Eclampsia: The term used to describe the condition when convulsions and/or coma develop in a pregnant or postpartum woman with pregnancy-related hypertension. The condition of preeclampsia becomes eclampsia whenever seizures or coma develop.

EDC: Estimated date of confinement. An older term that refers to the expected date of delivery (the date of a woman's "confinement"). *See* Pregnancy due date.

EDD: Estimated date of delivery. *See* Pregnancy due date.

Edema: Swelling due to an excessive amount of fluid in the tissues.

Effacement: The process of thinning of the cervix prior to and after the onset of labor.

Electrolyte: A substance that dissociates into ions when in solution (and thereby makes the solution capable of conducting electricity). Commonly refers to sodium, potassium, chloride, and bicarbonate in blood.

Embolus: A blood clot or other plug (such as an air bubble) carried by the blood from a larger blood vessel to a smaller vessel, where it lodges and obstructs the blood flow. Plural: emboli.

Embryo: Term used for the product of conception, from the time a fertilized egg is implanted until all major structures and organs are defined. In humans, this is the first 8 weeks of development. After 8 weeks and until birth, the term fetus is used.

Endocrine system: Refers to organs that release hormones into the blood.

Endometritis: Infection of the inner lining of the uterine cavity, the endometrium.

Engagement, engaged: Term applied during late pregnancy or in labor that indicates that the largest diameter of the presenting part is at or below the smallest diameter of the pelvis. Usually the presenting part is the fetal head, which is said to be engaged when a vaginal examination reveals the head to be at or below the ischial spines.

Environmental oxygen: *See* Inspired oxygen.

Epidural: A technique for providing anesthesia during labor. A hollow needle is inserted between 2 vertebrae in the woman's spine and a catheter is threaded through the needle and into the epidural space of the spinal column. A local anesthetic is then injected through the catheter into the epidural space. This eliminates all sensation for the nerve roots that the drug contacts. The greater the volume of anesthetic medication injected, the greater the number of nerve roots affected and, therefore, the larger the area of the body that is anesthetized. By anesthetizing only some of the spinal nerve roots, epidural anesthesia provides pain relief during labor but, at the same time, may also permit walking. As with spinal anesthesia, the anesthetic medication also blocks the sympathetic nerves leaving the spinal cord. Because of this, the blood pressure of the woman may decline and requires careful monitoring. (For this reason, a loading dose of 500 to 1,000 mL of normal saline may be given intravenously prior to the introduction of the anesthetic.)

Epigastric: Area immediately below the tip of the sternum in the center of the upper abdomen. Pain felt here is usually related to liver or gallbladder disease. Of most importance in pregnant women with preeclampsia, the onset of epigastric pain indicates the swelling of the liver capsule. This often precedes the onset of the first convulsion of eclampsia.

Epiglottis: The flap of cartilage that overlies the larynx. The epiglottis is open during breathing and closes over the larynx during swallowing to prevent food from entering the trachea.

Epinephrine: A natural body hormone that is released by the adrenal glands into the blood during stress. It may also be used as a drug during resuscitation to constrict the blood vessels and increase the blood pressure, and to increase the heart rate and volume of blood pumped.

Erb's palsy: The most common form of brachial plexus nerve injury in newborns.

Erythema: Redness of the skin produced by dilation of the smallest blood vessels. *Example:* The redness that occurs around an infected wound.

Erythroblastosis fetalis: A hemolytic anemia resulting from blood incompatibility between the fetus and the pregnant woman. A fetus with Rh-positive blood, whose mother is Rh negative, may develop erythroblastosis fetalis. Some of the fetal blood cells cross the placenta and enter the woman's blood. The pregnant woman then makes antibodies against these Rh-positive cells. The woman's antibodies may be transferred back to the fetus during this pregnancy, or during the next pregnancy, and react against the fetus's own blood cells. Many of the fetus's red blood cells are destroyed by the maternal antibodies, producing anemia. The antibodies against Rh-positive blood in the fetus will continue this destructive process after the baby is born, causing anemia and hyperbilirubinemia. Often the fetal blood cells will not enter the woman's bloodstream until the time of delivery. This usually spares the first Rh-positive baby from being affected. Following delivery or an episode of bleeding during pregnancy, Rh immune globulin (RhIG) is given to Rh-negative, unsensitized women to protect future pregnancies from the development of Rh disease.

Esophagus: The muscular tube that connects the throat and the stomach.

Etiology: The cause of anything. *Example:* Sepsis may be the etiology of hyperbilirubinemia in a newborn.

Exchange transfusion: Process during which a baby's blood is removed and replaced with donor blood so that when the exchange transfusion is completed, most of the baby's blood has been replaced by donor blood. Most often, exchange transfusions are used as a treatment for severe hyperbilirubinemia.

Expiration: (1) Period during the breathing cycle when the person is breathing out or exhaling. (2) The end of a period of usefulness, validity, and/or effectiveness, such as the expiration date for a product or medication, after which time the item should not be used. (3) Death.

Face presentation: The face is the presenting part. The chin (mentum) is the reference point, and it may rotate either anteriorly (mentum anterior), in which case vaginal delivery is likely if the pelvis is normal in size. When the chin rotates posteriorly into the hollow of the sacrum (mentum posterior), vaginal delivery is impossible unless the forces of labor or the use of obstetric forceps are successful in rotating the chin to the anterior position.

FAD: Fetal activity determination.

FAE: Fetal alcohol effects.

Familial: Used to describe a disease or defect that affects more members of a family than would be expected by chance.

FAS: Fetal alcohol syndrome.

Fat, brown: Fat tissue that has a rich blood and nerve supply. Babies have proportionally more brown fat than do adults and metabolize or "burn" it as their main source of heat production, while adults produce heat mainly by shivering. Extra oxygen and calories are used when brown fat is metabolized.

Fat, white: Type of fat that has few blood vessels and appears whitish. It is used mainly for insulation and as a reserve supply of energy and is not nearly as metabolically active as brown fat.

Fatty acids: Substances resulting from the breakdown of fat. Fatty acids decrease binding of bilirubin to albumin, thus increasing the chance of brain damage from hyperbilirubinemia.

FDP: Fetopelvic disproportion.

Femoral pulse: Pulse felt in the groin, over the femoral artery.

Fern test: A test for amniotic fluid in the vagina, used when rupture of membranes is suspected. When there is a pool of fluid in the vagina, a drop of it is smeared on a glass slide and allowed to dry in the air. The salt content of the amniotic fluid will dry in a typical pattern, resembling a fern, while other fluids (eg, urine) will not. If a fern pattern is seen, the membranes are ruptured.

Fetal activity determination (FAD): A noninvasive means to monitor fetal well-being that may be used by either low-risk or high-risk pregnant women. Approximately 80% of gross fetal movements observed on ultrasound are felt by the pregnant woman. Beginning at approximately 28 weeks' gestation, a pregnant woman records fetal activity daily according to one of several accepted protocols. Any significant decrease in activity warrants prompt (the same day) investigation of fetal condition.

Fetal alcohol effects (FAE): Some experts believe that effects of maternal alcohol ingestion during pregnancy may be seen in a baby without the baby having all the findings typical of fetal alcohol syndrome.

Fetal alcohol syndrome (FAS): Constellation of findings, including mental retardation, that may occur in fetuses of women who ingest alcohol during pregnancy, especially early in gestation.

Fetal distress: A term commonly used to describe non-reassuring fetal heart rate patterns. However, many fetuses labeled as being in distress during labor appear healthy at birth. Monitoring strips showing components that are worrisome are described as "non-reassuring," rather than labeled as showing fetal distress. The specific components, such as decelerations, variability, heart rate, etc, should then be described.

Fetal echocardiogram: An ultrasound technique that shows the movements of the walls and valves of the beating heart of a fetus. Certain valvular and other abnormalities of the fetal heart may be seen. Used only when there is some reason to suspect that the fetus may have an abnormal heart.

Fetal heart rate acceleration: Abrupt increase (at least 15 beats per minute) in fetal heart rate (onset to peak rate occurs in <30 seconds) that lasts at least 15 seconds but less than 2 minutes.

Fetal heart rate, baseline: Approximate average fetal heart rate during any 10-minute period that is free of accelerations, decelerations, and marked variability (>25 beats per minute [bpm]). The normal baseline range is between 110 and 160 bpm.

Fetal heart rate deceleration: A decrease in the fetal heart rate that then returns to baseline. There are 3 types of decelerations (early, late, and variable), which are defined by their shape and relationship to uterine contractions.

Fetal heart rate variability: Fluctuations in baseline fetal heart rate that are irregular in amplitude and frequency. Visual inspection is used to classify the peak-to-trough beats per minute (bpm) difference as absent (no detectable change from baseline), minimal (fluctuation of 5 bpm or less), moderate (fluctuation of 6–25 bpm), or marked (fluctuation of 25 bpm or more).

Fetal lung maturity: Analysis of a sample of amniotic fluid for the presence of surfactant components. The lecithin-sphyngomyelin (LS) ratio is one such test. The "FLM" test is another test of fetal lung maturity. *See* Pulmonary maturity.

Fetal membranes: The amnion and chorion.

Fetal monitoring, external: Refers to continuous electronic monitoring using a device strapped to the woman's abdomen to detect the fetal heart rate, periodic rate changes, and timing of the uterine contractions.

Fetal monitoring, internal: Refers to continuous electronic monitoring using a wire attached to the fetal presenting part to detect the fetal heart rate and a pressure transducer placed inside the uterus to detect the onset and intensity of the uterine contractions.

Fetal pole: A term used to describe the appearance of either end of the fetal body when the fetus is so small the head cannot be distinguished from the breech.

Fetopelvic disproportion (FPD): Condition in which the internal size of the maternal pelvis is too small and/or the fetal head is too large to allow vaginal delivery. Because exact measurements of the fetal head and the maternal pelvis cannot be made, this is a relative term.

Fetoscope: A specially constructed stethoscope used to listen to the fetal heart rate.

Fetus: After development of organ systems (after the first 8 weeks of pregnancy) an embryo is called a fetus until delivery.

F_{IO_2}: Fractional inspired oxygen. The percentage of oxygen being inhaled. An environmental oxygen concentration of 55% may also be written $F_{IO_2} = 55\%$. The F_{IO_2} of room air is 21%.

Flaccid: Limp.

Flexion: Bending of a body part. *Example:* Flexion of the arm occurs when the elbow is bent. By contrast, extension means the straightening of a body part.

Flip-flop phenomenon: Flip-flop is caused by lowering the environmental oxygen concentration too rapidly, or by allowing a baby requiring oxygen therapy to breathe room air for even a short period. In response, the arteries to the lungs constrict, thus limiting the amount of blood that can be oxygenated in the lungs. The baby then requires an environmental oxygen concentration even higher than that breathed previously to achieve the same arterial blood oxygen concentration.

FLM test: A standardized laboratory test of amniotic fluid used for rapid estimation of fetal lung maturity.

Foam stability index (FSI): A laboratory test of amniotic fluid used for rapid estimation of fetal lung maturity.

Foramen ovale: The opening between the 2 upper chambers (atria) of the heart in the fetus. It consists of redundant tissue in the interatrial wall that results in a functional closure of the opening when left atrial pressure exceeds right atrial pressure shortly after birth.

Forceps: Obstetrical forceps are 2 metal instruments, made in mirror image of each other, curved laterally to follow the shape of the fetal head and vertically to fit the curve of the maternal pelvis. Used to assist vaginal delivery of the fetal head and to shorten the second stage of labor, for either maternal or fetal reasons. They are made in a variety of sizes and shapes, including forceps designed to help deliver the after-coming head in breech presentations. When forceps are used, the delivery is classified as midforceps, low forceps, or outlet forceps, depending on fetal station and position when the forceps are applied.

Fundal height: During pregnancy, the fundus of the uterus can be felt higher and higher in the maternal abdomen. The distance between the fundus and the symphysis pubis (front pelvic bone) is the fundal height. It is used as an estimate of the gestational age of the fetus. There are several techniques to measure fundal height. Consistency in the technique used (preferably by the same examiner) throughout pregnancy is important for accurate results.

Fundus: The broad top two-thirds of the uterus.

Gastroschisis: A rupture of the abdominal wall during embryonic development, allowing the abdominal organs to protrude into the amniotic fluid. As opposed to omphalocele, there is no peritoneal sac covering the organs with gastroschisis.

GBS: Group B beta-hemolytic streptococcus.

General inhalation anesthesia: An anesthetic technique that produces loss of consciousness. The patient is usually given barbiturates and/or narcotics to induce anesthesia, followed by paralyzing drugs, endotracheal intubation, and artificial ventilation. Anesthetic gases are used to continue the anesthetic state until the surgical procedure is completed. Because the gases are quickly cleared from the blood by the lungs, the patient "wakes up" within a few minutes after the anesthetic gases are stopped. With this type of anesthesia the drugs and gases used can cross the placenta and may depress a fetus. Anesthesia provided to an obstetric patient must consider the unique physiological state of a pregnant woman as well as the potential effect drugs given to her may have on the fetus.

Geneticist: A person who specializes in knowing how genes are inherited by children from their parents and the association between certain genetic abnormalities and specific physical characteristics.

Genitourinary tract: Pertaining to the reproductive organs and urinary organs.

Glottis: The vocal cords and opening between them that leads to the trachea.

Glucose tolerance test (GTT): A test for abnormal glucose metabolism. A fasting patient is given a standard dose of glucose orally, with the blood level of glucose determined at standard intervals, usually 1 hour later, but may also be checked 2 and 3 hours later.

Glycogen: The main storage form of glucose in the body. It is changed to glucose and released to the bloodstream as needed.

Glycohemoglobin (A_{1C}): Glycosylated hemoglobin (HbA_{1c}) reflects circulating blood glucose for the previous 4 to 8 weeks. It is used as an indicator of long-term glucose control.

Gonorrheal ophthalmia, neonatal: Eye infection in newborn babies that results from gonorrhea bacteria acquired by a baby during the birth process, if the woman has gonorrhea. Silver nitrate drops or erythromycin ointment placed in the baby's eyes shortly after delivery prevents the development of this potentially damaging infection.

Gram stain: A specific stain for bacteria that separates gram-positive bacteria (which stain blue) from gram-negative bacteria (which stain red). These 2 categories of bacteria vary in the types of disease they cause and in their antibiotic sensitivity. Gram stain of an infected body fluid (urine, pus, amniotic fluid) may identify the type of organism causing the infection and allow appropriate antibiotic therapy to begin before culture and sensitivity studies can be completed.

Gravidity: The number of pregnancies a woman has had, regardless of pregnancy outcome. With her first pregnancy a woman is a primigravida. With her second pregnancy a woman is, technically, a secundigravida, and with her third or subsequent pregnancies, a multigravida. In practice, however, secundigravida is rarely used and multigravida is used to refer to any woman with her second, or subsequent, pregnancy. *See also* Parity.

Group B beta-hemolytic streptococcus (GBS): A type of streptococcal bacteria that can cause serious or fatal neonatal illness. Some women, without evidence of infection, have chronic GBS vaginal and/or rectal colonization, which may infect the fetus before delivery or the baby at the time of delivery.

Growth restriction: Formerly growth retardation. A small for gestational age baby shows growth restriction. Fetal growth restriction describes fetuses that, on serial examination, are significantly smaller than would be expected, with their growth falling below established standards for their gestational age.

Grunting: A sign of respiratory distress in a neonate. The grunt or whine occurs during expiration as a result of the baby exhaling against a partially closed glottis. The baby grunts in an attempt to trap air in the lungs and hold open the alveoli. Grunting sometimes may be normal immediately following birth; after 1 to 2 hours it is always abnormal.

GTT: Glucose tolerance test.

Habitual abortion: Term applied to the situation when a woman has had 3 (or more) consecutive spontaneous abortions.

HBIG: Hepatitis B immune globulin. Administration of HBIG soon after delivery is part of the treatment for newborns whose mothers are HBsAg-positive (test for hepatitis B).

HBsAg: Hepatitis B surface antigen.

Heart murmur, functional: A heart murmur that does not result from disease or an abnormality of the heart. A functional heart murmur is *not* associated with abnormal functioning of the heart.

HELLP syndrome: Hemolysis, elevated liver enzymes, low platelets. An uncommon and severe form of pregnancy-related hypertension.

Hematocrit (Hct): A blood test showing the percentage of red blood cells in whole blood. *Example:* An Hct of 40 means that 40% of the blood is red blood cells and 60% is plasma and other cells.

Hemoglobin (Hgb): (1) Blood test showing the concentration of Hgb in blood, (2) oxygen-carrying part of red blood cells.

Hemoglobinopathy: A genetic disorder that causes a change in the molecular structure of hemoglobin in the red blood cells and results in certain typical laboratory and clinical changes, frequently including anemia. Sickle cell disease is one type of hemoglobinopathy.

Hemolysis: The breakdown of red blood cells. Hemolytic anemia, therefore, is anemia that results from the destruction of red blood cells, rather than anemia that results from loss of blood or from inadequate production of red blood cells.

Hemorrhage: Bleeding; most often used to indicate severe bleeding.

Heparin lock: A technique used to prevent blood clot formation in an arterial or venous catheter, when a continuous infusion of fluids is not being used. A solution of intravenous fluids with a specific concentration of heparin is flushed through the catheter and then the stopcock is closed to the catheter.

Hepatitis B surface antigen (HBsAg): Term for the protein on the surface of the hepatitis B virus. Screening all prenatal patients for this antigen identifies those women who are carriers for hepatitis B, and therefore are at risk for passing the virus to their fetuses before birth. Such newborns should be given hepatitis B immune globulin and hepatitis B vaccine soon after birth.

Hepatitis: Serious inflammation of the liver usually caused by a viral infection. There are several forms of hepatitis, depending on the specific causative agent and the mode of transmission. Infection may be acute or chronic.

Hepatosplenomegaly: Enlargement of the liver and spleen.

Hereditary: Used to describe a condition that is transmitted by the genes, from parents to their children. *Example:* Cystic fibrosis is a hereditary disease, and eye color is a hereditary trait.

Heredity: Genetic transmission from parent(s) to child of traits and characteristics. *Example:* A baby with brown eyes can be said to have that color of eyes as part of his or her heredity.

Herpes: Refers to diseases caused by herpesvirus. Maternal herpes infection may have serious consequences for the newborn.

HIV: Human immunodeficiency virus. The virus that causes AIDS.

HPV: Human papillomavirus.

Human immunodeficiency virus (HIV): The AIDS virus that attacks and eventually overcomes the body's immune system.

Hyaline membrane disease: Older name for neonatal respiratory distress syndrome (RDS).

Hydatidiform mole: A pregnancy characterized by grossly abnormal development of the chorionic villi, which eventually form a mass of cysts. Usually, but not always, there is no fetus present. Excessive secretion from the trophoblast cells leads to very high levels of ß-hCG. Vaginal bleeding during the first trimester is common and may be the presenting sign. Uterine size usually does not correspond to expected size for the dates of a pregnancy: larger than expected in about 50% of cases and smaller than expected in about 30% of cases.

Hydramnios: Previously called polyhydramnios. Abnormally large amount of amniotic fluid. It may be associated with fetal abnormalities (particularly gastrointestinal tract abnormalities that prevent amniotic fluid from being swallowed into the gastrointestinal tract of the fetus) or certain maternal medical illnesses; however, in most cases, the cause of hydramnios is unknown.

Hydrocephalus: Enlargement of the head due to abnormally large collection of cerebrospinal fluid in the brain. It may be congenital or be acquired after birth. The accumulation of cerebrospinal fluid may be caused by a blockage in the normal flow of fluid around the brain and spinal cord or by a decrease in the normal absorption of the fluid.

Hydrops fetalis: Edema in the entire body of a fetus. Usually a result of severe hemolytic anemia caused by Rh disease or other isoimmunizations, but may (rarely) be caused by certain other serious in utero conditions or viral infections. In many cases the cause for hydrops is not clear.

Hyperbilirubinemia, physiological: Hyperbilirubinemia due to a baby's immature liver, which has a limited ability to excrete bilirubin from the body, rather than hyperbilirubinemia due to a disease process such as ABO incompatibility.

Hyperbilirubinemia: Excess amount of bilirubin in the blood.

Hyperkalemia: High blood potassium (K^+) level.

Hypernatremia: High blood sodium (Na^+) level.

Hyperosmolar: Used to describe a liquid with a higher concentration of particles than found in a physiological fluid. For example, an intravenous solution may be hyperosmolar compared to blood, or formula may be hyperosmolar compared to breast milk.

Hypertension: High blood pressure. In adults, generally defined as higher than 140/90 mm Hg.

Hyperthermia: High body temperature; fever. In adults, generally defined as greater than or equal to 38°C (100.4°F).

Hypertonic: Used to describe a solution that is more concentrated than body fluid and therefore will draw water out of the body's cells, causing the cells to shrink.

Hypocalcemia: Low blood calcium (Ca^{++}) level.

Hypoglycemia: Low blood glucose level.

Hypotension: Low blood pressure.

Hypothermia: Low body temperature.

Hypovolemia: Low blood volume.

Hypoxemia: Low level of oxygen in the arterial blood.

Hypoxia: A deficiency of oxygen and perfusion in the body tissues resulting in compromised metabolism and injured tissue.

IAI: Abbreviation for intra-amniotic infection.

Icterus: Jaundice.

Ileitis: Inflammation of the ileum, the distal portion of the small bowel (between the jejunum and cecum). Usually represents Crohn's disease, a chronic inflammation of the intestinal tract, most often affecting the terminal ileum (may also involve the colon). Cause is unknown, complications are frequent (abscess, obstruction, fistula formation), and recurrence after treatment is common.

Ileus: Obstruction of the intestines. Commonly used to refer to a dynamic or functional ileus where there is an absence of peristalsis resulting from postsurgical inhibition of bowel motility but frequently not associated with a mechanical blockage of the intestines.

Immune thrombocytopenic purpura (ITP): A disease of unknown cause in which the body destroys its own platelets, causing thrombocytopenia and resulting in clotting disorders and easy bruising. The fetus of a woman with ITP may also have thrombocytopenia. Formerly called idiopathic thrombocytopenic purpura.

331

In utero: Latin for "inside the uterus."

In utero resuscitation: Term applied to measures taken to improve fetal oxygenation when there is a non-reassuring fetal heart rate pattern during labor. These measures include provision of 100% oxygen by mask to the woman, correction of maternal hypotension (turn woman on her side or from one side to the other, give fluids, and/or elevate legs), and reduction of uterine activity (stop oxytocin, consider use of tocolytics).

Incompetent cervix: A condition in which the cervix (lower part of the uterus and entrance to the birth canal) dilates prematurely, causing a spontaneous abortion or preterm delivery. A woman with an incompetent cervix is at risk for a preterm delivery with each pregnancy. *See also* Cerclage of the cervix.

Infant death rate: The number of babies that die within the first year of life (365 days), per 1,000 live births.

Inferior vena cava: The major vein returning blood from the lower body to the right side of the heart.

Infiltration of intravenous fluids: Occurs when an intravenous catheter or needle in a peripheral vein perforates the wall of the vein and the intravenous fluids infuse into the surrounding tissue instead of into the bloodstream. Swelling and tenderness develop near the tip of the catheter. An infiltrated intravenous line should be removed immediately because some intravenous fluids can cause severe tissue damage.

Infusion pump: A machine used to push fluid at a controlled, preset rate into an artery or vein. All neonatal infusions should use a pump so that the volume infused can be controlled precisely. Some pumps infuse fluids by means of small, regular pulses, while other pumps, particularly syringe pumps, infuse continuously.

INH: Isoniazid hydrozide. Generic name for an antituberculosis medication.

Insensible water loss: Body fluid lost through the skin and respiratory passages.

Inspired oxygen: The oxygen concentration that is being inhaled (*not* the concentration in the blood). Also called environmental oxygen.

Intraamniotic infection (IAI): Also known as chorioamnionitis, or infection of the fetal membranes, which puts the fetus at risk for also becoming infected with the same organism.

Intracardiac: Inside the heart.

Intrapartum: Period of pregnancy during labor.

Intrauterine: Inside the uterus.

Intubation, endotracheal: Insertion of a hollow tube (endotracheal tube) into the trachea to suction foreign matter, such as meconium, from the trachea or to deliver air or oxygen under pressure directly into the lungs by assisted ventilation.

Iron: A mineral important for the formation of red blood cells. Iron deficiency is a common cause of anemia.

Isosmolar: Of the same particle concentration as body fluid.

ITP: Immune thrombocytopenic purpura.

IUGR: In utero growth restriction (formerly, growth retardation). *See* Growth restriction.

Jaundice: Icterus. The yellow coloration of the skin and mucous membranes resulting from hyperbilirubinemia.

Karyotype: The complete set of chromosomes of the nucleus of a cell. Also used to refer to the photomicrograph of the chromosomes arranged in a standard order. The process of identifying a karyotype uses a technique that stops cells in their reproductive cycle and causes the individual chromosomes to swell, thus allowing each chromosome to be identified and counted. This technique is used to identify conditions, such as Down syndrome (trisomy 21) or Turner syndrome (XO), that are caused by an excess or deficiency of one or more chromosomes. The technique cannot identify the individual genes that comprise each chromosome.

L/S ratio: A test of fetal lung maturity using the ratio of lecithin to sphingomyelin in a sample of amniotic fluid (obtained by amniocentesis).

Lactic acid: A by-product from one of the body's metabolic pathways. During periods of poor oxygenation, metabolism may be incomplete and lactic acid may build up, thus resulting in low blood pH or acidosis.

Large for gestational age (LGA): Refers to an infant whose weight is above the 90th percentile for infants of that gestational age.

Laryngoscope: An instrument used to visualize the glottis during endotracheal intubation.

Larynx: The area containing the vocal cords and located between the base of the tongue and the trachea.

Lecithin: One of the surfactant substances produced in the lung. The amount of lecithin produced increases with increasing gestational age of the fetus. Therefore, the ratio of lecithin to sphingomyelin (L/S ratio) in the amniotic fluid is used to estimate the lung maturity of the fetus.

Leopold's maneuvers: A method of systematically palpating the abdomen of a pregnant woman to determine fetal presentation and position.

Lethargy: Condition of diminished activity due to drowsiness, medication, or illness.

Lie: The relationship of the long axis of the fetus's body with that of the maternal spine (transverse, oblique, or longitudinal).

Lightening: The feeling of decreased abdominal distension a pregnant woman has as the fetus and uterus descend into the pelvic cavity during the last 4 weeks of a term pregnancy.

Macrosomia: Large body size. A newborn weighing more than 4,000 g (8 lb, 13 oz) at birth is considered macrosomic.

Maladaptation: Failure to adapt to the stresses of the environment.

Malformation, congenital: A defect that occurs during embryonic or fetal development. Used synonymously with congenital anomaly but not with deformation. *See* Deformation.

Maternal-fetal medicine (MFM): The subspecialty of obstetrics and gynecology that deals specifically with the care of high-risk pregnancies. This subspecialty is often, incorrectly, referred to as perinatology.

McRoberts maneuver: Used to relieve shoulder dystocia by elevating and flexing the woman's legs so that her knees and thighs are held as closely as possible against her abdomen and chest. This extreme flexion of the maternal hips rotates the pelvis in such a way that there is more room for the anterior shoulder to slip under the symphysis pubis, allowing delivery.

Meconium: The dark green-brown sticky material that makes up a baby's first stools. It is formed by the fetus in utero from intestinal secretions and swallowed amniotic fluid. The rectum may relax and release meconium into the amniotic fluid in post-term gestations and during periods of fetal stress. Meconium-stained amniotic fluid may be, therefore, a worrisome sign but does not always indicate fetal jeopardy.

Meningitis: Inflammation of the membranes that surround the brain and spinal cord.

Meningomyelocele: Congenital defect of the spinal column. Part of the spinal cord and surrounding membranes protrude through an opening in the spine and form a sac on the baby's back. The sac may be large or small, and located anywhere along the baby's spine. There may be various degrees of neurologic impairment occurring below the level of the meningomyelocele. It may be detected in the fetus by assessment of maternal serum alpha-fetoprotein.

Metabolism: All the physical and chemical processes that produce and maintain body tissue.

Methimazole: A mercapto-imidazole compound used to treat hyperthyroidism. This thyroid inhibitor may be associated with agranulocytosis. The more commonly used drug for treatment of this disease is propylthiouracil.

Morbidity: Any complication or damage that results from an illness.

Mortality: Death.

Motility: Movement.

MSAFP: Maternal serum alpha-fetoprotein. *See* Alpha-fetoprotein.

Multifetal gestation: More than one fetus. Multifetal gestation may be used to describe a pregnancy involving twins, triplets, quadruplets, quintuplets, etc.

Multigravida: Precise term for a pregnant woman who has had 2 or more previous pregnancies. Commonly used, however, to refer to a pregnant woman who has had one or more previous pregnancies. (Secundigravida is the precise term for a woman in her second pregnancy.)

Myometrium: The muscular wall of the uterus.

NaHCO₃: Sodium bicarbonate.

Naloxone HCl (Narcan): A drug that counteracts the depressant effects of narcotics. Naloxone may be given to a depressed baby whose mother received narcotic pain medication shortly before delivery. Adequate oxygenation with assisted ventilation, as necessary, should be provided *before* time is taken to give this drug. Naloxone should be used with caution if maternal drug addiction is suspected.

Narcan: *See* Naloxone HCl.

Nasal flaring: A sign of neonatal respiratory distress. The edges of the nostrils fan outward as the baby inhales.

Nasogastric tube: A pliable tube that is inserted through the baby's nose, down the esophagus, and into the stomach. It is used for feeding or to decompress the stomach by intermittent or constant suctioning of air and/or gastric juices out of the stomach.

NEC: Necrotizing enterocolitis.

Necrotizing enterocolitis (NEC): A serious disease in which sections of the intestines are injured and may die. Medical treatment may result in complete resolution, but in some cases portions of the intestines must be surgically removed. It occurs more often in preterm infants, but the cause is unclear.

Neonatal abstinence syndrome: Constellation of findings, including jitteriness, irritability, hypertonia, seizures, sneezing, tachycardia, difficulty with feedings, and/or diarrhea, often found in babies born to women who used heroin or methadone during pregnancy. These findings result from the baby's sudden withdrawal from maternal drugs following delivery.

Neonatal: Refers to the time period from delivery through the first 28 days.

Neonate: Baby from birth through the first 28 days of age.

Neonatologist: A pediatrician who specializes in caring for newborn infants, particularly at-risk and sick babies.

Nephrosis: General term used for any noninfectious disease of the kidney.

Neural tube defect: Used to describe any congenital defect in the brain or spinal cord (structures that developed from the neural tube of the embryo), including anencephaly, encephalocele, and meningomyelocele.

Neutral thermal environment: The very narrow environmental temperature range that keeps a baby's body temperature normal, with the baby having to use the least amount of calories and oxygen to produce heat.

Nitrazine: Trade name for phenaphthazine.

Non-hemolytic jaundice: Hyperbilirubinemia not resulting from an excessive breakdown of red blood cells.

Non-stress test (NST): One of several measures used to assess fetal well-being in high-risk pregnancies, during which spontaneous fetal heart rate accelerations in relation to fetal activity are monitored with an external electronic monitor. The pregnant woman is resting during the procedure and receives no medication.

npo (also written NPO): An abbreviation of the Latin phrase *nil per os*, which means nothing by mouth and is used to indicate that a person should not be allowed to eat or drink.

NST: Non-stress test.

Oligohydramnios: An abnormally small amount of amniotic fluid. It may be associated with abnormalities of the fetal kidney, ureter, or urethra (fetal urine is the primary component of amniotic fluid); certain fetal chromosomal defects; fetal growth restriction; utero-placental insufficiency; positional deformities (due to prolonged uterine pressure in the absence of a fluid cushion); and umbilical cord compression (particularly during labor). Oligohydramnios may also result from early, prolonged rupture of membranes.

Omphalocele: A congenital opening in the abdominal wall allowing the abdominal organs, covered with a peritoneal membrane, to protrude and form a sac outside the abdominal cavity. *See also* Gastroschisis.

Ophthalmia: General term for any disease of the eye.

Optical density: A measure of how well light passes through a substance. Optical density 650 (OD 650) is a test of the cloudiness of amniotic fluid and is used as an estimate of fetal lung maturity (cloudiness increases with increasing lung maturity).

Oral airway: A device that allows babies with blocked nasal passages to breathe through their mouths. It is inserted into the mouth and keeps the tongue forward, preventing it from obstructing the airway.

Orogastric tube: A pliable tube that is inserted through the baby's mouth, down the esophagus, and into the stomach. It is used for the same purposes as a nasogastric tube.

Orthopnea: Shortness of breath while lying down. It is usually caused by heart or lung failure and is characterized by the patient sitting up to sleep.

Osmolarity: The concentration of particles in a solution. Synonymous with osmolality.

Ovulation: The release of an egg, ready for fertilization, from an ovary.

Ovum: The female reproductive cell that, after fertilization and implantation, becomes an embryo.

Oximeter: A device that reads the color of blood and reports the percentage saturation of hemoglobin with oxygen (Sp_{O_2}). The probe of an oximeter emits a light that is sensed by a detector. *See also* Pulse oximetery

Oxyhemoglobin saturation: Hemoglobin is the oxygen-carrying component of red blood cells. The amount of oxygen attached to hemoglobin is measured as percent saturation and called oxyhemoglobin saturation (commonly shortened to "% sat" or "O_2 sat"). The degree of saturation can range from 0% to 100%.

Oxyhood: A small plastic box with a neck space designed to fit over a baby's head and allow precise control of a baby's inspired (environmental) oxygen concentration.

Oxytocin challenge test (OCT): *See* Contraction stress test.

Oxytocin: A hormone occurring naturally in the body and also used to induce labor, enhance weak labor contractions, and cause contraction of the uterus after delivery of the placenta.

Pa_{CO_2} or P_{CO_2}: Concentration of carbon dioxide in the blood ("a" specifies arterial blood).

Palate: The roof of the mouth. The structure that separates the oral and nasal passages. A cleft palate is one that is split from front to back, sometimes with an opening so deep that the mouth and nasal passages are connected.

Pa_{O_2} or P_{O_2}: Concentration of oxygen in the blood ("a" specifies arterial blood).

Parity: The condition of a woman with respect to having had one or more pregnancies reach a gestational age of viability. Parity is determined by the number of pregnancies that reached viability, whether the fetuses were live-born or stillborn, and not the number of fetuses. Twins, triplets, etc, do not increase a woman's parity. Nulliparity is the condition of having carried no pregnancies to an age of viability, primiparity of having carried one pregnancy to an age of viability, secundiparity of having 2 pregnancies reach viability, and multiparity of having had 3 or more pregnancies reach viability. In practice, however, secundiparity is rarely used and multiparity is used for any woman who has had 2 or more pregnancies reach an age of viability. *Example:* A woman whose first pregnancy ended in stillborn twins at 30 weeks' gestation, second pregnancy ended in a single, healthy fetus born at 39 weeks, and third pregnancy ended in spontaneous abortion at 10 weeks has a parity of 2. She is now pregnant for the fourth time, at 32 weeks' gestation, and therefore has a gravidity of 4. She may be described as a gravida 4, para 2. When she delivers the current pregnancy she will become a G4 P3.

Pelvis, contracted: Smaller than normal-sized pelvis. The pelvis may be too small to allow the vaginal birth of a baby.

Percutaneous umbilical blood sampling (PUBS): Also called cordocentesis. A highly specialized technique during which a needle is inserted through a pregnant woman's abdominal wall into the uterus and then directly into an artery or vein of the umbilical cord, usually near the base of the cord at the placenta. Ultrasound visualization of the fetus, placenta, and umbilical cord is used throughout the procedure. A sample of fetal blood is obtained. PUBS may be used to detect congenital infections, isoimmune diseases, and chromosomal defects (for chromosomal defects, fetal blood can yield results in a few days, while amniotic fluid cell culture may take several weeks). PUBS may also be used to give a direct blood transfusion(s) to a fetus in cases of severe anemia.

Perfusion: The flow of blood through an organ or tissue.

Pericarditis: Inflammation of the pericardium, the sac of fibrous tissue surrounding the heart. Pericarditis is sometimes caused by infection, other times by an inflammatory, noninfectious disease such as systemic lupus erythematosus.

Perinatal: The time surrounding a baby's birth, during the latter part of the prenatal period and the baby's first month of postnatal life. Technically, the perinatal period lasts from 20 weeks of gestation through 28 days of postnatal life.

Perinatologist: Technically, a subspecialist physician who cares for the fetus and neonate. Often used, incorrectly, to refer to an obstetrician with subspecialty training in maternal-fetal medicine.

Perinatology: The area of obstetrics and pediatrics that deals with the fetus during pregnancy and the infant after birth.

Periodic heart rate changes: Fetal heart rate accelerations and decelerations. Their occurrence and relationship to fetal activity or uterine contractions is used as an estimate of fetal well-being, for antenatal testing, and during labor.

Peripheral: The outward and surface parts of the body. *Example:* Peripheral circulation is the blood flow in the skin, arms, and legs.

PG: Phosphatidyl glycerol.

pH: Refers to the acidity or alkalinity of a liquid. A blood pH outside of the normal range indicates metabolic and/or respiratory disturbance.

Pharynx: The throat above the esophagus and below the nasal passages.

Phenaphthazine (Nitrazine): A pH-sensitive dye embedded in paper that, when dipped into fluids, estimates the pH of the fluid. Used primarily to distinguish amniotic fluid (which has an alkaline pH) from urine or vaginal secretions (which are acidic) in pregnant patients with symptoms of premature rupture of the membranes.

Phosphatidyl glycerol (PG): A chemical substance produced by the mature lung that passes into the amniotic fluid with fetal breathing. Its presence in the amniotic fluid is associated with a better than 99% chance that the baby will not develop respiratory distress syndrome.

Phototherapy: Use of fluorescent, tungsten-halogen, or fiberoptic lights to treat hyperbilirubinemia in neonates by breaking down bilirubin accumulated in the skin. The color of phototherapy lights ranges from nearly white to deep blue, depending on the type and brand of lights.

336

Pierre-Robin syndrome: *See* Robin syndrome.

Placenta accreta: Term used to describe a rare condition of implantation in which the implanting trophoblasts penetrate not only the endometrium but continue into the myometrium as well. This eliminates the normal cleavage plane in the decidua (endometrium during pregnancy) that allows normal spontaneous separation of the placenta following delivery. Attempts to remove a placenta accreta by manual separation usually result in excessive hemorrhage. Hysterectomy may be the only way to remove the placenta as separation from the myometrium may be impossible, and emergency surgery may be required if heavy bleeding begins.

Placenta previa: Abnormally low implantation of the placenta in the lower segment of the uterus. As the placenta grows with pregnancy, it spreads so that it partially or completely covers the internal cervical os at term. The resultant position of the placenta is in front of the fetus. Thus a vaginal delivery would require delivery of the placenta before the fetus. Painless vaginal bleeding during the third trimester is the most common sign of placenta previa. If not identified earlier, severe hemorrhage with maternal and fetal compromise may occur as the cervix dilates during labor. Whether placenta previa is identified prenatally or not until after labor has begun, cesarean delivery is required for the health of the woman and fetus. *Note:* Early in gestation a placenta may appear to be low-lying, but not be later in pregnancy. A diagnosis of placenta previa cannot be made until after 20 weeks' gestation, and should be reconfirmed at 26 to 28 weeks.

Placenta: The organ that joins the woman and fetus during pregnancy. The umbilical cord is implanted on one side while the other side is attached to the uterus. Maternal and fetal blood does not mix directly, but nutrients and waste products are exchanged across a thin membrane that separates maternal and fetal blood.

Placental perfusion: Blood from the uterine artery flows into the intervillous space, bathing the placental villi that protrude into this space with nutrients and oxygen. The flow of blood through the intervillous space allows perfusion of nutrients and oxygen into the fetus from the maternal blood and waste products of fetal metabolism to pass from the fetus to the maternal circulation. Fetal and maternal blood does not mix. The nutrients and waste are exchanged across the thin membrane of the placental villi.

Pneumonia: Inflammation of the lungs. Neonatal pneumonia has many possible causes, such as bacterial infection, aspiration of formula, aspiration of meconium, etc.

Pneumothorax: Rupture in the lung that allows air to leak outside the lung, form a collection of air between the lung and chest wall, and thereby compress the lung so it cannot expand fully. Often when a pneumothorax develops, a baby suddenly becomes cyanotic and shows signs of increased respiratory distress. There are decreased breath sounds over the affected lung. Insertion of a tube or needle into the chest is required to remove the air pocket and allow the lung to re-expand. Plural: pneumothoraces (rupture in both lungs).

Polycythemia: Abnormally high number of red blood cells. It is more common in infants of diabetic women and in newborns small for gestational age.

Polyhydramnios: Term synonymous with hydramnios, although hydramnios is now the preferred term for this condition.

Position, fetal: Relationship of the fetal presenting part to the maternal pelvis. In vertex presentations, the posterior fontanel is the reference point. With breech presentations, it is the tip of the fetal sacrum; with face presentations, the chin; with brow presentations, the anterior fontanel. Position is not the same as presentation. A fetus in vertex presentation may be in any of several positions. *Example:* Left occiput anterior position indicates that the fetal occiput, as determined by the position of the posterior fontanel, is located on the left side of the anterior part of the woman's pelvis.

Positive-pressure ventilation: Artificial breathing for a person by forcing air and/or oxygen into the lungs under pressure by bag and mask, bag and endotracheal tube, T-piece resuscitator, or mechanical ventilator.

Post-term: Refers to a fetus or baby whose gestation has been longer than 41 completed weeks (longer than the first day of the 42nd week).

Postnatal: The time after delivery, used in reference to the baby.

Postpartum: The time after delivery, used in reference to the mother.

Potter syndrome: A rare, fatal congenital malformation with characteristic facial appearance and absent or hypoplastic kidneys. Oligohydramnios may be noted in the mother. These babies are often born at term, are frequently small for gestational age, and may have hypoplastic lungs.

Precipitate labor: Labor lasting less than 3 hours from the first contraction to delivery. The rapidity of labor carries risks of trauma for the woman and the fetus.

Preconceptional: Before conception. Refers to counseling women or families *before* conception regarding the risks of various problems during pregnancy. This is particularly important when (1) a woman has a disease known to affect pregnancy or fetal development or a family history of such problems or (2) pregnancy carries increased risks for a woman because of an illness or condition she has.

Preeclampsia: A more severe form of pregnancy-related hypertension.

Pregnancy due date: The expected date for the onset of labor. On average, the date of delivery will occur 280 days, or 40 weeks, after the first day of the last menstrual period. The normal range of variation is 2 weeks before or after the calculated due date. Babies delivered between 37 and 42 weeks' gestation are considered term. Babies delivered prior to the onset of the 37th week are designated preterm, and those delivered after the end of the 42nd week (the completion of the 42nd week or later) are considered post-term. Inaccuracies can occur with calculating the due date because the date of the menstrual period may not be recalled correctly or because there are variations in the length of the pre-ovulatory phase of a menstrual cycle. In some women with irregular periods, the pre-ovulatory phase may be prolonged several weeks or even months.

Premature rupture of membranes (PROM): Rupture of the membranes ("bag of waters") before the onset of labor.

Prenatal: The time during pregnancy and before the birth of the baby. Synonymous with antenatal.

Presentation: Refers to that part of the fetus that is in the birth canal and will deliver first. The normal presentation, near term and during labor and delivery, is vertex (head-first). Any other presentation at that time is considered abnormal.

Preterm: Refers to that part of pregnancy prior to the start of the 37th week (eg, preterm labor, preterm rupture of the membranes, or an infant born before 37 weeks' gestation, etc).

Primary infection: The first episode of a given infection. Some infections, such as cytomegalovirus or herpes, remain latent, without symptoms, in a person but may recur from time to time. The primary infection, however, is the most severe and likely to be the most damaging to a fetus or newborn. Other infections, such as syphilis or gonorrhea, may be cured but if reinfection occurs, it will be as severe as the first infection.

Primigravida: A woman pregnant for the first time. *See also* Gravidity.

Primipara: A woman who has had one pregnancy carried to viability. *See also* Parity.

Prodromal labor: Refers to a patient having contractions, but without sufficient cervical changes to make the diagnosis of true labor.

Prodrome: The time before a disease or process reaches its full strength. *Example:* The prodrome of a herpes infection may be mild itching in the area where the vesicles will later appear. This could be described as prodromal itching.

Prognosis: A forecast of the most likely outcome of an illness.

Prolapse: The falling out of a viscus. For example, an umbilical cord that slips through the cervix ahead of the fetus is a prolapsed cord, or a uterus that falls partially or completely into the vagina has prolapsed.

Prolapsed cord: Premature expulsion of the umbilical cord during labor and before the fetus is delivered. This is an emergency situation because a prolapsed cord is likely to be compressed, which may cause severe fetal compromise.

Propylthiouracil (PTU): The principal antithyroid agent used to treat hyperthyroidism during pregnancy. In the non-pregnant woman, radioactive iodine would normally be used, but during pregnancy, the radioactive iodine will enter the fetus and destroy its developing thyroid gland and may cause further malformation due to radiation injury. Maternal treatment with PTU may cause fetal goiter, however, from the antithyroid agent crossing the placenta and suppressing fetal thyroid activity.

Proteinuria: Condition in which proteins from the blood are present in the urine. Also called albuminuria.

Psychosis: Any major mental disorder when the person loses contact with reality and is deranged.

PTU: Propylthiouracil.

Pudendal block: Nerve block by injection of local anesthetic agent into the area of the pudendal nerve. Used primarily for anesthesia of the perineum for delivery.

Pulmonary hypoplasia: Underdevelopment of the fetal lungs, usually related to in utero compression of the fetal chest or lungs that prevents appropriate growth. This is seen with diaphragmatic hernia and with severe oligohydramnios, such as may occur with Potter syndrome.

Pulmonary maturity: Refers to the relative ability of the fetal lungs to function normally if the fetus were to be delivered at the time a test for pulmonary maturity is performed. As the lungs mature, various chemicals produced by the fetal lungs appear in the amniotic fluid. Lecithin/sphingomyelin ratio, phosphatidyl glycerol detection, and/or FLM test, etc, may be performed on a sample of amniotic fluid to assess fetal lung maturity.

Pulmonary: Refers to the lungs.

Pulse oximetry: Uses a noninvasive device that allows continuous measurement of the saturation of hemoglobin with oxygen. Hemoglobin changes color from blue to red as it becomes increasingly saturated with oxygen. A pulse oximeter uses a tiny light to shine through the skin and a light detector to measure the color of the light coming through the skin. The color of the light coming through the skin is determined by the amount of oxygen carried by the hemoglobin in the red blood cells. From this the percentage of saturation is calculated (SpO_2). The percentage of saturation is not the same as a PaO_2 value, which measures the amount of oxygen dissolved in plasma.

Quickening: The first time fetal movements can be felt by the pregnant woman. This usually occurs between 16 to 20 weeks of gestation. Quickening generally occurs later in pregnancy for a primigravida than for a woman who has had a previous pregnancy.

Radiant warmer: A servo-controlled heating device that is placed over a baby and provides radiant heat to keep body temperature normal.

Respiratory distress syndrome (RDS): Formerly called hyaline membrane disease. A disease mainly affecting preterm infants, due to immaturity of the lungs and lack of surfactant. Without surfactant the alveoli collapse during exhalation and are difficult to open with the next breath.

Resuscitation team: This concept refers to the fact that more than one person is needed to provide resuscitation. At least 2, preferably 3, health care professionals, skilled in the techniques of resuscitation, are needed for each resuscitation.

Resuscitation: The process of restoring and/or supporting cardiac function, blood pressure, and respiration so as to provide adequate oxygenation and perfusion to a baby, child, or adult who is apparently dead or near death. For newborns, resuscitation is needed most often in the delivery room; for adults, resuscitation may be needed after any of a number of life-threatening events.

Reticulocyte count: Estimation of the number of newly formed red blood cells (reticulocytes) in a blood sample.

Retinopathy of prematurity (ROP): Abnormal blood vessel growth in the eye that may lead to detachment of the retina and partial or complete blindness. The blood vessel changes may result from many factors including excessively high arterial blood oxygen levels for a period that can be as short as a few hours. The more preterm a baby, the more likely the baby is to develop ROP. Often ROP resolves spontaneously, but if permitted to proceed unchecked, scarring may occur and the retina may detach. It is critical that babies with ROP be followed by an ophthalmologist trained in examining babies so that laser therapy may be used to check the progression.

Retractions: A sign of respiratory distress. These occur with each breath as the skin is pulled inward between the ribs as a baby tries to expand stiff lungs.

Retrolental fibroplasia (RLF): The scarring phase of retinopathy of prematurity.

Rh blood type: Besides the major blood groups of A, B, O, and AB, there are a number of minor groups, of which the Rh system is the most important for perinatal care. Prevalence of the Rh factor varies by ethnic and racial groups. In Caucasians, 85% have the Rh antigen and are said to be Rh-positive, while 15% lack the Rh antigen and, therefore, are Rh-negative. Regardless of ethnic or racial heritage, persons who lack a blood antigen can make antibodies against that blood group. This means that Rh-negative persons can make antibodies against Rh-positive blood, if their immune system has been exposed to that blood (from external transfusion or transplacental transfer). Persons who have developed such antibodies are said to be isoimmunized, or sensitized to that blood group. *See also* Rh isoimmunization and Erythroblastosis fetalis.

Rh disease: *See* Erythroblastosis fetalis.

Rh isoimmunization or Rh sensitization: (1) The development of antibodies by an Rh-negative woman pregnant with an Rh-positive fetus. The antibodies cross the placenta into the fetus's blood, thus causing hemolysis of the fetus's red blood cells. (2) The development of antibodies against the Rh-positive red blood cells following a transfusion of Rh-positive blood accidentally given to an Rh negative person.

RhIG: Rh immune globulin (formerly called Rhogam). The antibodies from sensitized Rh-negative persons can be harvested, purified, and prepared for safe injection into another Rh-negative, but unsensitized, woman. The product is called Rh immune globulin, or RhIG. The injected antibodies contained in RhIG prevent isoimmunization by reacting with the antigens on the few Rh-positive blood cells that may have escaped from the fetus into the maternal circulation. Rh-negative, unsensitized women should receive RhIG at 28 weeks' gestation and again following delivery. Rh-negative, unsensitized women should also receive RhIG within 72 hours of an abortion or an episode of vaginal bleeding during pregnancy. Protection lasts for 12 weeks. Therefore, depending on the course of the pregnancy, subsequent doses may also be needed. Use of RhIG protects fetuses in future pregnancies from Rh disease.

Rhinitis: Inflammation of the mucous membranes of the nasal passages, causing a characteristic runny or stuffy nose. Although generally uncommon in newly born infants, rhinitis is frequently found in babies with congenital syphilis.

RLF: Retrolental fibroplasia. *See also* Retinopathy of prematurity.

Robin syndrome: A group of congenital anomalies that include a small jaw, a cleft palate, and backward displacement of the tongue. Babies with Robin syndrome may have great difficulty breathing and/or eating.

ROP: *In neonatal care,* retinopathy of prematurity. *In obstetric care,* an abbreviation for a specific position (right occiput posterior) of a vertex presentation during labor.

Rotation (of the fetal head): Gradual turning of the fetus during labor for the fetal head to accommodate the size and shape of the maternal pelvis as the fetus descends through it.

Rubella syndrome: A group of congenital anomalies resulting from an intrauterine rubella infection. Anomalies commonly include cataracts, heart defects, deafness, microcephaly (abnormally small head), and mental retardation.

Rubella: A mild viral infection, also called German measles. A rubella infection in a pregnant woman during early pregnancy may result in infection of the fetus and cause the rubella syndrome.

S-thal (sickle-thalassemia) disease: Sickle cell disease and thalassemia are genetically transmitted anemic diseases caused by abnormal hemoglobin. *See* Hemoglobinopathy.

SBE: Subacute bacterial endocarditis.

SC (sickle-C) disease: A hemoglobinopathy similar to sickle cell anemia.

Scalp stimulation test: Test in which fetal heart rate response to mechanical stimulation of the fetal scalp (by examiner's gloved finger or sterile instrument) is assessed. Used as an estimate of fetal well-being during labor.

Scaphoid abdomen: Sunken or hollow-looking abdomen, occurring when there is a diaphragmatic hernia, which allows the intestines to slip from the abdomen through a hole in the diaphragm and into the chest cavity.

Secondary infection: Recurrent infection. *See also* Primary infection.

Sepsis: Infection of the blood. Also referred to as septicemia.

Serum bicarbonate: Also called blood or plasma bicarbonate. The concentration of bicarbonate in the blood. Bicarbonate is the main body chemical responsible for the acid-base balance of the blood.

Servo-control: A mechanism that automatically maintains skin temperature at a preset temperature. A thermistor probe is taped to the baby, registers the skin temperature, and in turn activates a radiant warmer or incubator to continue to produce heat, or to stop heating.

Sexually transmitted infection (STI): An infection that is transmitted from one partner to another during sexual activity. Many infections can be transmitted in this way, but certain STIs can have significant impact on the fetus or newborn, including syphilis, gonorrhea, *Chlamydia*, HIV, etc.

Shake test (also called bubble test): A bedside test of amniotic fluid, formerly used for rapid estimation of fetal lung maturity and now largely replaced by more refined tests.

Shock: Collapse of the circulatory system due to inadequate blood volume, inadequate cardiac function, and/or inadequate vasomotor tone. *In babies*, the causes are most often hypovolemia, sepsis, or severe acidosis. The symptoms are hypotension, rapid respirations, pallor, weak pulses, and slow refilling of blanched skin. *In pregnant women*, the cause is most often hemorrhage. Because of the expanded blood volume of pregnancy and the vasoconstrictive capabilities of most (young, healthy) pregnant women, blood loss may be severe before symptoms of shock (hypotension; weak and rapid pulse; rapid respirations; anxiousness or confusion; and cold, clammy, pale skin) become evident.

Short bowel syndrome: A syndrome of weight loss and dehydration related to having less than the normal length of intestine. The less intestine a baby has, the less well formula and other nutrients can be absorbed. Short bowel syndrome may result from a baby being born with an abnormally short bowel, or may be the result of a portion of the intestines having been removed for treatment of certain types of bowel disease.

Shoulder dystocia: Situation in which the baby's shoulders become wedged between the maternal symphysis and sacrum after delivery of the fetal head. The head may be pulled back against the perineum as the woman relaxes her push that delivered the head (the "turtle sign"). Various procedures may be tried to free the shoulders. Severe asphyxia or fetal death can occur if there is significant delay in delivery of the shoulders and trunk.

Shunt: A diversion of fluid from its normal pathway. (1) *Blood:* In some sick babies, blood will be shunted from the right side of the heart to the left (baby will be blue); in other babies, the shunt will be from the left side of the heart to the right (baby will be in congestive heart failure). Commonly seen in babies with congenital heart disease or severe lung disease where the result is that the blood cannot be normally oxygenated. (2) *Cerebrospinal fluid:* An artificial pathway for the flow of cerebrospinal fluid when there is a blockage in the normal pathway resulting in hydrocephalus. Typically, cerebrospinal fluid is shunted through a one-way valve from the ventricles into a small tube that is tunneled under the skin and empties into the abdominal cavity. This is called a ventriculoperitoneal, or V-P, shunt.

Siamese twins: Former name for conjoined twins. *See* Twins, conjoined.

Sickle cell anemia: *See* SS disease.

Sims position: The patient rests on one side, with the upper leg drawn up so that the knee is close to the chest. Often used with an emergency delivery in bed or outside the hospital. This position does not allow for much assistance by an attendant, but has the advantage of placing less tension on the perineum during delivery and, therefore, may result in fewer lacerations.

SLE: Systemic lupus erythematosus.

Small for gestational age (SGA): A baby whose weight is lower than the 10th percentile for infants of that gestational age.

Sniffing position: Proper position of a baby's head during bag-and-mask ventilation or endotracheal intubation. The head and back are in straight alignment, with the chin pulled forward as if sniffing. This position is different from the one used for endotracheal intubation of an adult because the relative size and relationship of the anatomical structures is different between babies and adults. The neck is *not* hyperextended (bent backward to an extreme degree) during endotracheal intubation in babies.

Sodium bicarbonate (NaHCO$_3$): Drug used to counteract metabolic acidosis. After being given to a baby it rapidly changes to carbon dioxide (CO$_2$) and water (H$_2$O). Therefore, it should be given only to babies who are breathing adequately on their own or who are receiving adequate assisted ventilation. These babies can "blow off" the excess CO$_2$ formed. If sodium bicarbonate is given to a baby with a high Paco$_2$, it will make the Paco$_2$ go even higher and thereby worsen the acidosis.

Sonography: Also called ultrasonography. Technique used to visualize the fetus and placenta by means of sound waves bounced off these structures. The sound waves are then turned into a picture outline of the structures. Used to assess fetal growth, fetal well-being, congenital abnormalities, multifetal gestation, placental location, location of structures during percutaneous umbilical blood sampling and amniocentesis, and volume of amniotic fluid.

Sphingomyelin: One of the chemical substances in the lungs; the amount of sphingomyelin remains fairly constant throughout gestation. Using amniocentesis, a sample of amniotic fluid is obtained and the ratio of lecithin to sphingomyelin is compared to estimate the pulmonary maturity of the fetus.

Spinal (block): An anesthetic technique in which a local anesthetic is introduced into the subarachnoid space of the spinal canal through a hollow needle placed (temporarily) in the spine. It is technically easier to perform the placement of an epidural catheter because spinal fluid in the subarachnoid space will flow out through the hollow needle and, thereby, identify proper placement of the needle before injection of the anesthetic. Because the anesthetic medication also blocks the sympathetic nerves leaving the spinal cord, the blood pressure of the woman may decline. (For this reason, a loading dose of 500–1,000 mL of normal saline may be given intravenously prior to the introduction of the anesthetic.) Spinal anesthetics are not ordinarily given until the second stage of labor has begun because the anesthetics used do not remain effective for longer than 2 hours.

Spo$_2$: The percentage of saturation of hemoglobin by oxygen as detected by a pulse oximeter, which reads and reports how red the blood is. Fully saturated hemoglobin appears bright red, while desaturated hemoglobin appears blue.

SS disease (sickle cell anemia): A genetic hemoglobinopathy causing chronic anemia. Crises, resulting from infarction of various body areas clogged by the sickled cells obstructing small blood vessels, may occur periodically. Management during pregnancy is particularly complicated.

Sterile vaginal examination: Vaginal examination with a speculum, using sterile technique. In this situation, sterility obviously cannot be ensured. When a woman is pregnant and rupture of membranes is known or suspected, the goal is to minimize the risk of introducing bacteria during the examination.

Sternum: The breastbone. The chest bone that joins the left and right ribs.

STI: Sexually transmitted infection.

Stopcock: Small device with 3 openings and a lever to close any 1 of the 3 openings. One of the openings is designed to fit the hub of an intravenous catheter, umbilical catheter, etc. The other 2 openings are designed to connect with a syringe or intravenous fluid tubing.

Stylet: Slender metal probe with a blunt tip that may be inserted inside an endotracheal tube to make the tube stiffer during intubation. Also, the solid, removable center within certain needles.

Subacute bacterial endocarditis (SBE): Endocarditis is an infectious inflammatory process in which the infecting bacteria form growths on the heart valves and/or endocardium. The process may have an acute or subacute course. Diagnosis is usually made during the subacute, longer-lasting stage. Heart tissue is permanently damaged and the infection can be difficult or impossible to treat effectively. Patients with heart valve malformations are particularly prone to develop these infective growths on the abnormal valves and the surrounding endocardium.

Succenturiate lobe of placenta: A malformation of the placenta in which the placenta has a second lobe, with the umbilical blood vessels traversing the membranes between the main placenta and the accessory or succenturiate lobe. The umbilical vessels between the 2 lobes may lie over the cervical os (creating the condition known as vasa previa) and can be torn, particularly if the membranes are ruptured artificially. Also, the succenturiate lobe may produce a placenta previa if it lies over the os, even though a previous ultrasound may have reported a normally placed placenta, which may be accurate for the main portion of the placenta.

Superimposed preeclampsia: The development of preeclampsia in a woman who already has chronic hypertension. Sometimes it is difficult to tell if the increase in blood pressure is due to poor control of existing hypertension or to development of preeclampsia. If the blood pressure increases and there is increasing proteinuria, superimposed preeclampsia is most likely. This complication increases the risk of the development of eclampsia.

Supine hypotension: In late pregnancy, the enlarged uterus may compress the vena cava when a woman lies on her back. This reduces the return of blood to the heart and, thus, reduces cardiac output. This then causes a reduction in blood pressure and a reduction in the perfusion of body tissues. The woman may feel faint. Most pregnant women lie on their sides to sleep. During labor it may be helpful to have a woman lie on her side as much as possible. If supine hypotension develops with a woman resting on her back, uterine blood flow may be affected, which might result in a non-reassuring fetal heart rate pattern. One measure to take if a non-reassuring fetal heart pattern occurs during labor is to turn a woman onto her side (if on her back) or from one side to the other to relieve pressure on the vena cava.

Supine: Position of a person when he or she is flat on his or her back.

Suprapubic puncture: A technique used to tap the bladder of a newborn. A needle is inserted into the center of the lower abdomen, above the pubic bone, and into the bladder to obtain a sterile urine specimen for culture.

Surfactant: A group of substances, including lecithin, that contributes to the compliance (elasticity) of the lungs by coating the alveoli and allowing them to stay open during exhalation. Without surfactant the alveoli collapse during expiration and are difficult to open with the next breath.

Symphysis pubis: The connection between the right and left hip bones in the front of the body, in the pubic area.

Systemic: Refers to the whole body.

Tachycardia: Rapid heart rate. (1) *Fetal* tachycardia is considered to be a sustained heart rate faster than 160 beats per minute. (2) *Neonatal* tachycardia is considered to be a sustained heart rate faster than 180 beats per minute while a baby is quiet and at rest.

Tachypnea: Rapid respiratory rate. In a neonate, tachypnea is considered to be a sustained breathing rate faster than 60 breaths per minute.

Tent: Small cone-shaped device made of material that can expand. Used to dilate an orifice or keep a wound open. In obstetrics, tents may be used for cervical ripening and may also be called osmotic dilators.

Teratogen: A substance that causes malformations in the developing embryo. Certain medications are known teratogens and should not be taken during pregnancy. Most congenital malformations, however, cannot be traced to a teratogen but are instead due to unknown factors (most common) or to hereditary factors.

Thalassemia: Any one of several hereditary hemolytic anemias caused by abnormal hemoglobin.

Thermistor probe: A small sensing device that measures temperature continuously and is able to detect very small changes. Servo-control devices operate by a thermistor probe attached to the baby and then to the radiant warmer or incubator.

Thrombocytopenia: Abnormally low number of blood platelets.

Thrombophlebitis: Inflammation of a vein associated with the formation of a thrombus. In a superficial blood vessel a thin red streak will form in the skin directly over the path of the blood vessel and the area will feel warm to the touch. Thrombophlebitis may develop at the site of a peripheral intravenous catheter, in which case the catheter should be removed and the intravenous line restarted into another vein. Further treatment is rarely needed. If thrombophlebitis develops in deep veins, however, it is a serious condition, generally requiring treatment with intravenous heparin.

Thrombosis: The process involved in the formation of a thrombus (blood clot in a vessel).

Thrombus: A blood clot that gradually forms inside a blood vessel and may become large enough to obstruct the blood flow. If a thrombus separates from the blood vessel and is carried in the blood, it becomes an embolus. Plural: thrombi.

Thyroid stimulating hormone (TSH): A protein secreted by the anterior pituitary gland that stimulates thyroid function.

Thyroid stimulating immunoglobulin (TSI): An antibody produced by lymphocytes that, for unknown reasons, stimulates the thyroid to release thyroxin. These antibodies may cross the placenta and cause hyperthyroidism in the fetus.

Thyroid storm: A sudden worsening of adult hyperthyroidism, usually triggered by trauma or surgery and characterized by marked tachycardia and fever.

Tocolysis: Administration of a drug to stop uterine contractions.

Tonus: The amount of continuous contraction of muscle. Uterine tonus refers to how tightly the muscle of the uterus is contracted between labor contractions. With an internal monitor, it is measured as the resting pressure in the uterus between contractions. Hypertonus refers to a uterus that remains excessively tense and does not relax normally between labor contractions.

TORCHS: Toxoplasmosis, other, rubella, cytomegalovirus, herpes, and syphilis. A specific group of infections that can cause in utero fetal infection (usually resulting in severe damage) or, in the case of herpes, life-threatening neonatal infection. The "other" category includes less common, serious infections such as varicella, coxsackievirus B, HIV, etc.

Toxemia: Term formerly used to refer, collectively, to all forms of pregnancy-specific hypertension.

Toxoplasmosis: Disease caused by a type of protozoa (a type of microscopic one-cell animal). Toxoplasmosis in a woman may go unnoticed but may infect the fetus, thus causing congenital toxoplasmosis. Congenital toxoplasmosis damages the central nervous system of the fetus and may lead to blindness, brain defects, or death.

Trachea: The windpipe or tube of stacked cartilaginous rings that descends into the chest cavity from the larynx and branches into the right and left bronchi, which branch further into smaller bronchioles inside the lungs.

Transfusion, fetal-fetal: Situation that may occur, in utero, between fetuses of a multifetal gestation, when there is a connection between an artery of one fetus's placenta and a vein of the other fetus's placenta. The fetus on the arterial side becomes a chronic blood donor to the fetus on the venous or recipient side. When born, the donor twin may be pale, severely anemic, and small for gestational age. The recipient twin may be red, polycythemic and, occasionally, large for gestational age.

Transfusion, fetal-maternal: Situation that may occur in utero if an abnormal connection develops between the fetal and the maternal circulation in the placenta. The reverse direction of maternal-fetal transfusion apparently does not occur. The newborn may present with findings similar to the "donor" fetus described in fetal-fetal transfusion. To diagnose this condition, the woman's blood can be tested for the presence of fetal cells with the Kleihauer-Betke test.

Transverse lie: The body of the fetus lies horizontally across the maternal pelvis and, hence, across the birth canal entrance. A cesarean section is required for safe delivery of a fetus in transverse lie.

Trendelenburg position: A position of the body that may be used for surgery or examination. The patient lies supine on an inclined surface, with the head lowered below the level of the feet.

Trimester: A period of 3 months. The time during pregnancy is often divided into the first trimester (first through third month), second trimester (fourth through sixth month), and third trimester (seventh through ninth month).

Trisomy: Chromosomal defect in which there is an extra (third) chromosome of one of a normal pair of chromosomes. The most common is trisomy 21 (three #21 chromosomes), which is also called Down syndrome. Other trisomies also occur, such as trisomy 13 (three #13 chromosomes) and trisomy 18 (three #18 chromosomes), both of which have a characteristic set of multiple congenital anomalies.

TSH: Thyroid stimulating hormone.

TSI: Thyroid stimulating immunoglobulin.

Turner syndrome: A chromosomal defect in which there are 45 chromosomes instead of the usual 46, with the sex chromosomes identified as XO (O stands for absent) instead of XX (female) or XY (male), and may be accompanied by physical abnormalities including webbed neck; low hair line; and certain skeletal, urinary tract, lymph system, and cardiac abnormalities. The baby will have female external genitalia but the ovaries may be completely absent and sexual development will be severely impaired.

Twin-twin transfusion: *See* Transfusion, fetal-fetal.

Twins, conjoined: Formerly called Siamese twins. Twin fetuses joined together, usually at the chest or abdomen but may be at almost any site, and sharing one or more organs. This results from incomplete separation during the process of twinning of single ovum (which, if completely split, would have become identical twins). The greater the degree of organ sharing, the less likely one or both twins can survive surgical separation.

Twins, fraternal: Two fetuses created from the fertilization and implantation of 2 separate ova.

Twins, identical: Two fetuses created from the division of one fertilized ovum.

Ultrasonography: *See* Sonography.

Urine drug screen: Commonly available test in which the metabolic breakdown products of recently taken drugs can be identified in the urine.

Uterine atony: Failure of the uterine muscle (myometrium) to contract in the immediate postpartum period. A leading cause of postpartum hemorrhage.

Uterine dysfunction: Abnormal progress of labor due to uterine contractions that are inadequate in strength or occur in an uneven, uncoordinated pattern.

Uterine fibroids: Tumors of the uterus made up of fibrous connective tissue and smooth muscle. Also called leiomyomas. These myomas may become very large, occasionally interfering with implantation. Other risks, although uncommon, include placenta previa, obstructed labor, preterm labor, postpartum hemorrhage, and endometritis.

Uterine inertia: Inadequate labor caused by uterine contractions that are too short, too weak, and too infrequent to produce adequate progress.

Uteroplacental insufficiency: An inexact term suggesting a placenta that is functioning poorly, with inadequate transfer of nutrients and oxygen to the fetus, and used to explain some cases of in utero growth restriction and/or fetal distress during labor.

Uteroplacental: Refers to the uterus and placenta together as a functioning unit.

Uterus: A hollow, muscular organ in which the fetus develops, often called the womb.

Vacuum extractor (VE): An instrument used to assist delivery, in which a plastic cup is placed over the fetal occiput, suction is applied so that the cup is sealed to the scalp, then traction is applied to the cup. There are risks, benefits, and specific indications for use of vacuum extraction.

Vagus nerve: A major nerve with branches to the heart and gastrointestinal tract. Something that stimulates one branch of the vagus nerve may also affect another branch. *Example:* Suctioning deep in the back of a baby's throat directly stimulates part of the vagus nerve to the gastrointestinal tract and indirectly may affect the branch to the heart and cause bradycardia (termed reflex bradycardia).

Varicella-zoster (chickenpox): The virus that causes chickenpox in children. Adults who were not infected as children and, therefore, did not acquire immunity may also develop chickenpox, which, in adults, can cause life-threatening pneumonia. Infection in a pregnant woman early in pregnancy can cause severe fetal malformations and serious neonatal illness at term. *Note:* Reactivated infection in adults is herpes zoster. This occurs in a small percentage of individuals who had chickenpox as children, and causes pain and the formation of vesicles along specific nerve tracks. These symptoms are known as shingles.

VariZIG: Varicella-zoster immune globulin. Specific antibodies to the varicella-zoster virus obtained from persons who have had the disease. Principally used to attenuate infection in the newborn of a mother who has the infection.

Vasa previa: An abnormality of placental development. Instead of joining together at a point over the placenta, the vessels that form the umbilical cord join some distance from the edge of the placenta. The vessels lie on the membranes and, if the vessels lie across the cervical os, are exposed when the cervix dilates. This is a dangerous situation because when the membranes rupture or are artificially ruptured, the vessels may tear open. The fetal hemorrhage that results is often fatal.

Vasoconstriction: Tightening of the blood vessels, allowing less blood flow through the vessels. For example, when a significant volume of blood is lost, the small blood vessels in the skin will constrict, thus allowing the remaining blood to be directed to the brain and other vital organs.

VBAC: Vaginal birth after cesarean. When an indication for cesarean section other than a previous cesarean section is not present in a subsequent pregnancy, labor with vaginal delivery may be successful. VBAC is the term used to describe this situation.

Vein: Refers to blood vessels that return blood to the heart. In most veins, this blood is dark red because it has a low oxygen concentration because most of the oxygen from the arterial blood has been transferred to the body's cells for metabolism. The pulmonary veins, however, carry oxygenated blood as it flows from the lungs to the heart.

Vertex: Top of the head. A fetus in vertex presentation is head-first in the maternal pelvis. This presentation is identified on vaginal examination by palpation of the posterior fontanel in the center of the birth canal.

Vital signs: Refers to the group of clinical measures that includes respiratory rate, heart rate, temperature, and blood pressure.

Vitamin E: A vitamin important for maintaining red blood cell stability. When a baby is deficient in vitamin E, the red blood cells may break down more rapidly than normal and the baby may become anemic.

Volume expander: Fluid used to replace blood volume, and thereby increase blood pressure, in cases of hypotension thought to be due to hypovolemia. Blood or normal saline are examples of volume expanders.

Woods maneuver: The maneuver for management of shoulder dystocia in which the fetus is rotated 180° so the posterior shoulder becomes the anterior shoulder.

Zavanelli maneuver: The maneuver for management of shoulder dystocia in which the fetal head is replaced into the vagina and a cesarean delivery is done.

Index